Medical
Information Systems

The Laboratory Module

Medical Information Systems

The Laboratory Module

Ralph R. Grams

Medical Systems Division
University of Florida
Gainesville, Florida

Springer Science+Business Media, LLC

Library of Congress Catalog Card No.: 78–71496
  Grams, Ralph R.
    Medical Information Systems: The Laboratory Module
  Clifton, N.J.:
  432 p.
  7902   781113

ISBN 978-1-4757-1424-1   ISBN 978-1-4757-1422-7 (eBook)
DOI 10.1007/978-1-4757-1422-7

© 1979 Springer Science+Business Media New York
Originally published by The HUMANA Press Inc. in 1979
Softcover reprint of the hardcover 1st edition 1979

Dedication

The long-range system plan to be described and given a thorough critique in this volume was designed for the improvement of patient care at Shands Teaching Hospital, University of Florida, Gainesville. The concepts and the final product are a direct result of the dedicated effort of the faculty and staff of the Department of Pathology under the leadership of Dr. Richard T. Smith, chairman, and Mr. Wayne Herhold, the previous executive director of the hospital.

Acknowledgments

During the past five years, it has been my personal privilege and challenge to work with an enthusiastic group of professionals in the Department of Pathology at the University of Florida in the creation of a distributed processing network for our teaching hospital. This document will more than adequately testify that many thousands of hours have been used to delineate the needs, highlight the inconsistencies, and project the future for a hospital and medical school interested in operating under a communication system concept. Over the years, we have depended very heavily on certain key people who have provided ideas, time, and personal effort to establish the necessary criteria for success. Special recognition is due Mr. Ed Pastor who came to the department as an experienced laboratory data processing manager and extended our knowledge well beyond the capabilities of our initial group. His contributions to the pages of this document and the final system configuration were invaluable.

It is certainly apparent to me that our initial decision to create a team to make this program a reality was the correct one and has proven to be the sustaining resource. Neither the hardware nor the software are productive or creative without the cheerful, instructive, concerned activity of our special faculty and staff who deal with the problems of

system control and maintenance. A special and sincere thanks goes to Mrs. Ann Brooks for her valuable assistance in coordinating nursing floors and hospital administrative requirements with the needs of the laboratory. Mrs. Margaret Gruver deserves special commendation as chief computer operator. She has borne the burden of bringing the system in and training new operators in the language and technology of hospitals, computers, and pathology. She has engendered the respect and sincere gratitude of the house staff through her devotion to patient problems and their personal resolution through her hands.

Mrs. Linda Litzkow is singly responsible for the flow charting and documentation, as well as the final manuscript organization. Her contribution as an analyst and editor is sincerely appreciated.

As a test of the state-of-the-art, this book was written on an IBM 370 using an IBM/ATS program for text editing and revision. Ms. Pat McDonough and Mrs. Georgina Peck were responsible for this project and the final revisions.

As a principal investigator in this program, I must give my sincerest thanks to Dr. Richard T. Smith for his steadfast belief in the project. His personal support and confidence created a stable team which sustained the program during initial scrutiny from the clinical staff.

An undertaking such as this is totally impossible without the concerted support of individual divisions and faculty members within the department who daily interact with the system, having aided in the development of the primary parameters during the design phase. Dr. Jack Gudat in Clinical Chemistry, Dr. Perry Teague in Immunology, Dr. Herman Baer in Microbiology, Dr. Kenneth Pierson in Anatomic Pathology, and Dr. Lynn Flory in the Blood Bank represent these clinical interfaces. All have contributed greatly to the development of the test files and the specific subsystems to be described. As further evidence of the teamwork necessary for such an undertaking, the involvement of each technologist and medical student within Shands Teaching Hospital, in retrospect, represents a sincere effort to improve patient care. Under periods of stress and system malfunction, when the odds seemed virtually impossible and the barriers immense, this group sustained the effort and the belief that the project could be accomplished. As we perceive it at this time, they were correct and the systems survived and continue to grow.

The challenge presented by the problems and systems which we have used affected every individual in our hospital in a different way. To all those who have been involved, I can only say thank you for your help. From my vantage point, this project exemplifies what can be accomplished through combined efforts toward a common goal.

Preface

This book represents the working papers, discussion, and critique of an operating hospital communication system centrally housed in the clinical laboratory. The programs were designed to function in the intense environment of a tertiary-care teaching hospital. The system is now three years old and continues to grow in service capacity. The ideas and concepts presented have been tested and validated by numerous students and faculty who have evidenced their concern over the years. The detailed design of the system is provided for the reader so that those areas which have proven to be painfully insufficient in our hands can be recognized and avoided by others in the future. New design criteria which would be desirable will be presented. We have tried to review our material and experience in implementing a hospital communication system so that others may be better equipped to deal with the complications of such a venture and the pitfalls to be expected in today's health care environment.

The book presents a detailed description of an existing system. This is necessary because of the critical nature of the design and the need for specific documentation before formal programs are proposed and implemented. Mistakes are all too often not published, but left for others to

repeat. Here, we will try to highlight where we made initial errors and what had to be done to correct these. The discussion in the text emphasizes the difficulty of achieving a communication system within an active health care community and the necessity of a highly trained staff to handle the day-to-day problems that occur during periods of stress.

This book should be of value to all those who are involved in hospital data processing. Such active participants as medical system designers, hospital directors, laboratorians and pathologists, and systems contractors and consultants are often asked for advice on, and must make proposals for new hospital systems. To serve as a reasonable point of departure for critiques of these systems, the major effort of the text is geared toward understanding the application programs and formats, with detailed programming steps omitted. Human engineering and the techniques of staff- and physician-interface are highlighted. The emphasis is placed on the obvious fact that any system must be sold to the community of potential users, and sustained and nourished as a continuing commitment if successful performance is to be realized.

The concept of a communication system centered around the clinical laboratory is presented from an historical standpoint covering the necessary steps to achieve a final product. Elements related to planning, installation, and testing are discussed. The detailed files are reviewed and described. Each area of the hospital is analyzed to show what programs and systems were necessary, along with an appropriate critique of our current design. The analysis and discussion of each of the subsystems is based on more than three years of experience and staff input. Hospital departments, such as Admissions, Emergency Room, Outpatient, and, of course, the nursing station present unique problems to the designer of both procedures and hardware. Special emphasis is placed on the topics of laboratory ordering and specimen handling, which are unique in each laboratory system operating in a communication mode. For those in the clinical laboratory, each major section is reviewed so that existing systems can be analyzed and future systems applications projected.

Along with a review of current operating procedures, the text examines the unique aspects of a computer center organized around patient care. The manual backup system is detailed since it stands as a ready reserve in case of hardware failure. Special topics such as billing, system archives, and departmental requirements for hospital administration are reviewed. A chapter is devoted to our implementation and an anecdotal review of problems that occurred as we jumped into the abyss in November, 1975. The last chapter deals with the long-range plans for

our communication system and what the future may hold as the state-of-the-art continues to change.

Readers have the option of following the historical viewpoint in reviewing each system as it progressed in our hands, or individually reviewing sections of primary interest for reference to working systems.

This book is intended as an initial volume in a series of related texts centered around the concept of hospital information systems. Additional modules for admissions, medical records, scheduling, pharmacy, and so on are planned for the future. These modules are referenced in the introduction and will be topics of review as these systems are constructed, implemented, and finally evaluated.

Contents

Dedication   v

Acknowledgments   vii

Preface   ix

Part 1: Fundamental Concepts and Developmental Planning

Chapter 1.   Distributed Processing Network   3

Introduction   3
Hardware   5
Software   9
The University of Florida's Distributed Processing Network   11
Current Data Processing Developments   20

Chapter 2.   The Modular Concept   22

Description   22
Real Data   22
Not An Mis—Yet   23
Commercial Interest   23
Objectives   23

Chapter 3.   Historical Background   25

When   25
The Study   28
   System Objectives   30
Specifications   31

Contract Criteria   31
Contracting Is A Tricky Business   32

Chapter 4.   System Planning   34

Forms   34
Supplies   34
File Construction   35
Pert Charts   35
System Inspection   37
Contract Monitoring   37

Chapter 5.   Installation   38

UPS   38
Hospital Cabling   41
Central Evaluating   42
Software Evaluation   43
Staff Required   45
Videotape Production   47

Part 2 : Laboratory and Reporting Mechanisms

Chapter 6.   Shands Lis Documentation   51

Overview   51
File Structure   51
General File—Room Numbers   53
General File—Terminal Function Matrix   54
Master Test File   55
Master Test/Subtest   55
Master File—Age/Sex Range Table   56
Expanded Test File   56
Special Files   59
Instruments   59
Doctors   60
Laboratory Areas   60
Work-Sheet Programs   60
File Maintenance   61

Chapter 7. Admissions   63

Introduction   63
Format   64
Programs Required   67
On-Line Operation   68
Admits   68
Bed Control   69
Unique Problems   69
  How to Identify a Patient   69
  Admission Orders   70
  Terminal Location   70
  Hardcopy   71
  Failure to Transfer   71
  Failure to Discharge   72
Constant Monitor   72
Outside Demands   72
Admissions Critique   73

Chapter 8. Emergency Room   75

Introduction   75
Forms   76
Audit Trails   76
Chart Handling and Data Retrieval   76
Terminal   77
Daily Reports   78
Special Problems   78
  Speed   78
  Personnel   79

Chapter 9. Ordering Procedure   ·   80

Introduction   80
On-Line Versus Off-Line   80
Forms   81
Ordering Process   86
Message Files   90
Audit Trails   90
Signatures   90
Physician Interface   91
Nursing Station Operation   91
Critique   92

Chapter 10.   Laboratory/Nursing Station Interface   95

Introduction   95
Terminal   96
Orders   97
Chart Operation   97
Blue Cross Approval   97
Reports   98
   Ward Reports   98
   Daily Charts   98
   Seven-Day/Final Charts   99
   Census   102
   Inquiry   102
   Archive   106
Specimen Handling   107
Problems   107
   Crowding   107
      Overutilization   108
   Sabotage   108
   Audit Trail   109
   Space   109
   Sound   110
Design Criteria For a Nursing Station Terminal   110
Ideal Terminal   111
   Printer   111
   Cathode Ray Tube (CRT)   111
   Keyboard   112
   Communications   112
   Terminal Design   113
   Cart or Mounting Media   113

Chapter 11.   Outpatient Operation   116

Introduction   116
Outpatient Admissions   116
Order Forms   117
Result Entry   117
Chart Reporting   117
Problems   118
   Terminals   118
   Transport   118
   Data Accuracy   118
   Remote Operation   118

Chapter 12. Specimen Handling   119

Key System   119
Protocols   119
    Stats   119
    Expedites   120
    Routines   120
Specimen Screening   120
Check-In and Timing   121
Specimen Audit   123
Specimen Number Assignment   124
Label Production   124
Training Area   125
Problems   126
    Improper Specimens   126
    Wrong Numbers   126
    Incomplete Orders   126
"Ideal" Specimen Number Program   126
Label Speed   127
Coordination with a Central Processing Unit   127
Central Communications for The Lab   128
Specimen Acquisition   128
    Blood Drawing   128
    Specimen Check-In   128
    Doctor Draws   128
Credits   129
Stat Specimens   129
Special Orders   130
Outpatient Specimens   130

Chapter 13. Chemistry System   131

Introduction   131
Forms   132
Specimen Preparation   132
Special Orders   132
Work Sheets   133
Input Terminals   134
Smac Interface   135
Unfinished Test Report   136
Abnormal Test Report   137
Chart Reports   139

Staffing and Organization 140
Quality Control 141
Referral Labs 141
Mark-Sense Card 141
Critique 141

Chapter 14. Hematology   144

Introduction 144
Forms 144
Specimen Preparation 145
Special Orders 145
Work Sheets 145
Input Terminals 146
Unfinished Test Report 148
Abnormal Test Report 148
Chart Reports 148
Staffing and Organization 150
Quality Control 151
Mark-Sense Cards 152
Critique 152

Chapter 15. Microbiology   154

Introduction 154
Request and Source File 154
Specimen Preparation 155
Input Terminals 158
Unfinished Test Report 159
Chart Reports 159
Staffing 161
Mark-Sense Cards 164
Epidemiology Input 164
Critique 164

Chapter 16. Immunology   165

Introduction 165
Request Forms 165
Specimen Preparation 166
Work Sheets 166
Input Terminals 166
Unfinished Test Report 168

Abnormal Test Report 168
Chart Reports 168
Staffing and Organization 169
Quality Control 169
Mark-Sense Cards 169
Critique 171

Chapter 17.   Blood Bank   **172**

Introduction 172
Request Form 173
Specimen Handling 173
Input Terminals 173
Unfinished Test Report 174
Chart Reports 174
Staffing 175
Mark-Sense Cards 175
Critique 179

Chapter 18.   Anatomic Pathology   **180**

Introduction 180
Request Form 181
Input Terminals 181
Unfinished Test Report 181
Chart Report 183
Critique 183

Chapter 19.   Computer Center Operation   **184**

Introduction 184
Personnel 184
Schedules 186
Training 186
Functions 187
System Control 187
    Census 187
    Reports 187
Halts 191
Loops 191
Physician Problems 192
File Handling 192
Specimen Handling 192

Report Distribution 194
Service 195
New Programs 195
Noise 196

Chapter 20. Equipment and Configuration   197

Description 197
Reliability 197
Service 199
Down Time 201
Spare Program 201
Software Maintenance 201

Chapter 21. Back-up System   203

Introduction 203
Hardware Rotation 203
Scheduling of Spare Parts 204
Service Contract 204
Manual Systems 205
    Less Than 24 Hours 205
    Greater Than 24-Hour System 206
    Limitations 206

Chapter 22. System Reports   208

Ward Reports 208
Daily Charts 208
Seven-Day or Final Charts 209
ADTL 209
Abnormal Test Report 209
SMAC Sequential Multiple Analyzer with Computer . . . 209
Disc Copy 210
Doctor Reports 210
Correcting The Patient's Data Files 211
Work Sheets 211
Census 212
Archive Input 213

Chapter 23. Billing   214

Introduction 214
Tape Handling 214
Interface 216

Chapter 24. Archive Retrieval   **217**

Introduction   217
Inputs   217
Output   218
Microfilm Processing   219
Microfilm/Computer Interface   219

Chapter 25. Departmental Requirements   **224**

Introduction   224
Organization   224
Control and Monitoring   225
Start-up and Training   225
House Staff Orientation   226
Know Your Company   226
Corporate Problems   227
The Marriage Contract   229

Chapter 26. Hospital Implementation   **230**

Introduction   230
    Staff 230
Case History   231
Additional Problems   237
    System MD Challenges   237
    Reverse Education   238
House Staff Orientation   239
Inservice Education   239

Chapter 27. Future Plans   **240**

Introduction   240
Additional Horsepower   241
On-Line Versus Off-Line   241
Library Capability   241
"Normal Value" Statistics   242
Terminals   242
What Has Been Accomplished?   243

Chapter 28. Comparative Systems   **244**

Bibliography   **247**

Appendix 1.   The System Contract   **250**

Introduction   250
Lease Agreement   250

Appendix II.   File Building Procedure   **259**

Introduction   259
Laboratory Procedure Documentation   259

Appendix III.   The Shands System Flowcharts   **262**

Introduction   262
System Symbols   264
The Problem Statement   265
Operations Statements   267

Appendix IV.   The Shands System Files   **412**

Introduction   412
Master Test Files   412
Test Files   413
Expanded Test Files   414
Expanded Test Files   415
Message File   416
Room File   416
Room File   417

Appendix V.   The Emergency File   **419**

Introduction   419
Manual Laboratory System Plan A   419
  Outpatient Clinic   420
  Inpatient Blood Drawing   420
  Emergency Room   421
  Medical Records   421
Manual Laboratory System Plan B   421
  Outpatient Clinic   421
  Inpatient Blood Drawing   421
  Emergency Room   422
  Medical Records   422
Manual Laboratory System Plan C   422
  Outpatient Clinic   422

Inpatient Blood Drawing   422
Emergency Room   423
Medical Records   423

Index   **425**

PART 1

FUNDAMENTAL CONCEPTS AND DEVELOPMENTAL PLANNING

1

Distributed Processing Network

INTRODUCTION

Large medical computer systems can be visualized and designed in at least two practical configurations. Using a "central" concept predicates a large host computer in which a single data base is maintained for interaction with a number of terminal users (Fig. 1) [1, 2]. In this configuration, the major expense is the central system itself, and the speed and access to the files are dependent on the data-base managing software. The obvious limitations of this design relate to the lack of failsafe redundancy and the high cost of the initial investment.

A second approach is a distributed processing and distributed data-base "network," which accomplishes as much computing as possible at the source. This "network" communicates only data that are absolutely essential to the operation of a higher level or parallel processor (Fig. 2). The realization of distributed processing networks has only been possible since the advent of minicomputers and microprocessors, devices that offer great utility and feasibility for source processing at a reasonable price [3–6].

3

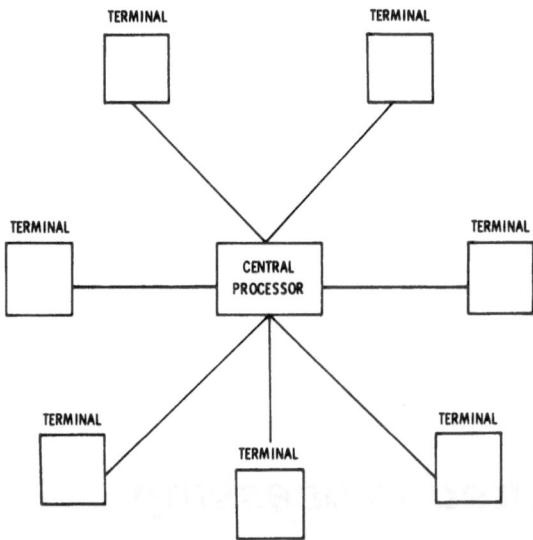

FIG. 1   The traditional central processor is the primary supporting unit in a customary star configuration utilized for multiple terminal installations. Any failure in the central processor or communications link usually terminates service at the individual terminals.

There are many examples of large, centralized medical-computer systems with multiple terminals [7–9]. Distributed networks, however, are new and as yet undefined in the medical environment. Our current configuration marks the first implementation of this new

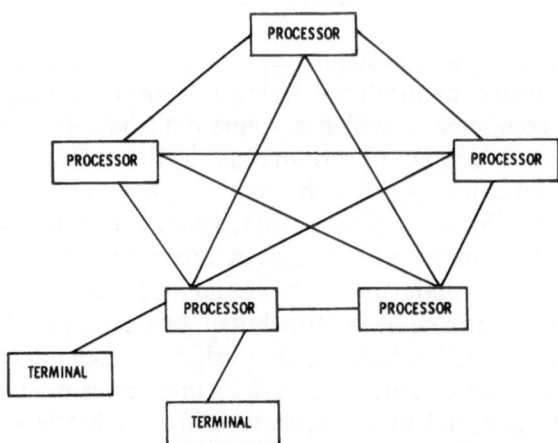

FIG. 2   In a multiprocessor environment, as the number of individual processors increases, the complexity of internal communications increases to the point at which a highly sophisticated operating system is required to decipher interprocessor communication.

network philosophy for our institution and will require several years to complete.

HARDWARE

In order to achieve a distributed data-base communication system, all hardware must be totally compatible and meet a number of stringent requirements.

1. For medical purposes, the hardware must optimize real-time speed and communication with the individual user so that response time and access are optimal (usually less than one second). Achieving this transaction speed insures that the terminal users will accept the system and participate in an active and constructive manner.

2. The modular approach must offer flexibility to hospital administration, which may need time to build its staff to support a new system. Using a distributive hardware network, the individual hospital is allowed to select the most appropriate module for implementation and install this in isolation from others that might be more futuristic.

3. The cost/performance criteria of management must be promoted by a distributed network, since each individual subsystem will include only that software and hardware necessary to accomplish its particular operation. One should not need to buy excess hardware and capability for future use.

4. The distributed network must provide hardware and software that is both upward and downward compatible, so that each processor has the ability to integrate into any other level. This hardware requirement makes it imperative that the manufacturer contemplating development of such architecture start at the user terminal and carry the concept all the way through to the central multiplexing/concentrating processor in which the individual distributive functions are switched (Fig. 3). A comparison of Figs. 2 and 3 illustrates the "network" simplification that can be achieved by centralizing all intranetwork message switching. This eliminates the need for multiple lines between CPUs.

5. The distributed processing network requires a "smart" terminal able to perform significant remote processing at the user's request. This polyfunctional terminal will contain a microprocessor or a set of micros, and sufficient hardware and firmware to accomplish defined functions. As an example, nurses' notes and vital statistics on

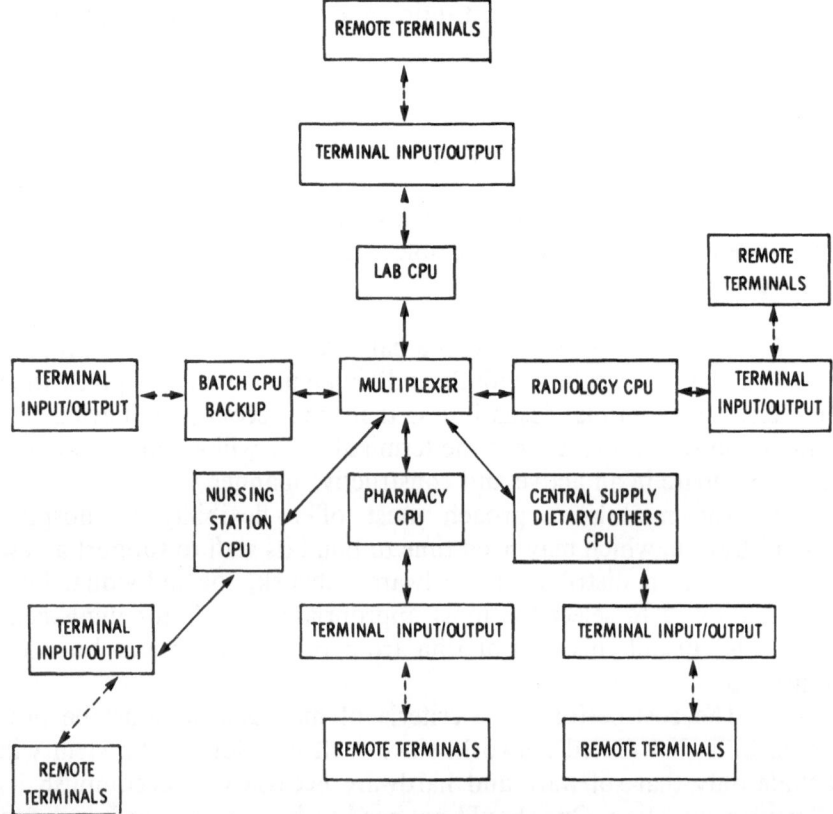

FIG. 3   To eliminate the endless lines of communication among processors, a configuration can be drawn in which one central multiplexer/concentrator is used to handle the high speed communication among processors. In this particular design, remote terminals are supported on dedicated processors and linked to other major subsections of the hospital communications network through the central hub. Unfortunately, the software and hardware capable of handling this type of configuration are extremely limited. An additional problem is that any failure in the central multiplexer will bring down the entire interprocessor communication network.

patients might be retained in the memory of "smart" nursing terminals without hampering the next level processor (which really does not need to handle or store this type of information).

6.   The final element of a distributed network should provide the individual user with total control over the work environment. In the field of medicine, this calls for the use of portable, hand-held entry devices, which will soon become a part of the physicians' and paramedics' armamentarium (Fig. 4). Such a unit will be carried on rounds

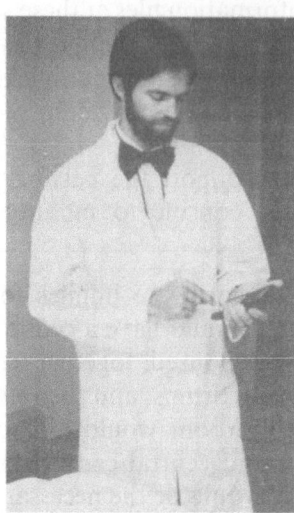

FIG. 4   The remote processor mentioned earlier will someday evolve into highly portable small devices which will allow an individual physician or health care specialist to encode the significant patient information for subsequent transmission into a local "smart" terminal and, therefore, to a central storage media.

to collect patient information on a real-time basis. These portable terminals will then have access, review, and edit entry through the remote intelligent terminals to the entire distributed network that will ultimately store, process, and transmit the collected information. A new generation of medically-applicable remote portable-entry devices is just beginning to appear. State-of-the-art, low-power, electronic technology permits such terminals to retain large data-storage capacities over long periods on very limited battery power [10].

7.   The distributed network must allow for either batch or real-time access to a large-scale computer which can handle complex file manipulation and massive sorts and merges. This can be accomplished by removable magnetic media (such as tapes or discs), or through a hardwire connection with another large machine. Using this type of arrangement, it is possible to strip off all the accounting and memory-consuming functions from the real-time system and relegate them to the batch environment while still maintaining full real-time control and operational integrity.

8.   In order to maintain the hardware configuration on a real-time basis, the distributed processors must be able to communicate operational intelligence with each other at extremely high speeds, and further

be allowed to transfer information files at these same speeds. To do this, there must be direct "tie-lines" (memory-to-memory) between the CPUs operating through a master multiplexer/concentrator. Spare "tie-lines" in this central module provide protection if partial failure should occur.

9. The hardware to support the network must have switchable peripherals and a master console to monitor overall network performance.

This configuration of hardware implies four levels of allocation (Fig. 5). First, the hospital should have a central data-processing room in which all CPUs would be housed, together with the central magnetic storage media, such as discs, drums, and their associated teleprocessing communication lines. This room would also contain the high-speed printers, magnetic tapes, and central control facilities. Located at the next physical-system level would be the necessary hardware and control

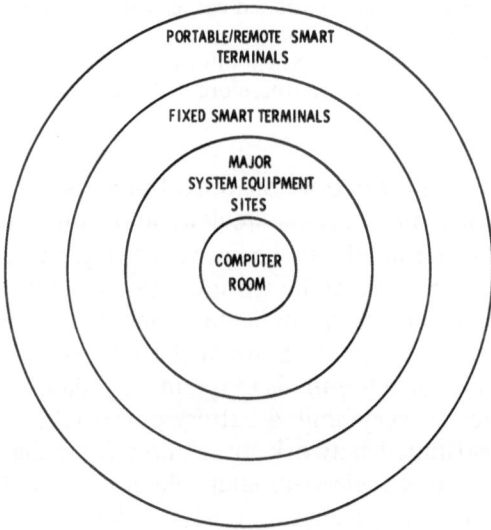

FIG. 5 Looking at the areas of interface, one finds that the central computer is the hub of all activity surrounded by the major equipment sites, which might be located in the laboratories or admissions section. Dependent on that major equipment are the fixed "smart" terminals which are able to carry on a high degree of interactive dialog in and of themselves and eventually process the information through the major system equipment sites and into the central computer room. As a fourth level of interactive terminal control, we are predicting the availability of hand-held "smart" portable terminals which will be personal data entry devices such that the physician or health care specialist will have a personal mode of inquiry and input on hand at all times.

equipment to maintain the viability of each individual network subsystem. For example, the clinical laboratory would have its own line printer, card reader, and associated control facilities sufficient to generate the work sheets, labels, and reports necessary to maintain laboratory processing integrity. Such hardware would most probably be located remote from the central computer room, and could be positioned anywhere within the hospital.

The third physical level of network hardware is the "fixed" remote terminal or input device. This could be a nursing station terminal or a laboratory terminal for data gathering within a special area.

The fourth level of system access would be the primary users' hand-held terminals. These portable data collection devices will extend coverage to virtually all levels of staff. Figure 3 shows this nesting of hardware within the range of a distributed hospital data processing network.

SOFTWARE

The past five to ten years have seen great emphasis on the development of software for minicomputers to allow the implementation of a number of specific medical systems. Each package has been geared to its own processor and written in the language supported by the equipment manufacturer. In almost every case, using a 16-bit or smaller machine, the ability of a given processor to handle large files and to perform complex functions on large data bases has been severely limited. It appears that for those routine functions in constant demand within the hospital, it is most appropriate to program the applications in an "assembler" language in order to make them as small and as efficient as possible. In the same context, the distributed network will require the development of a "parent–child" relationship among system files (Fig. 6). For an admissions package, the primary data base (or "parent" file) would be held on the admissions processor. A copy, however, might be transferred to laboratory, pharmacy, x-ray, or other distributed subsystem so that rapid access to the proper patient data set for departmental processing is possible. This type of file "housekeeping" is a significant problem and must be approached directly as the files are built and the system developed. For the "parent" file, one would functionally like to lock and unlock this area, offer input and output as well as compare, and have a defined security level for access.

To communicate information within the network, software conversion must be established for all intranetwork message traffic.

FILE STRUCTURE

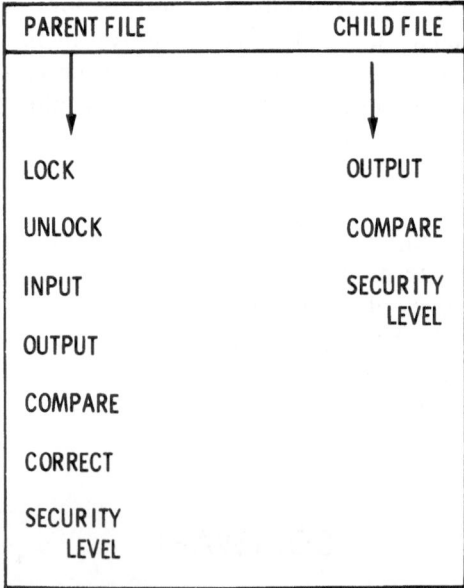

FIG. 6   To support an interprocessor communication network, it will be necessary in certain hardware configurations, to postulate and to configure a "parent" and "child" file structure in which certain functions are available to multiple processes and programs.

Figure 7 describes a standard message segment. After the start code, a user terminal processor identification is attached. The originating software determines the location to which the message will be sent and appends the location to which the answer will be routed. All data would be packaged and followed by an end code. By keeping this message envelope uniform throughout the network, each processor and its software can be treated separately and in isolation from all other entities.

As an added feature, the distributed data base and the distributed

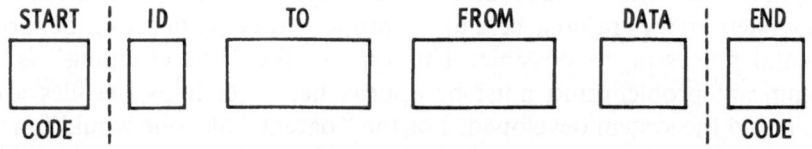

FIG. 7   For the communications network to have a standardized format for transmitting information between processors, a type of structure and coding will be necessary so that each individual processor can unpackage and repackage information as it is handled.

software network create a truly modular system which allows for redundancy and protection in the event of a subsystem failure. Even though the admissions package may be holding the "parent" file, the secondary files are able to support each of the modules until the primary file can be repaired and the faulty element brought back on-line. Alternate software can be maintained in the network to take over "parent" file control and support the other subsystems.

THE UNIVERSITY OF FLORIDA'S DISTRIBUTED PROCESSING NETWORK

Figures 8–13 show our five-year plan to achieve the distributed network for our medical information system. The system started with one computer supporting admissions, laboratory, and nursing stations. Phase II segments the nursing station load and increases terminal capacity. "Smart" terminals replace existing teletype terminals in Phase III. Phase IV carries admissions and maximally uses the tie-line communication arrangement. Phase V illustrates the multiplexer and the addition of pharmacy. The final step (Phase VI) creates a number of modules around the periphery supporting such subsystems as pharmacy, x-ray, dietary, central supply, laboratory, admissions, and eventually the patient's medical record. The terminals utilized in this network are "smart" terminals that incorporate a wide range of capabilities. Such terminals include facilities for accessing and handling microprocessor input from hand-held units and, of course, can fully integrate with the next level of processor. The hub of the network is the "traffic manager" which handles the high-speed "memory-to-memory" links between the CPUs and makes certain each important system function is transferred to the appropriate processor. Additionally, the central unit supports consolidation of peripheral equipment within the main computer room and allows switching of tape drives, printers, card readers, and other peripherals. This provides for economy of hardware and "back-up" protection in case any single element fails.

Our five-year plan was initiated with the concept of laboratory, admissions, and nursing stations integrated into a single processor. A "parent" and "child" file is maintained for the admissions data and was the initial start in the distributed data-base network. The second computer module added to the network isolates the nursing station and admissions function, and is a direct memory link to our laboratory processor. Each CPU is configured with 64 communication lines with core resident buffers for each terminal. The operating system on each

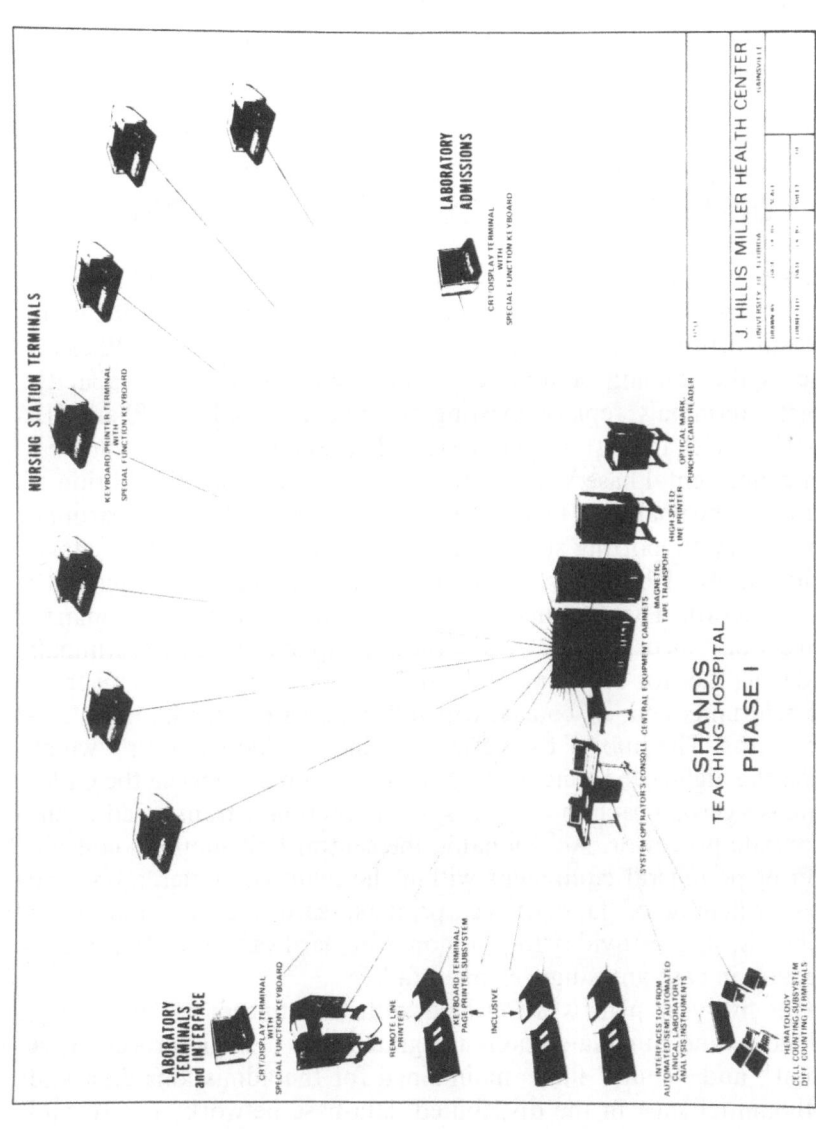

FIG. 8 Phase I of Shands Teaching Hospital Communication System involved the clinical laboratory, nursing stations, and all the laboratory terminal interfaces required to maintain a full service environment. This project was initiated in 1975.

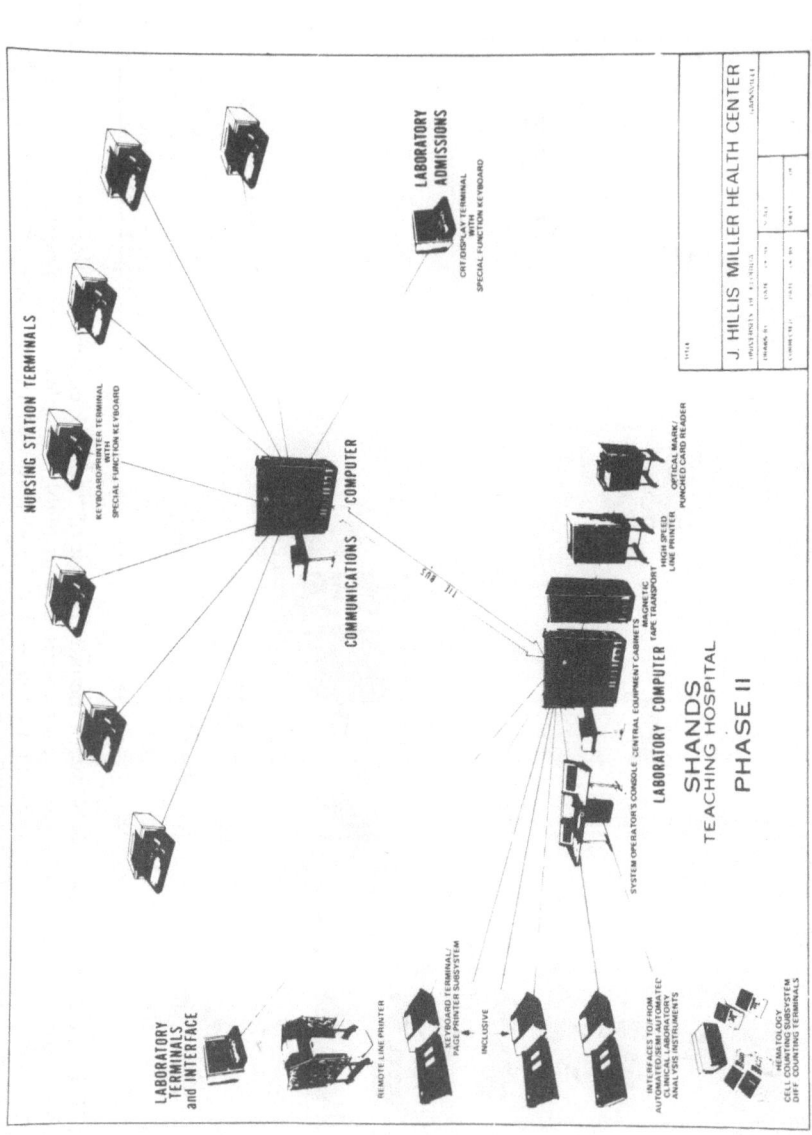

FIG. 9 Phase II in the Shands Teaching Hospital Communication Network evolved into a two processor network using a tie-bus to communicate between the two processors at memory speeds and allowing processor A to handle the clinical laboratory and processor B to handle admissions and the nursing stations. This project was completed in June 1977.

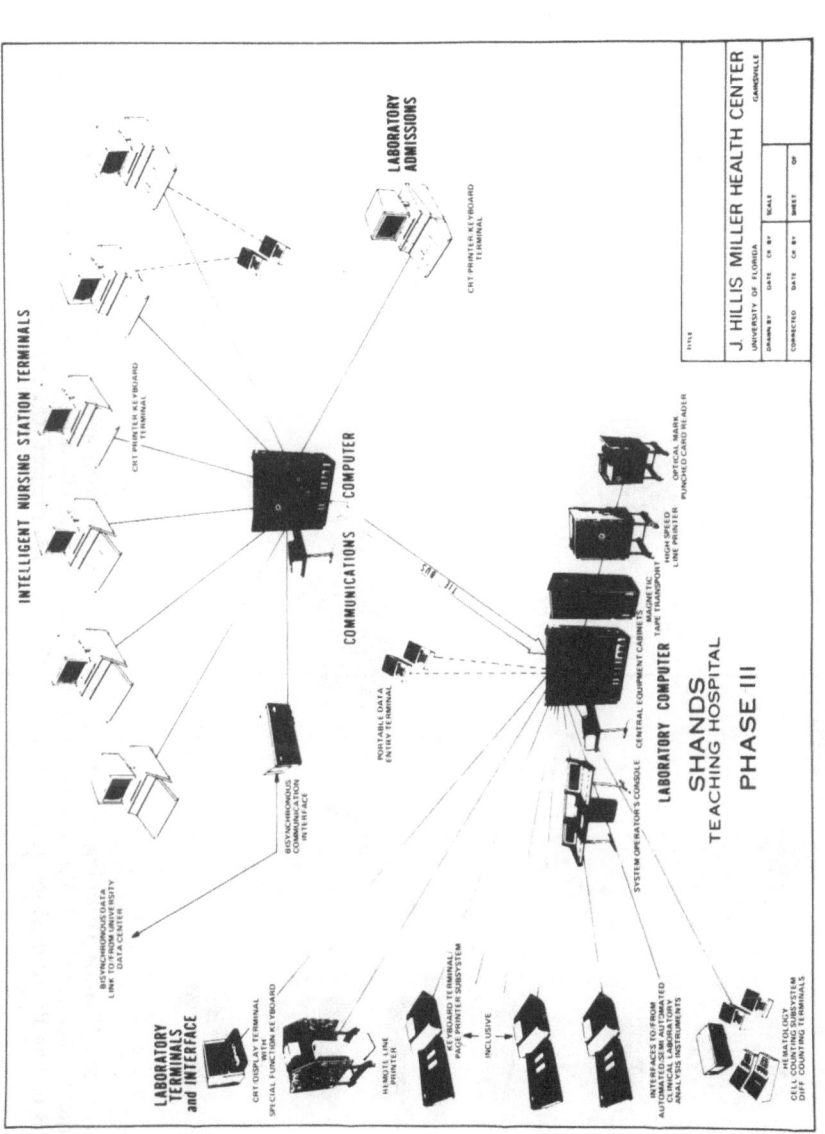

FIG. 10 Phase III in the Communications Network includes the use of "smart" communication terminals for nursing stations specifically designed for the speed and sound requirements in that highly complex environment. In addition, a synchronous communication mode is shown to a remote computer as well as hand-held battery entry devices available for both the clinical laboratory and the nursing station. This project was completed in October 1977.

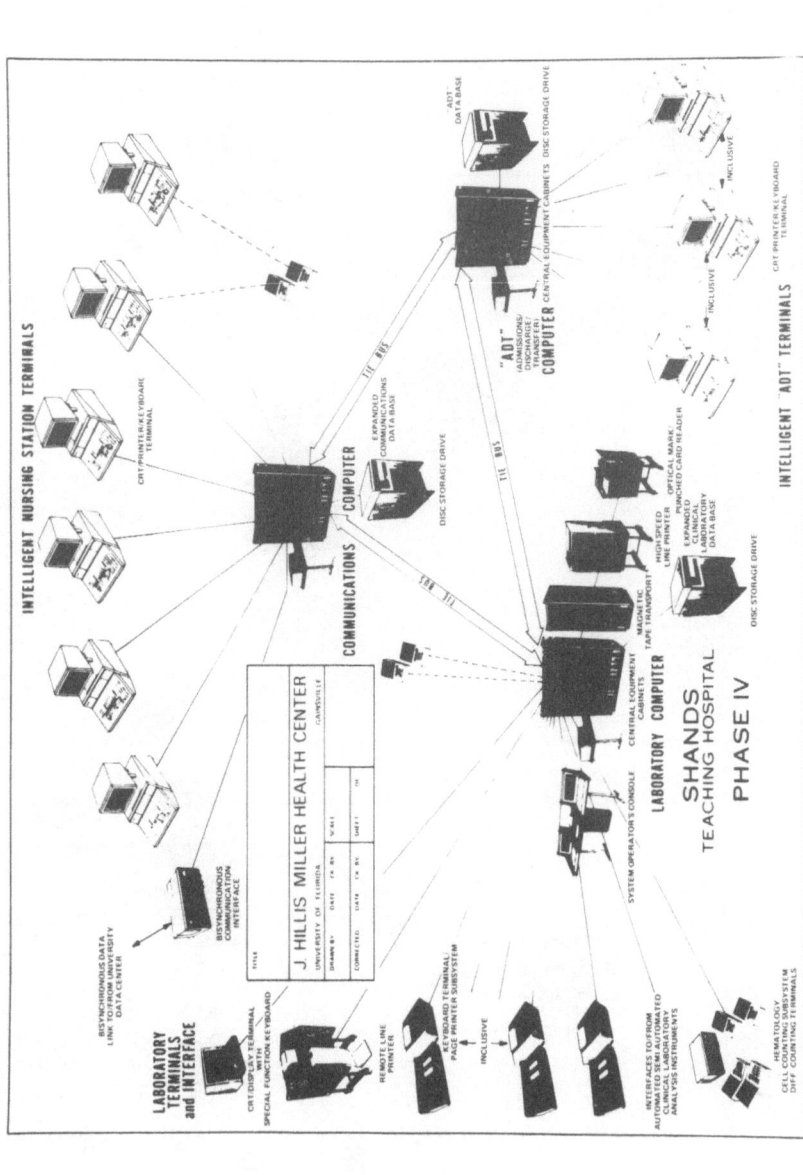

FIG. 11   Phase IV of our communication network is yet to be built and involves the addition of a full admissions package to handle all the insurance and third party reimbursement information necessary for patient accounting.

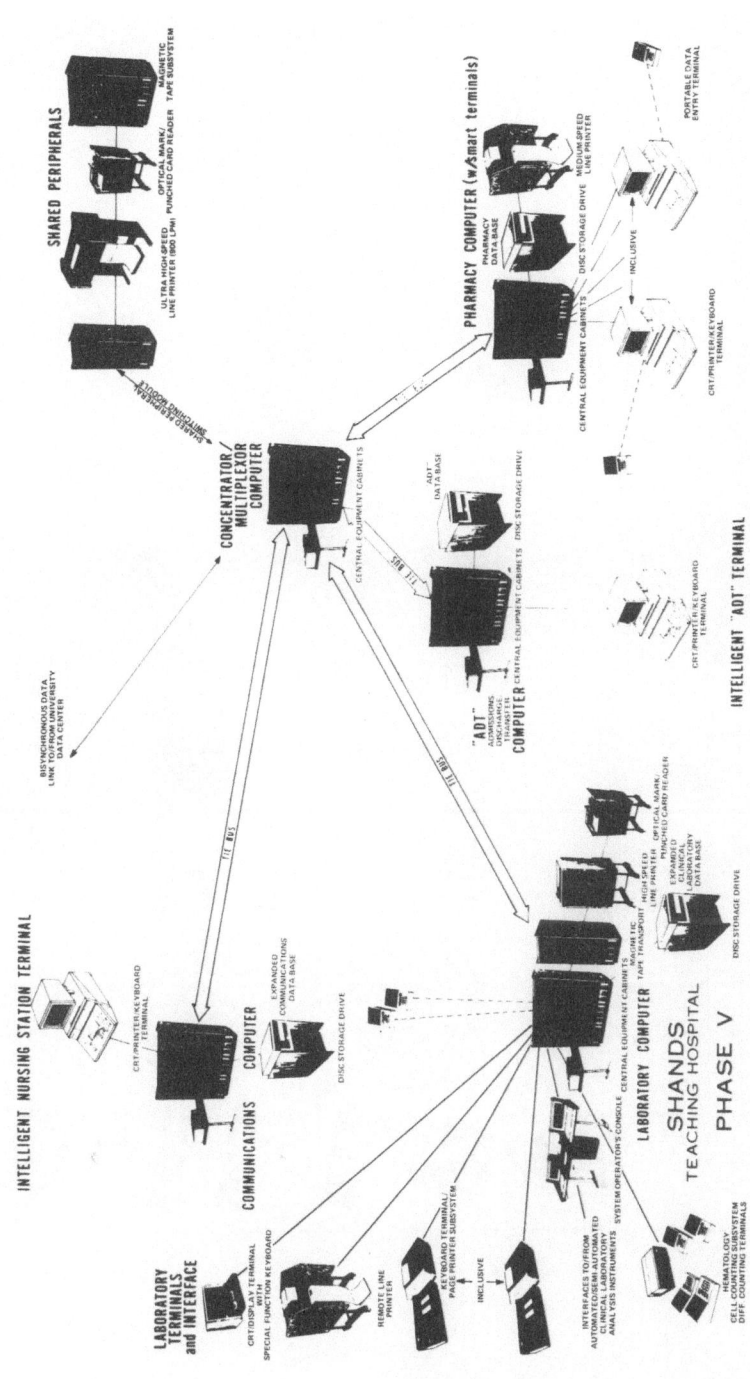

FIG. 12 Phase V allows the introduction of a central multiplexer with the addition of the pharmacy system and shared peripherals among processors. The pharmacy module and multiplexer are yet to be built.

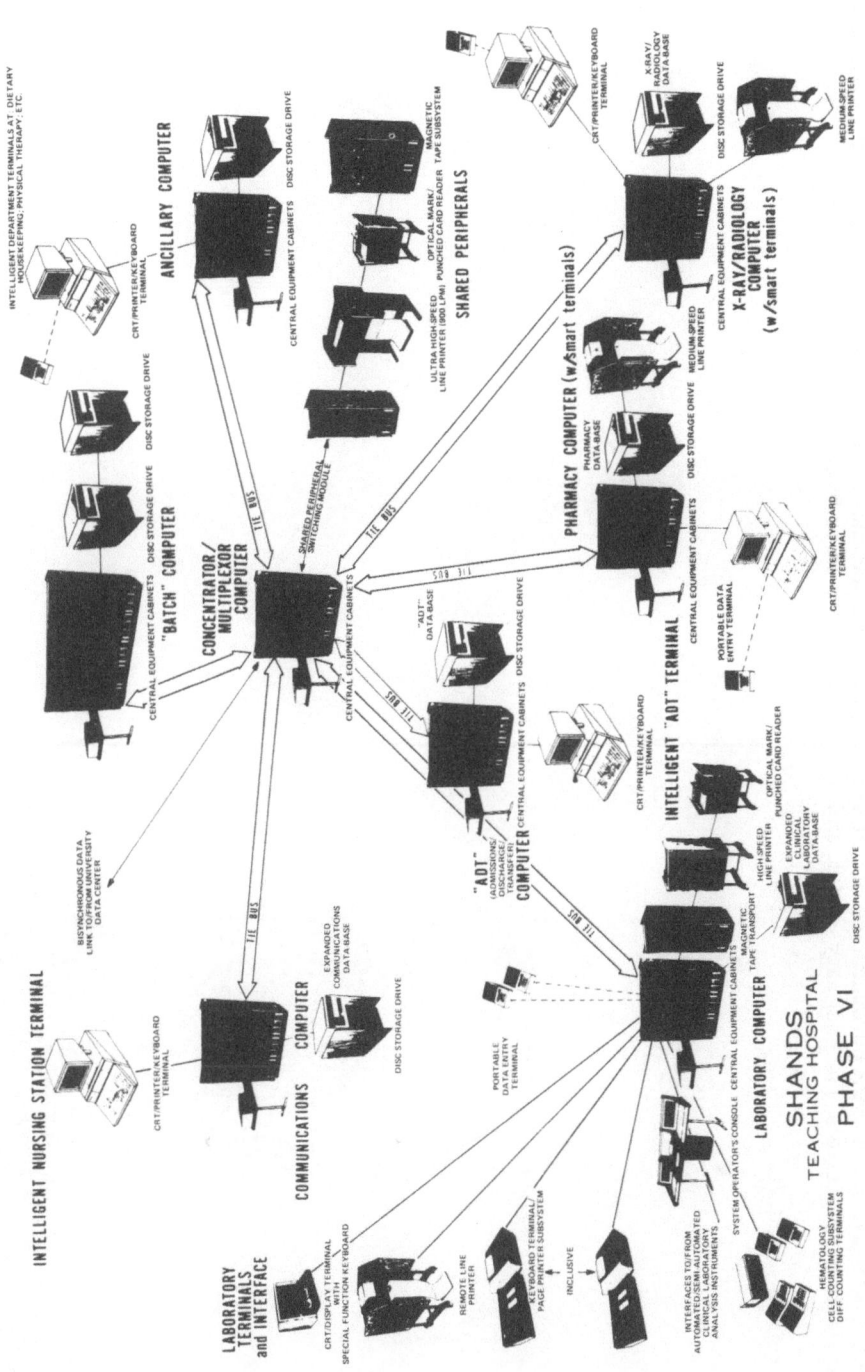

FIG. 13   Phase VI of the Shands Communication Network includes the addition of a batch computer system usable for patient accounting, financial reporting, and other batch functions, an ancillary computer allowing the capture of charges at the nursing station along with a complete inventory system for the entire hospital, and the addition of a full radiology computer network for patient care.

module allows for a priority of software input and a selection process by which the queueing of programs is accomplished. Once the network exceeds three processors, the central multiplexer/concentrator module becomes a necessity because of the intermixture of memory-to-memory (tie-line) cables.

Our first module consisted of only a single computer. It had to encompass the capability to handle nursing stations and admissions, together with operation of the clinical laboratory. This is the key link in moving between individual systems and a coordinated network. Once the nursing stations are brought on-line, it is a natural progression to upgrade the hardware to offer more capability, speed, and service. Suggestions will be made regarding the necessary elements for information system integration as well as the criteria selected for hardware improvement. At this date, Phase III is completed and Phase IV and V are being contemplated.

CURRENT DATA PROCESSING DEVELOPMENTS

Since the conceptual framework of our system was elaborated in 1974, there has been little progress in developing the necessary sophistication of both hardware and software to carry the configuration beyond the three-processor state (Phase IV). Although the modules are structurally sound and practically obtainable, the multiplexer and controller concept for multiple minicomputers has not matured sufficiently to perform the high-level functions necessary in a hospital system. Although one could envisage an operating system able to handle multiple processors, the facts seem to indicate that these technical skills of the computer program would eventually reach a limit, and that the final product would resemble a large main-frame system with its many inherent disadvantages. The features which seem most important for hospitals are:

1. Modularity—the ability to install the right package at the right price.
2. Upward compatibility—freedom to grow without interrupting or destroying what has been achieved.
3. Speed—response times at the terminal site of one or two seconds for transaction processing.
4. Protection—nonstop operation with many levels of hardware, software, and system redundancy.
5. Support—hardware and software stability sufficient to retain product integrity now and in the future.

With our experience to date, it seems impractical to pursue the traditional unicomputer network philosophy. We have worked for over two years to achieve a two CPU system and it still falls short of our five critical objectives. The question of design must really return to the primary computing machine. Instead of incorporating standard mini-computers as the building block, one must postulate the creation of a new machine capable of reaching the hospital information system objectives.

Product development in hospital systems has always been a very minor consideration for hardware manufacturers. The largest market has always been in the business sector, which can tolerate many more system limitations than can hospitals. An interesting change has occurred in recent years with the expansion of real-time business data processing. Suddenly, the batch oriented mainframes are being asked to operate in a nonstop environment. Industry has discovered that real-time systems can create business (24-hour computer banking), promote efficiency (inventory control), and assist in the daily management of corporate offices.

Whenever such a market arises, there are those who are perceptive enough to anticipate this need. Such is the case for the Tandem Corporation in Cupertino, California. Their hardware, software, and system architecture are totally consistent with hospital needs for modularity, upward compatibility, speed, protection, and support. Others will certainly follow in this fertile marketing sector as the demand for real-time support increases.

Perhaps hospitals will always remain an EDP step-child to business, but at long last computers are moving out of the batch environment and into the challenges of nonstop transaction processing. This appears to be the necessary incentive to release technology sufficient for real-time hospital operation. If we can take this development as given, then the rate-limiting step to apply our new technology now becomes medical systems design, validation, and management. Our systems plans, as projected through Phase VI for a modular design, can be directly transferred to this new type of hardware architecture. Such a potential is the exciting possibility for the future.

2

The Modular Concept

DESCRIPTION

The laboratory and hospital communication module which will be described and evaluated in detail was designed in 1973. It represents a collection of single systems and subsystems encompassing the operation of our pathology specialities (Chemistry, Microscopy, Hematology, Immunology, Microbiology, Blood Banking, and Anatomic Pathology), admissions, bed control, and remote hospital-terminal control and communication.

Since our financial resources were limited, all functions were placed on one computer. This obviously represents the bare minimum starting module for a distributed network.

REAL DATA

The information presented in this document is actual on-site material experienced by the author and co-workers of this project. It is extremely important for those who will become involved in expanding

information systems within the hospital environment to appreciate the magnitude and complexity of integrating a complicated facility with only the rudimentary skills and basic capabilities found in a computer. Such an undertaking is often underestimated at the outset, oversimplified during negotiations, and most certainly destined to a fate less than optimal during implementation.

NOT AN MIS—YET

The system to be described includes pathology, the nursing station, and admissions. Contained within the confines of this discussion will be: the input of real-time admission data, central bed control, nursing station operation for ordering and retrieval of information regarding laboratory work, maintenance of an outpatient clinic laboratory through remote terminal input, a modular testing and reporting facility for all pathology data, and the integration of an emergency room through peripheral terminals. The coordination of these diversified areas and remote terminal input represents a dramatic change in respect to the standard isolated laboratory computer system [11–13]. Those principles which appear to be unique for laboratory communications will be highlighted and described in a critical manner to delineate any areas of initial miscalculation which were made during the design and development phase of the project. It is hoped that this information, along with detailed accounts of some of our experiences, will help those who wish to participate in creating a similar environment for their hospital.

COMMERCIAL INTERESTS

This publication is in no way intended to promote the wares of any specific vendor. We believe that after reading the full discussion you may have as many questions regarding the proclivities of individual vendors as we do at this point.

OBJECTIVES

This document presents a comprehensive discussion of a live ongoing hospital/laboratory communication module which is based upon a systems study of a patient care facility with approximately 500 beds and an active and growing Outpatient Clinic and Emergency Room service.

The long-range distributive network previously described serves as the focal point for system design and hardware selection. The information presented will reflect many of our current assumptions based on the elements which we must face daily. Since our system has grown in complexity and additional demands have been made for more highly skilled activity, it has become apparent that there is a basic minimum number of systems which must be designed correctly if any similar communication network is to survive. These areas will be highlighted during the discussions and alternate approaches which appear feasible will be presented.

Historical Background

WHEN

The initial thrust to establish a computer-based laboratory system was formulated in 1970. The departmental faculty had been exposed to other laboratories in which computers were being utilized. They believed the hospital would be better served using this type of report-generating system. At that time, the hospital employed a cumulative record system in which each one of the laboratory areas had a separate report card (Fig. 14) [14]. The data was written in columns headed by date and time and kept in divisional baskets for copying on a daily basis. The entry mode of the laboratory system used an IBM "Port-a-Punch" card for requests (Fig. 15). Following laboratory use, the cards were then sent to an IBM 370 computer system for charging. Those same cards, submitted without specimens during the day, created blood-drawing lists and work sheets in batch mode. A great dissatisfaction with the port-a-punch card system arose because many difficult manual transactions were required in the handling of the cards and manipulation of the data files. Since the system offered no reporting capabilities, there was little benefit to the laboratory, other than the preparation of labels in the

CLINICAL PATHOLOGY LABORATORIES
University of Florida Hospital and Clinics
CUMULATIVE REPORT

Presumptive Diagnosis: Date Reported: Clinical Chemistry

CHEMISTRY

Analysis	Normal Values	Date:											
CO_2 Content mEq/l.	24 – 30												
Chloride mEq/l.	98 – 109												
Sodium mEq/l.	135 – 145												
Potassium mEq/l.	3.1 – 5.3												
Calcium mg/100 ml	Adult 9.0 – 11.0 Child 9.0 – 11.6												
Magnesium mg/100 ml	1.8 – 2.8												
Total Base mEq/l.	140 – 153												
Blood pH units	Art. 7.34 – 7.48 Ven. 7.31 – 7.45												
Blood pCO_2 mm Hg	35 – 45												
Inorganic Phosphorus mg/100 ml	Adult 3.0 – 4.5 Child 4.0 – 7.0												
Alkaline Phospharase K-A units	Adult 4 – 13 Child 13 – 20												
Acid Phosphatase K-A units	0 – 4.0												
Amylase Somogyi units	60 – 160												
Lipase units	<1.0												
Lactic Dehydrogenase units	80 – 120												
SGO Transaminase units	10 – 40												
SGP Transaminase units	5 – 35												
Aldolase units	3 – 8												
Bilirubin Total mg/100 ml	0.1 – 1.2												
Bilirubin Direct mg/100 ml	0.0 – 0.2												
B.S.P. % retained at 45 min	0 – 5												
Cephalin Flocculation Hanger units	0 – 2+ (48 hr)												
Thymol Turbidity S-H units	0 – 5												
Total Proteins gm/100 ml	6.7 – 8.3												
Albumin gm/100 ml	3.7 – 4.9												
Fibrinogen mg/100 ml	200 – 500												
Triglyceride mg/100 ml	10 – 140												
Cholesterol mg/100 ml	Age 20 – 30 130 – 230												
Creatinine mg/100 ml	0.6 – 1.2												
Urea Nitrogen mg/100 ml	8 – 18												
Uric Acid mg/100 ml	Male 3.4 – 7.8 Female 2.5 – 6.2												
Glucose, Fasting: mg/100 ml	65 – 110												
Glucose Tolerance Test mg/100 ml	Date: Time:							Date: Time:					
Serum Iron mcgm/100 ml	75 – 150												
T.I.B.C. mcgm/100 ml	250 – 350												
Iron Saturation percent	20 – 55												
Plasma Hemoglobin mg/100 ml	0 – 5.0												
Oxygen Saturation percent	Art. 94 – 100 Ven. 60 – 85												
Protein Bound Iodine mcgm/100 ml	3.7 – 7.6												
Plasma Cortisol mcgm/100 ml	6 – 25												

Key to Symbols:

A. Laboratory accident
B. Confirmed
C. Clotted
D. Moderate
E. Recollect specimen
F. Physician notified
G. 2 hr. p.c. glucose
H. Hemolysis
J. Xanthochromic or Icteric
K. Marked
L. Lactescent
M. Minimum
N. Not done if total bilirubin is normal
P. Patient not available
Q. Quantity insufficient
R. Improper labeling
S. Improper specimen
T. To follow
U. 45 min. BSB-sample not received
X. Test cancelled by physician

CLINICAL PATHOLOGIST

FIG. 14 Prior to the installation of the communication network, a cumulative report was used on which each of the major laboratories recorded its information manually by date and time.

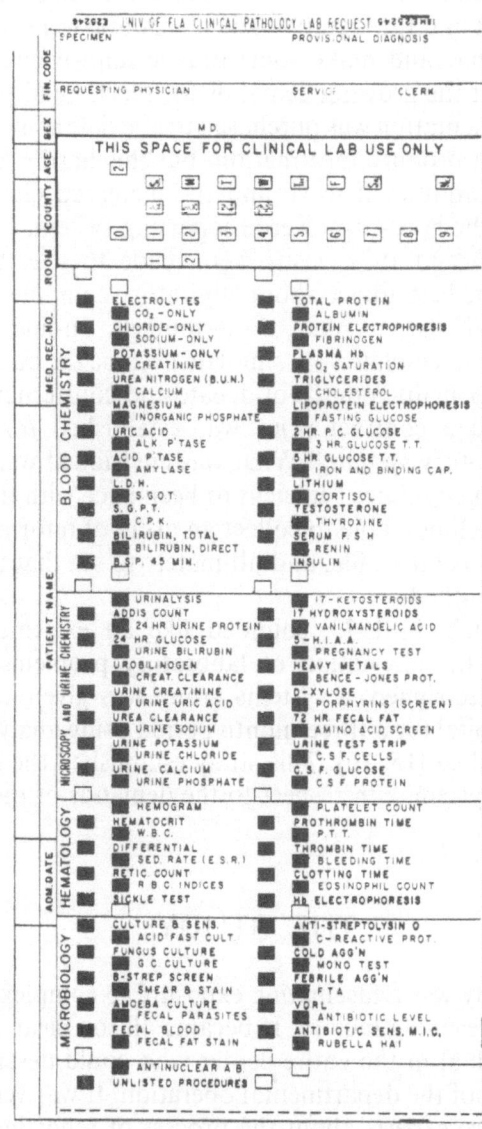

FIG. 15   As part of the communication network, a port-a-punch card was used for laboratory ordering. Holes were frequently lost and errors commonly occurred in punching.

morning. As the requests for stat testing increased at an exponential rate, the port-a-punch card system became quite useless and more of a burden than a productive tool. The complaints and concerns of the staff were evident and the faculty made it very apparent that the laboratory had to change and make some drastic improvements in its performance to meet the growing demands for service and productivity.

New instrumentation was purchased to alleviate some of the manual effort required to produce information, but this hardly kept pace with the demand for additional work and the increased clerical workload associated with the hard-copy Xerox reporting system.

During 1970 and 1971, visits were made to selected sites in an effort to solicit the best advice about laboratory computers. Such words as in-house, out-house, turnkey, do-it-yourself, on-line, off-line, real-time, batch process, emulate, and simulate became the buzz words of the department. After many months of debate and consternation, a vendor was selected and a contract price was established for a "standard intramural laboratory system." What was envisioned was a high-speed report-generating computer sufficient to keep pace with the demands of the hospital and clinics, able to collect an array of information and put the significant facts into a file, and ultimately to see that the billing was properly accomplished.

This approach, in 1973, sounded like an extremely reasonable prescription for the alleviation of laboratory problems. Before final specifications were signed, a systems group was given an opportunity to study the hospital for a three-month period using analytic techniques previously described [15, 16]. This study established the needs and criteria for a new system with respect to the demands of the hospital and the laboratory.

THE STUDY

The systems study was a fascinating exposure to complex departmental operations in a teaching facility. It became all too clear that there was no single individual in the entire center who could describe, in detail, any major phase of the departmental operation. It was very common to ask administrative experts about the process of reporting, billing, and requesting, only to discover a partial or incomplete answer. Manual systems were used and grossly abused by faculty and staff without any appreciation of the repercussions for the patients. Our initial task was to bring these manual computer systems conceptually together using flow charts and exhibits so that one could adequately explain what was

Table 1

Serious Laboratory Problems and Associated Areas of Resolution

Nature of problem	Lab only	Administration + lab	Communication system
Too many phone calls			×
Redundant requests for data			×
Lost reports	×	×	×
Lost requests		×	×
Lost charges	×	×	×
Lost or misplaced specimens			×
Lost historical data		×	×
Inaccurate patient identification		×	×
Inadequate outpatient reporting	×	×	×
Inaccurate blood drawing lists		×	×
Illegible orders			×
Incomplete ward training			×
90% stat orders			×
Need for primary doctor		×	×
Reporting paperwork bottleneck		×	×
Totals	3	9	15
% Resolution	20	60	100

actually happening. The problems that were encountered in looking over the systems and interviewing technologists, nurses, hospital administrators, and departmental faculty related to 15 critical areas within the hospital complex (Table 1) [17]. In an honest evaluation of the problems and what could be accomplished, the standard isolated laboratory system, at best, could look forward to the resolution of only 60 percent of its problems with a long-term highly coordinated effort between hospital administration and the laboratory services.

As a recap of approximately 200 persons interviewed over three months, the following conclusions were reached:

1.   The increased number of employees used to operate the manual systems had become counterproductive, and there was no commensurate increase in management and supervisory personnel (all of which were insufficient and unavailable).

2.   No single individual or group understood the operations of the Department of Pathology and its interaction with the hospital.

3.   Systems outside the territorial boundaries of pathology were the major limiting factors—nursing service, couriers, floor clerks, medical records, etc.

4. The timely communication of information was the key ingredient missing in the service function equation required for successful laboratory operation.

These conclusions were further supported by the data derived from the system's flowcharts, which showed that approximately 30–40% of all problems involving laboratory/patient services resulted from demands outside the control of the Department of Pathology.

It was quite apparent at that point that only through the use of a communication system would the department ever achieve anywhere close to a 100% success in solving the critical problems uncovered during the system's review. After contemplating this information and presenting it to the executive faculty, a decision was made to develop a communication system in which we would integrate a turnkey laboratory data-handling package of known capability with a fully-developed remote-terminal order/retrieval system of unknown and unproven capability.

What we really needed was a modular medical information system in which pathology could communicate through a network of terminals connected to the nursing stations, clinics, and emergency room on an interactive channel to provide the information each needed for optimal patient care. Since the initial design, our modules have solidified into specific packages which can now be configured for a distributed-data processing system. Technology has provided the tools for this important step and opened the door for more flexible and responsive systems at a very competitive price.

System Objectives

After the initial study, another three months was spent writing specifications to support a contract to develop and deliver our laboratory communication module. Some of the fundamental criteria for system success dictated at the outset were:

1. A mandatory 24-hour per day operation.

2. The response times from any of the individual terminals had to be less than three seconds.

3. Terminal operation had to be interactive so that both the system and the user could accomplish complex constructive tasks.

4. The system had to be designed to give to those who participate something of interest and value to sustain their efforts. As an example, the cooperation of admissions in gathering the information should supply them with an on-line census to help them with bed allocations.

5. Hardcopy audit was considered essential on all terminals of the system to eliminate any ambiguity or mishandling of data because of its highly integrated nature.

6. Special checks and balances were designed into the system to guarantee successful operation and to eliminate the possibility of system error. As an example, patients who are not admitted to the proper beds cannot have laboratory work ordered. By this simple function, one can control patient movement within the hospital and guarantee that laboratory work will return to the proper patient at his correct location when it is completed.

7. Human engineering was to take a dominant role in the evolution of the software, in the application of the programs, and in file maintenance functions. Both the hardware and software must seem simple and obvious so that our untrained clerks and secretaries could assume the role of computer operator and adequately maintain the system [18, 19].

SPECIFICATIONS

Approximately 300 pages of detailed specifications were written for the system in flowchart format delineating each step of the way and each function that was to be performed by the software. All selectable functions were described and each file sized and parametrically defined. This set of specifications was then sent to the vendor for implementation and required approximately one year of programming and construction before initial installation.

CONTRACT CRITERIA

Appendix I contains many of the details of our state-negotiated contract. This particular document required one year and heroic efforts to negotiate. The pain and agony of contract bargaining almost exceeds description. When such a function becomes involved with the constraints of a state bureaucracy, all questions and their answers become philosophical and elusive. An initial view of the document will show that it is a performance contract that starts payment only when acceptance is achieved. It is designed as both a lease and a purchase agreement so that the state (the customer) has the option of a direct buy out at a pre-negotiated time. There are a number of specific clauses which relate to system acceptance and a number of definitions of delivery dates and

times which may be of value for others involved in negotiations. Probably the most useful function of the contract is to demonstrate the level of preliminary planning expected of both parties for successful implementation. For no other reason, a well-written contract will stimulate proper consideration by both customer and vendor of the requirements of a particular project before its programmatic conclusion.

CONTRACTING IS A TRICKY BUSINESS

To be a good consumer, one must know the market, the products, and the ultimate plan before purchase. This is why we strongly recommend a systems study first, then a detailed list of priorities for the future, followed by a documented plan of action. Calling a vendor in before the plan is completed is self-defeating. Only when you know what you want and how the systems are to be implemented can you adequately judge a vendor.

The idea that the company knows best, or will do it for us, is wishful thinking. Vendors are in business to make a profit, and long design and planning programs are usually not profitable. Therefore, select your vendor from your systems plans and your priorities. Large companies in the computer business do not like this method because it requires preparation of custom software and systems. They are looking for a high-profit package deal and the opportunity to sell hardware.

The smaller companies specializing in hospital communications will probably be more responsive. They too have standard packages, but will usually modify these for an additional cost. A search through industry journals will produce the names of several companies in this category.

Write the vendors you have selected, state your objectives, and provide your plans. Ask for their specifications in regard to your project, and their costs and projected delivery date. Solicit a current list of customers, and while they are preparing your bid, start calling. You will have to do your own detective work when investigating companies— the corporate turnover rate has been high. Armed with facts and figures you must make your own decisions, but before signing the contract there are two steps you should employ for self-protection.

First, hire the best legal specialist in computers you can find and have him review the contract, equipment, and software. Determine ownership of each element and liability. Make sure the payment schedule enforces performance and not merely the arrival of hardware.

Second, hire a systems consultant in your area of interest to evaluate your plan and proposal. This can usually be accomplished in one to two days and will uncover many hidden problems which might otherwise lead to costly repairs. Consultants are usually considered expensive and unnecessary; however, in this situation, one is not asking for designs, but analysis. The detection of serious deficiencies before contract completion is a necessary cost of system design. If properly used, the system consultant can provide that service.

After a protracted period of contract negotiation, we celebrated the signing of the final lease–purchase document with champagne and began making plans for the next stages of the program.

4

System Planning

FORMS

One of the most tedious tasks in the computer field is the development and planning of the forms, cards, paper, and print-outs required for complex systems. This is a very detailed job which demands a long period of concentration and a sincere tenacity to ensure that every last element is accurate and complete. Our order forms and other documents were reviewed dozens of times only to discover irritating and persistent misprints or errors. Some of the obvious forms we required were those for the ordering of laboratory tests, the basic computer forms for the print-out of the charts and reports expected from the system, labels for stats as well as morning blood drawing, and special types of form paper for the laboratory control sheets required to maintain daily operations.

SUPPLIES

Supplies for any hospital-based computer system include a list of hundreds of elements starting with paper and ending with printer

ribbons. Most vendors will supply such a list of materials necessary to maintain their hardware and usually an address, a price, and possibly even forms on which these can be ordered. Additional efforts will have to be made in terms of determining whether these items are on a state or central purchasing contract. We have found it extremely dangerous to rely on a central storehouse for many primary hardware items since inventories can mysteriously fall to critically low levels and resupply may take weeks to achieve. In order to solve this perplexing problem, we maintain a secondary warehouse to store approximately one week's worth of supplies. These are not touched in normal operation. These supplies are kept as a ready reserve in the event that the central warehouse should default on any of our orders and place us in a position of back-order.

FILE CONSTRUCTION

The construction of files for the pathology system was the most time-consuming operation in the entire development process. What was required was the traditional laboratory data for all procedures, along with the complete information necessary for ordering and proper specimen control. A standard work sheet was used (Appendix II) which allowed us to collect the basic information on each procedure performed in the laboratory. This amounted to more than 700 primary test items covering all areas. The file data was then transcribed from the hand-written forms onto keypunch sheets and sent to the vendor for insertion into our computer library. This process took one year and, of course, is an ongoing program since the files are constantly changing owing to the appearance of new methodologies and daily experience with old procedures and new information.

PERT CHARTS

To maintain some semblance of order in the organization during the initial phases of systems planning, we used a PERT chart to coordinate our efforts (Fig. 16). Each major stage was graphed and a deadline was set for completion. This was monitored weekly to make sure adequate planning was done in all areas and that the facility would be ready for

the scheduled delivery date. Attention to detail becomes one of the key factors in the successful planning and development stages of complex systems. Without an adequate staff to meet these demands, less than optimal results can be guaranteed.

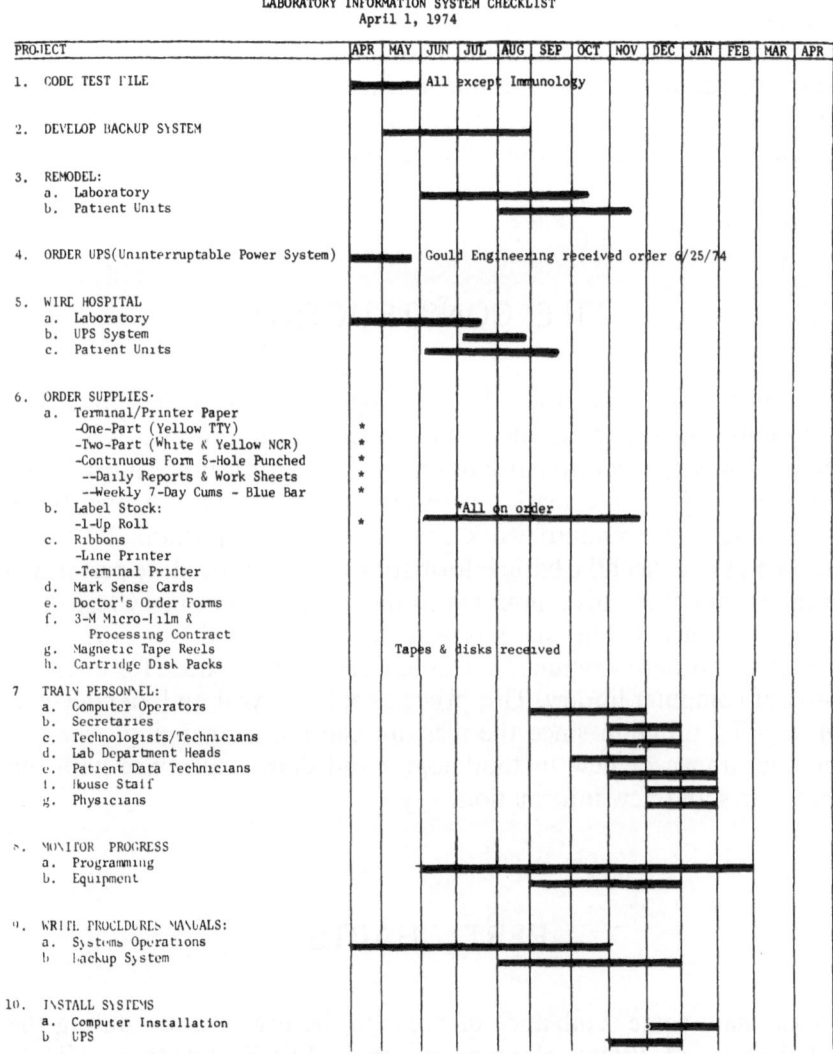

FIG. 16 A Program Evaluation Review Technique (PERT) was used during the design and installation phases to guarantee that each one of the projects was completed on time with adequate material for review and evaluation.

SYSTEM INSPECTION

Approximately six months after the signing of the contract, the systems group visited the vendor for the review of the hardware and software. At that time, the specifications which were in flowchart format were compared with the programming documentation to make sure that every step was being accomplished. The entire system review was completed in three days and delineated those areas in which the programmers were deviating from the specifications and could be creating new problems downstream. In other areas, discussion showed why some of the requirements which we had initially anticipated were actually inappropriate to the system and its configuration at the time of programming. In all cases, a negotiated settlement was reached on each of the major logical points so that the programmers could continue and we could return with the assurance that the system was on course and on schedule.

CONTRACT MONITORING

Following the initial site visit by the department, monthly contact was kept with the programming team and documents were exchanged regarding software to ensure that each stage was completed according to specification.

5

Installation

UPS

After one year of experience in the hospital laboratory at the University of Florida, it was apparent that the electric power systems in Gainesville were totally predictable and one could almost set a watch by the flicker of the lights at one, two, and four o'clock in the afternoon.

Investigation revealed that the power companies were switching sources at these times, and there was nothing they could do to eliminate the occasional flickers. The house power was monitored and showed surges and drops in current and voltage which were incompatible with our new computer. The only solution to this type of problem was the installation of an uninterruptable power supply (UPS). Such a system stands between the electric company and the individual computer to provide a buffer in case of failure. Any lack of power is automatically covered so that the computer recognizes only one steady continuous source of electricity.

Bids were sent out for the selection of a UPS and the final unit chosen provided us with 10 kiloVolt-amps (kVA) of power coming from 60 lead acid batteries under constant charge (Fig. 17). The system func-

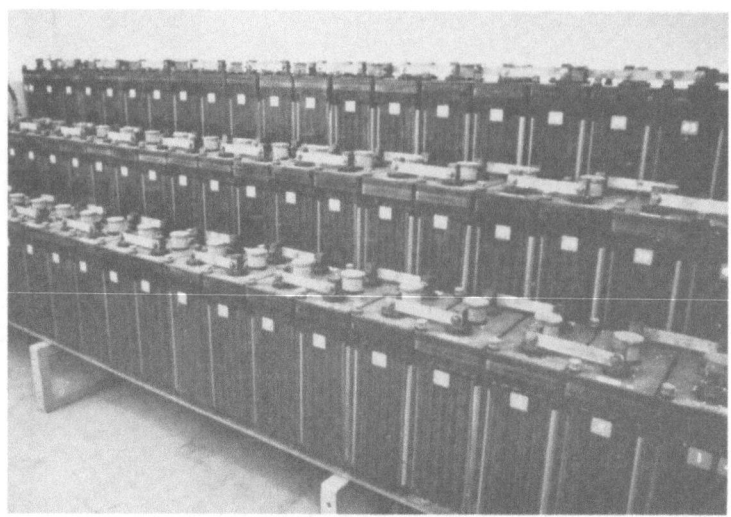

FIG. 17   Because of the frequent power failures and surges in the hospital electrical lines, an uninterruptable power supply (UPS) was required and is shown with a bank of 60 lead acid batteries necessary to maintain the computer on a continuous battery power supply.

tions very much like a car battery, except that an inverter is put on the output side of the batteries and changes the DC voltage to AC and sends that up to the computer (Fig. 18). With this system, if all power is cut off, the batteries continue to send 110 AC power to the computer until they are totally discharged. For our particular system, this means approximately eight to ten hours of continuous operation without any 110 AC incoming power from either the emergency generators or alternate sources within the state of Florida. If our hospital is ever down that long, we certainly will not have to be concerned about the laboratory, or the computer for that matter.

There is a great comfort in having a UPS system installed, since one of the most common ploys of any vendor in this business is to blame the hardware and/or software problems on the power supply. We went through this little shell game initially when the system was installed and were told many times that there was nothing wrong with the software; it was the hardware which was reacting to the uncontrolled 110 AC power supplied to the system. The individual customer cannot attack this kind of argument since the vendor can always claim there is a transient spike in the power line and that is what is destroying the main system. From the time our UPS system was installed, we have had

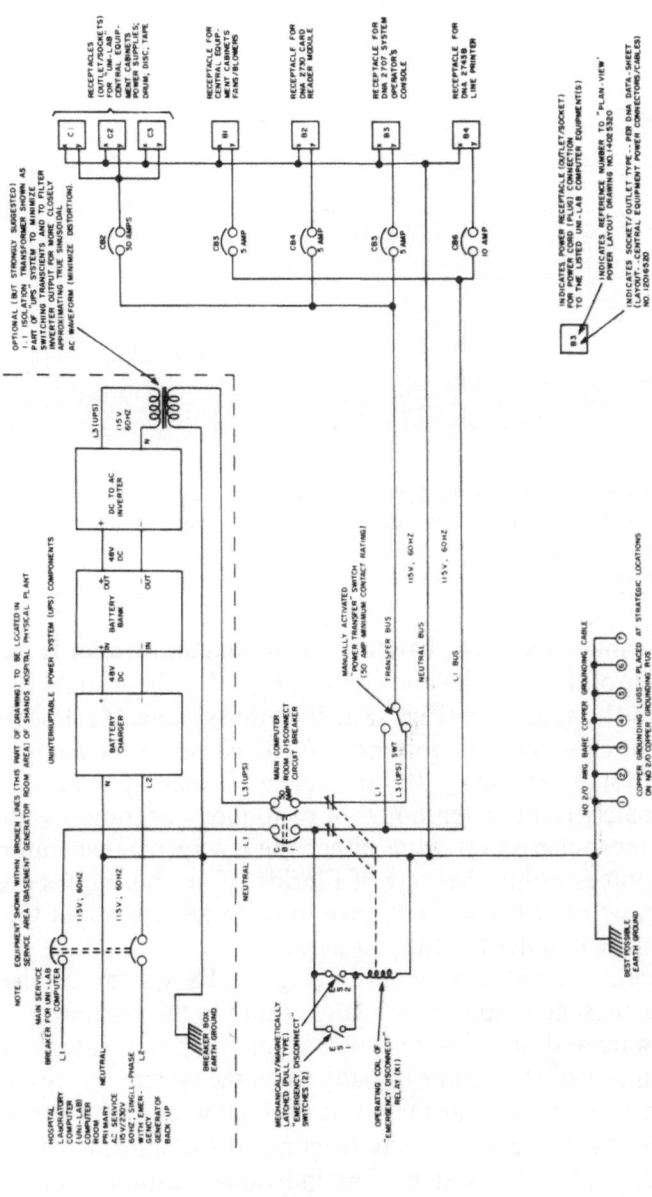

FIG. 18 The battery power system allows the computer to continually draw off the battery on a DC to AC convertor while continually charging the batteries on an AC to DC convertor.

flawless and uninterrupted power and never a moment's concern when the lights dim and the whole hospital goes black. We have had brown-outs and blackouts for periods up to a half an hour, and during that time, the little light of the computer continued to wink while the hospital was in a state of spasm. Such a level of security and protection, in my estimation, is an absolutely essential element for the installation of any communication system or computer operating for patient care purposes.

HOSPITAL CABLING

During our initial planning, the size of the hospital dictated the installa-tion of at least 32 channels of communication from the central computer to serve adequately the various areas. Our health center facilities stretch for about one mile, tip to tip, and include a total of nine floors over this range. Initially, the hospital electricians were contacted and their response was not encouraging. How could they ever get wire through this entire complex to meet our requirements? We made a very intelli-gent (lucky) decision after many frustrating attempts: call the telephone company. Southern Bell Telephone promptly arrived, and they were able to give us a specific plan, time of installation, and cost estimate for the entire program. They pulled communication buses in the hospital to suffice for many, many years of expanded growth and development. We are currently wired for 256 possible terminals which can reach all floors in the hospital and any remote customer in the future. The phone company charges only for the lines that are being used and will guaran-tee the continuity of those connections from the computer room to the peripheral location, service those lines if problems develop at any time of day or night, and maintain these same lines during construction and remodeling. This last feature is something that stretches far beyond the range of control for the pathology department or even the hospital on a normal day-to-day basis.

It is my opinion that the telephone company is the best choice to handle the establishment of the communication lines in the hospital. Our system uses the standard four-wire telephone cable and does not require coaxial lines or special wire for operation. This should be a serious consideration when an LIS or MIS is evaluated since cabling is expensive and special wire may be outside the limits of telephone company service.

Once the communication lines are terminated in the computer room, a junction box is necessary to mate the incoming lines with recognized computer-communication hardware. Special electrical boxes exist which

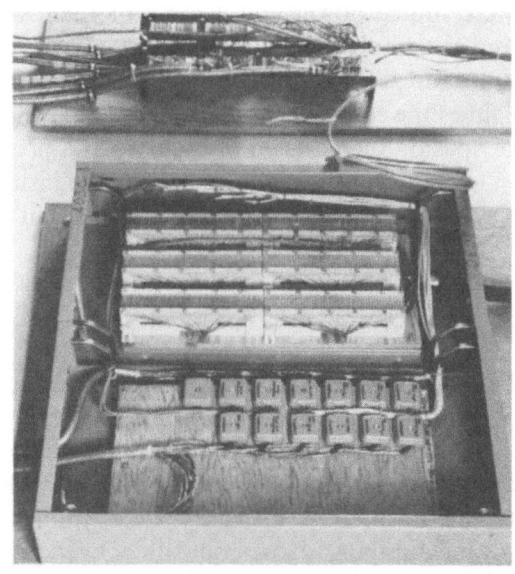

FIG. 19   To house the many communication lines necessary to handle the nursing stations and remote terminals, a central communication network was established which would allow patching of various circuits to the computer. This was our initial design and has been subsequently replaced by a patch board manufactured and installed by the telephone company.

allow one easily to change lines when terminals are moved or disabled. Ease of transfer and flexibility are key factors in the selection of such a utility box. Our current system uses a matrix board and small gold-plated pins to connect compatible circuits (Fig. 19). Better arrangements now commercially available use open-faced lugs that are screwed into a terminal board. The phone company offers a switchboard panel for remote terminals on a rental basis. These units are larger in size, yet permit more access and flexibility.

CENTRAL EVALUATION

During the initial installation of the computer system, it was contractually important to determine the total effectiveness of all the peripheral stations. We housed the terminals in a central location so that the response time could be evaluated for all functions run simultaneously on the 32 communication channels. Since the software to do this kind of time-sharing had not been used before, it was extremely important to

evaluate this capability before the terminals were placed on the floor and the nurses and clerks were allowed to make an initial judgment.

During the trial run, 16 people pushed buttons, ordered tests, canceled items, and generally utilized the terminals simultaneously to determine the response times. Initially, the results were very discouraging, since the delays were in the magnitude of 20–30 s, which was totally unacceptable. After some software changes and adjustments, a response time of 3–5 s was achieved in the worst case.

It is important to test thoroughly the initial installation before hospital release, since the ultimate success of the unit will be judged as soon as it is placed on the floor and is turned over to the nursing staff. The failures and dirty laundry should be kept within the confines of the development group, and should not be propagated to the active hospital staff unless it becomes absolutely essential. The psychology involved is critical and highly predictable. If the system does not work at first, it becomes an easy target for hostility and active resentment. After that, the project becomes a joke and will be ridiculed and destroyed by those who discovered the initial malfunction. Such antagonistic behavior can be circumvented by careful screening of every program and system before it is released to the floor. A positive, realistic attitude must be maintained by hospital personnel, and this comes only from well-planned, functioning hardware and software.

SOFTWARE EVALUATION

The system we are describing does not require the physician to use a computer terminal, but places the ward clerk at the terminal for normal data entry. We had neither the money, nor the hardware to support a physician/computer-interfaced system such as has been used in other hospitals [20]. Our faculty believed there were enough problems without having to change the entire working schedule of the teaching staff. Thus, the designers elected to interface the physician with a form that would be extremely simple to complete and would be placed in the chart and handled by the clerks on a prescheduled basis (Fig. 20).

To evaluate this design, a prototype station was established on the internal medicine floor of the hospital. In this area, intensive ordering occurs over a short period of time for a wide variety of patients. The second test module was located in the emergency room where a high volume of stat orders is anticipated on a crisis-oriented schedule. If the system could accept these two areas successfully using the specified software and hardware, it should be ready for the rest of the hospital.

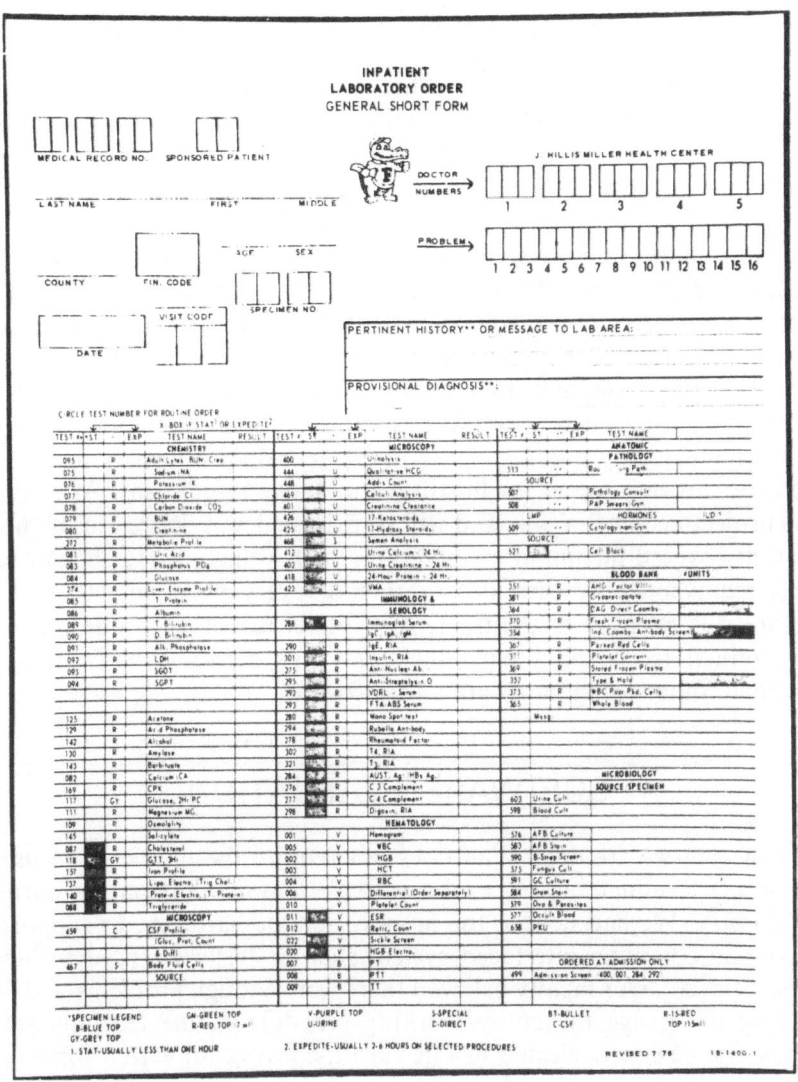

FIG. 20 The general short form of the laboratory order includes those things which are predominantly requested by all services in the hospital. A special area is allowed for addressograph input in the left upper corner in half-tones and special areas for physician numbers and patient problems are allowed on the right upper margins. A circle or an "x" is all that is required to identify what procedure is required. The type of specimen and special information regarding stat orders is provided.

Initially, these two sites operated synchronously for one week. On the first evaluation, many unsuccessful items were identified. The specifications were modified and the programming was changed (Table 2). The methodology, the forms, and the procedures were changed to meet the expectations of the staff in the limited time frame of routine services. After about three months of additional work, the prototype areas were retested. The second pass was much more successful and, of course, took advantage of a great deal of training with the nursing staff in both areas. Two more months were dedicated to adjustments in the system to iron out some of the procedural problems. At last, a viable system was ready for total hospital operation.

STAFF REQUIRED

The research and development required during installation of the laboratory module could never have been accomplished without the staff and day-to-day assistance of our systems group in the department. It is essential to any information system to have a specialist in ward and clerk operations who can speak directly with the individual floor supervisors to work out problems and to delineate areas of deficiency. We call this individual a "patient unit coordinator." All problems related to floor operation are referred to this individual for evaluation and program planning. In addition, a computer operator with a background in pathology is required for training individuals to handle the upgrading of existing staff and to maintain the system on a 24-hour schedule. Currently, our operation uses six computer operators plus a supervisor to handle the system on continuous coverage. All of our initial computer operators were taken from clerical and secretarial staff who had previously been used to complete our cumulative report forms. Although no additional staff was added, it is appropriate to mention that many of the initial clerical people have since quit to take employment elsewhere after being placed on a rotating schedule which maintains 24-hour coverage. Certain types of individuals easily acclimate to a computer system and, of course, others find this extremely difficult. The computer operators form a critical part of the information system in the laboratory operation and therefore should be selected very carefully at the outset. These persons must learn the entire operation of laboratory specimen handling and be able to resolve the on-line problems that develop among physicians and staff. It is natural to become frustrated and infuriated by the comments made by some of the overanxious physicians. A positive attitude toward the patients and the facility is required for responsive operation.

Table 2

First Prototype Evaluation of the LIS

___

Hardware
  Nursing terminal is too noisy.
  Halt-sound alarm is required to alert computer operator of system failure.

Software
  We are facing a problem with clinic and floor orders which are generated at the
    site, yet are not STATS—the number and label system becomes confused.
  Blood drawing lists should be called by individual wards.
  Need more detailed ADTL lists.
  Need SMAC software for paper-tape reader.
  Bed numbers on all reports should include letter designator.
  Patient test files must be 48 tests in length.
  Sample check-in needs the immediate date and time entered in the test file.
  Chart report forms should be changed to 6 columns.
  Differential for Hematology should be in proper sequence.
  Every test must be given a work sheet except for Microbiology.
  Expand stat test number area to 0–999.
  Need page up and down for CRT since it overflows on reports.
  Stat results should not interrupt lab order sequence.
  ADTL times must be time of transaction.
  Message segment must have time and station sending.
  Archive data entry should be one pass and should be done into a buffer before
    changing cartridge.
  All specimens—stat or routine—should be checked in before answers allowed.
  All labels must have test # plus description.
  Order cancel should be specimen number and test number activated.
  Billing report should have MR# and problem on all entries.
  Name field should be 21 characters.
  Test file must allow 999 tests as well as work sheets for all tests.
  Inquiry by patient and ward report should show doctor #'s and names.
  The magnetic tape should be programmed to store all seven-day and discharge
    reports for future statistical analysis.

Operational Problems
  File write over.
  The Alpha search not working properly—not locating proper Alpha area.
  ADTL halts.
  Clock problems at check-in at midnight 00:00—for any specimen checked in
    at midnight (± 15 min) should read 24:00.
  Printers are over printing on lines since data fields are greater than 72 characters.
  Stat morphology reports to floor should be compressed (too many spaces).
  The incomplete test report needs to show patient room number.
  Ward report has no paging.
  Usage report should be updated if patient is credited.
  Master work sheet should be a complete list of tests by patient for each lab area.
  Sometimes on admission entry there is no "entry accepted" returned.

VIDEOTAPE PRODUCTION

At the outset it was apparent that the message that we had to tell about the system was lengthy and detailed, and would exhaust our resources eventually if we did not have some means of communication other than the spoken word and written page. Approximately three months before our system inauguration, the chairman of the Department of Pathology and two other members of the systems group produced three videotapes which were subsequently used for the training and orientation of the faculty and staff of the hospital. These videotapes have proven to be invaluable for in-service training of nursing personnel, floor clerks, medical technology students, residents, and medical students as they interact with the hospital and begin to use the hospital system for patient care. Additionally, training manuals for the computer operators and medical technologists have been written showing the major functions the system provides in each of their areas, along with the format and system criteria for successful operation. Such documentation is essential if the program is to be maintained and training is to be available for continuous operation.

PART 2

LABORATORY
REPORTING MECHANISMS

PART 2

SPORTING MECHANISMS

6

Shands LIS Documentation

Linda Litzkow, M.A.,
Medical Systems Analyst

OVERVIEW

The complete flowcharts for our current laboratory information module are provided in Appendix III. The overview flowchart in this chapter (Fig. 21) displays the basic systems. The subsystems are delineated in detail under the appropriate Appendix headings [21, 22]. Every step of the operation can be reviewed by the use of this particular document. Exhibits and off-page connectors are used for convenience as the reader looks at details associated with each step. Those particular sections referenced as the major divisions of the laboratory are discussed in greater detail in the following chapters. For step-by-step reference to procedure or protocol, Appendix III should be consulted.

FILE STRUCTURE

A computer system is certainly no more intelligent than its files. During the development stage, a great deal of effort was spent delineating those

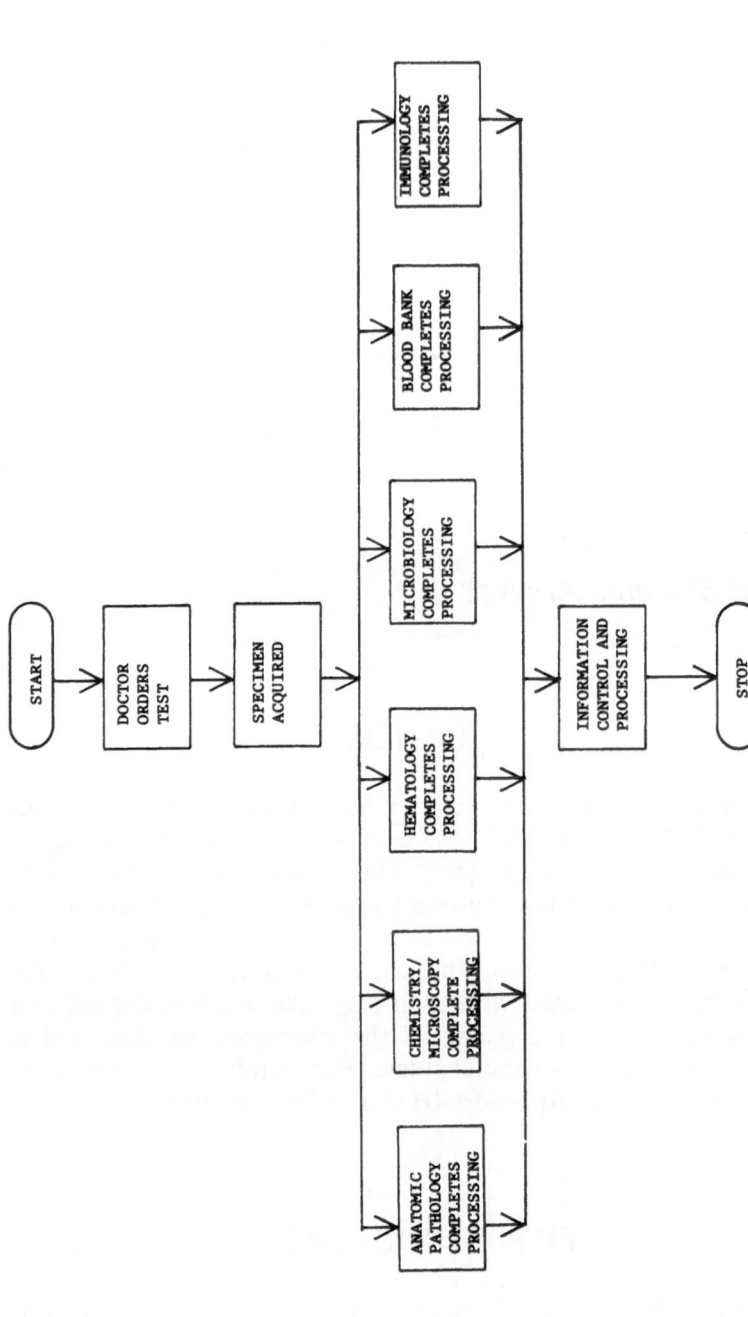

FIG. 21 The overview flowchart for the communication system begins with the physician order and specimen acquisition. From that point the specimen passes to each one of the major laboratory areas for processing. The information is then sent to a central controlling source which is the computer and subsequently distributed through hospital Terminals.

factors essential to the resolution of our high priority problems. The items described in the various file elements are those believed to be most essential for proper integration of both physician and laboratory, and ultimately of the reporting and audit functions of the hospital.

The basic test files for the system are stored on punch cards and kept in decks to be loaded into the system at initiation. Subsequent changes in the file, in most cases, can be made on-line through one of the remote terminals. Special codes and dialog are employed to insure that only authorized users are allowed access to the files. In addition, a new card is made for the master card deck with every on-line change, so that if the system should require an emergency reload, the card files would accurately represent the system at the last moment before it went down. Four basic files are employed: (1) a general laboratory data file, (2) a master file, (3) an expanded test file, and (4) a message file.

The data contained within these files has taken several work-years to accumulate and could be useful for others looking for ideas. Appendix IV presents this information in compact form for reference.

General File—Room Numbers

Every room and clinic in the hospital must be defined by ward, room number, and maximum allocated beds. The algorithm we used states: two times the number of normal patients in the area plus one equals the total number of allocated bed spaces. This allows for some overlap in case patients are not discharged before others are admitted. An "a, b, c, d" through "z" bed designator is used in each room, but is not an exclusive category, so that more than one patient can be in an "a" bed. In the outpatient and discharge area 256 patients can be admitted before file overflow. The emergency room file currently holds a maximum of 156 patients.

Each ward or clinic is additionally identified by a cost center code for workload analysis. Eight cost centers are used currently.

Warning—do not underestimate your hospital, clinic, and out-patient potential for growth. Since our system was designed, the hospital has added 150 new beds, increased the Emergency Room volume by a factor of three, and multiplied the clinic volume by a factor of seven to ten. Such rapid growth eventually destroys any system, and in consequence we are currently unable to provide full service to all areas of the hospital. In projecting growth, use the most optimistic figure possible and hope that it will be sufficient—do not underestimate.

General File—Terminal Function Matrix

A special file exists to activate and deactivate each terminal in the network. Figure 22 shows the functions assigned to each of our current peripheral stations. These can be changed on-line by appropriate central commands.

	TERMINAL #	GENL ADMIT	STAT ADMIT	TRANSFER	DISCHARGE	CORR PT ID	DR UPDATE	UNABLE TO DRAW	SEND MESSAGE	INQ ARCH	INQ DOCTOR	INQ PATIENT	INQ SPECIMEN	WARD REPORT	CENSUS REPORT	LAB ORDER	ORDER CANCEL
LABORATORY	12	X	X	X	X	X	X	X	X	X	X	X	X	X	X	X	X
ADMISSIONS	13	X	X	X	X	X	X		X	X	X	X	X	X	X	X	
5-WEST-OPTH.	14						X	X	X	X	X	X	X	X	X	X	
EMER. ROOM	15	X	X	X	X	X	X		X	X	X	X	X	X	X	X	
3rd FLOOR	16						X	X	X	X	X	X	X	X	X	X	
4th FLOOR	17						X	X	X	X	X	X	X	X	X	X	
5th FLOOR	18						X	X	X	X	X	X	X	X	X	X	
6th FLOOR	19						X	X	X	X	X	X	X	X	X	X	
7th FLOOR	20						X	X	X	X	X	X	X	X	X	X	
SURG. I.C.U.	21						X	X	X	X	X	X	X	X	X	X	
3rd AMB.	22						X	X	X	X	X	X	X	X	X	X	
PEDS I.C.U.	23						X	X	X	X	X	X	X	X	X	X	
OPC LAB	24	X	X	X	X	X	X	X	X	X	X	X	X	X	X	X	
OR/REC/R	25	X	X	X	X	X	X	X	X	X	X	X	X	X	X	X	X
M.I.C.U. 4th FLR	26						X	X	X	X	X	X	X	X	X	X	
ANATOMIC PATH.	27	X	X	X	X	X	X	X	X	X	X	X	X	X	X	X	
N.I.C.U. 3rd FLR	28						X	X	X	X	X	X	X	X	X	X	
6-WEST	29						X	X	X	X	X	X	X	X	X	X	
LAB-CRT-1411	30	X	X	X	X	X	X	X	X	X	X	X	X	X	X	X	X
ALL TERMINALS	00																

FIG. 22   For each of the terminals in the hospital, a matrix exists for enabling the various functions within the communication system. This is handled under software control and can only be changed by the chief computer operator and customer engineer.

Master Test File

A.   A three-digit unique number identifying each test is stored for reference (same as expanded test file element A).

B.   A two-digit code is used to reference the result units which are indexed on the message file.

C.   A single digit is used to indicate the placement of the decimal point in the final answer.

D.   A high normal limit can be specified by age and sex ranges for a procedure.

E.   A low normal limit can be specified by age and sex ranges for a procedure.

F.   The high-maximum rejection limit is stored by procedure.

G.   The low-maximum rejection limit is stored by procedure.

H.   A one-digit code is used to identify the laboratory area in which the test is performed: e.g., Chemistry, Microbiology, etc.

I.   Two digits are used to indicate the type of specimen to be processed for this particular procedure.

J.   A sixteen character name identifies the test on file.

K.   One digit (yes–no) codes the test for listing on the blood drawing report and specimen collection label routine.

L.   Two digits code the type of specimen collection tube to be used.

M.   Two digits code the tube volume needed for specimen collection.

N.   Two digits code for a master test.

O.   Two digits code for a test using controls, e.g., prothrombin time.

P.   Two digits code for a charge-only procedure.

Master Test/Subtest

In the organization of the test file, it is possible to put in a complex test such as the Coulter S and delineate the subtests under this particular order. This means that a single order can integrate any number of possible results depending on how the subtests are organized. Our major need for master test/subtest arrangement comes from: the Coulter S, hematology differential count, urinalysis, SMAC test batteries, admission profile, organ profiles, and timed procedures such as clearances and various RIA tests.

Master File—Age/Sex Range Table

In most procedures it is extremely important to have age and sex ranges established. Table 3 shows our selected age and sex ranges. When creating the test files, it is possible to use correct limits on each procedure by making up the appropriate card with the proper limit pointer and selected ranges required.

Table 3
Laboratory Age/Sex "Normal" Range[a]

Male		Female	
Limit pointer	Age range[b]	Limit pointer	Age range[b]
0	0–0 Fetal	16	0–0 Fetal
1	1–7 Days	17	1–7 Days
2	7 Days–1 month	18	7 Days–1 month
3	1–6 Months	19	1–6 Months
4	6–12 Months	20	6–12 Months
5	1–3 Years	21	1–3 Years
6	3–6 Years	22	3–6 Years
7	6–15 Years	23	6–15 Years
8	15–19 Years	24	15–19 Years
9	20–29 Years	25	20–29 Years
10	30–39 Years	26	30–39 Years
11	40–49 Years	27	40–49 Years
12	50–59 Years	28	50–59 Years
13	60–69 Years	29	60–69 Years
14	70–79 Years	30	70–79 Years
15	80–Plus years	31	80–Plus years

[a] The age/sex range table consists of age ranges for both male and female. Sixteen (16) ranges are allowed. Test results with multiple limits use this range table. If multiple limits are not used, this table is not completed.

[b] Age ranges may be supplied in days, months, or years.

Expanded Test File

The following data is collected on each of the procedures:

A.   A three-digit unique test number is used during the ordering sequence by the clerk or physician.

B.   A special bit is set either to zero or one and is called the "done" bit. When the bit is set to zero, only a stat or expedite order will produce

```
**READY
LAB ORDER, USER ID:          00,   09:11   06/08/77,   STATION 21



MR#  097022      OK?  Y
NAME:  WXXXXX, EDWARD OPCLI   00,   09:13   06/10/77         OK?  Y
DR#:  607
PROBLEM:  NOT GIVEN  OK?  Y
T#  071  URIC AC MG/DL  OK?  Y  STAT:  Y
U DRAW 3ML RT TB
ENTRY OK?  Y                                 0096              DONE
T#  070
DATA ERROR
T#  070  CREATININE MG/DL   OK?  Y  STAT:  Y
U DRAW 5ML RT TB
ENTRY OK?  Y                                 0096              DONE
```

FIG. 23 During a routine laboratory order, the date, time, and station number is output, followed by a request for the medical record number. This is validated with a "yes," and the name, location, time, and date, and are checked for accuracy. If this is valid information, the system then displays the doctor number that is currently listed for that patient along with the current problem. The system allows a change of problem if appropriate. Following this, the test number is requested from the user. This is followed by the name of the test. If it is a stat test, stat instructions are provided along with a stat specimen number. The "DONE" to the right of the page is used for the nursing staff to initial and time the completion of that particular order on the medical record. The subsequent order shows the correct entry for creatinine clearance. An instruction is shown for a stat order along with a stat specimen number. For those areas in chemistry, the same stat specimen number is applied for each of the tests requested.

a specimen number along with a "done" printed on the right side of the page. If the bit is set to one, a specimen number and "done" will appear on a routine, expedite, and stat order sequence (Fig. 23).

C. A logical terminal number is put in the files which will trigger a message to be printed during the ordering sequence (Fig. 24). This allows the user to send a message for a particular order directly to the logical terminal number designated. Zero set in this area means no message is acquired or sent.

D. A specimen type is used for the specimen prep sheets during subsequent splitting and sample handling (Fig. 25).

E. A two-digit specimen volume is used to indicate quantity of specimen needed for subsequent testing after spin down.

F. One digit indicates the number of labels required during the splitting process.

G. A CAP workload unit number is stored by test for subsequent workload reporting by cost center.

```
MR#:   305067   OK?  Y
NAME:  BXXXXXXX, ANNA  OPCLC  00,  09:55  06/18/76  OK?  Y
DR#:   591
PROBLEM:  NOT GIVEN  OK?  Y
T#  469  MISC ROUTINE CUL  OK?  Y  STAT:  N  EXP#  Y
EXPEDITE TRANSPORT-- ONLY FOR UNLISTED SOURCE-LABEL SOURCE+TYPE MSG
MSG:  SINUS TRACK - L BREAST
ENTRY OK?  Y                              1158           DONE
T#
```

FIG. 24   For a routine culture, the order begins with patient identification, verification of the problem, and the input of an expedite request. The type of transport media is shown and a message is requested to locate the source. Again, a specimen number is assigned before additional tests are allowed.

H.   A series of nine four-digit numbers are used as pointers to an eight-character message file which strings together message segments that can be employed during the printing of a routine or expedite order (Fig. 26).

I.   Another string of nine four-digit numbers is used to signify the

FIG. 25   Mini-labels can be prepared by the system for transfer tubes and small testing samples and vessels in the clinical laboratory. These are produced following blood drawing.

```
LAB ORDER , USER ID:  22    14:30        10/02/76   , STATION   12

MR#  1198649     OK? Y
NAME:   GXXXXXX, LINDA      WF02    22 , 14:30    10/02/76      OK? Y
  DR#:    250 260
PROBLEM:   LOW FEVER     OK? Y
T#  023    CRYOGLOB  OK? Y STAT:  N   EXP#  Y
CALL  4185 TO SCHEDULE-LAB WILL PICK UP- **LS-ND*
MSG:  PATIENT FEBRILE
ENTRY  OK? Y                          2253            DONE
  T#
**READY
```

FIG. 26   A routine laboratory order in immunology validates name and problem and shows that for an expedite order the individual requester should call 4189 to schedule so that the laboratory can make the pick-up. The LS-ND indicates that at low staffing this procedure is not performed. The input process allows for a message to be sent to the immunology laboratory telling the technologists that the patient is currently febrile. After verification, the specimen number is assigned and another test can be entered.

print-out which will be used during that stat order sequence, and puts together the same maximum number of eight messages taken from the message file (Fig. 27). The maximum message length is 72 characters for either the stat, the routine, or the expedite order.

```
MR#: 280638  OK?  Y
NAME:  PXXXXX, LUCY M.  OPCLP 00,  09:54 06/19/76     OK?   Y
DR#:   785
PROBLEM:  RENAL  OK?  Y
T#  008  PT  SEC  OK?  Y STAT:   Y
U DO COLLECTION:  5ML BT TUBE RQ;PEDS-USE BT TUBE RQ 2.7ML BLOOD

ENTRY OK?  Y                       0078              DONE
T#
```

FIG. 27   A hematology order begins with patient and problem verification. In this particular case, a stat protime is requested and the system instructs the user to collect 5 ml in a blue-top tube before transmitting it to the laboratory. For pediatrics, 2.7 ml of blood is required in a blue-top tube. After verification, a stat specimen number is assigned.

Special Files

Instruments

A special series of files was established for autoanalyzers, which require programming input to ensure that the machine will properly handle the data and use the appropriate run summary at the end of a batch.

Doctors

A special section of the message file contains the names and numbers of those doctors who have been designated by the chief of staff as practicing physicians in the hospital. This allows the laboratory to identify the individual doctor responsible for the patient and route the appropriate reports to that physician in a convenient fashion.

Laboratory Areas

One section of the files delineates the lab areas and the maximum number of tests allowed for each section. Table 4 shows this organization for our facility.

Table 4

Tests Allocated for Laboratory Areas

Lab name	Number of tests
Hematology	001–074
Chemistry	075–274
Clinical immunology	275–349
Blood bank	350–399
Microscopy	400–499
Anatomic pathology	500–574
Microbiology	575–706
Spare	706–999

Work-Sheet Programs

Work sheets are available for each of the divisional lab areas to help technologists organize their day and provide them with a special measure of assistance following blood drawing, when a great surge of tubes and production is expected. Work-sheet programs are called following blood drawing and are organized to provide a convenient document for the technologist. In some cases the forms have headers across the top which will allow for the input of time, dates, and volumes. In other cases, the work sheets may represent multiple tests across the top and individual specimen numbers down the side (Fig. 28, 29).

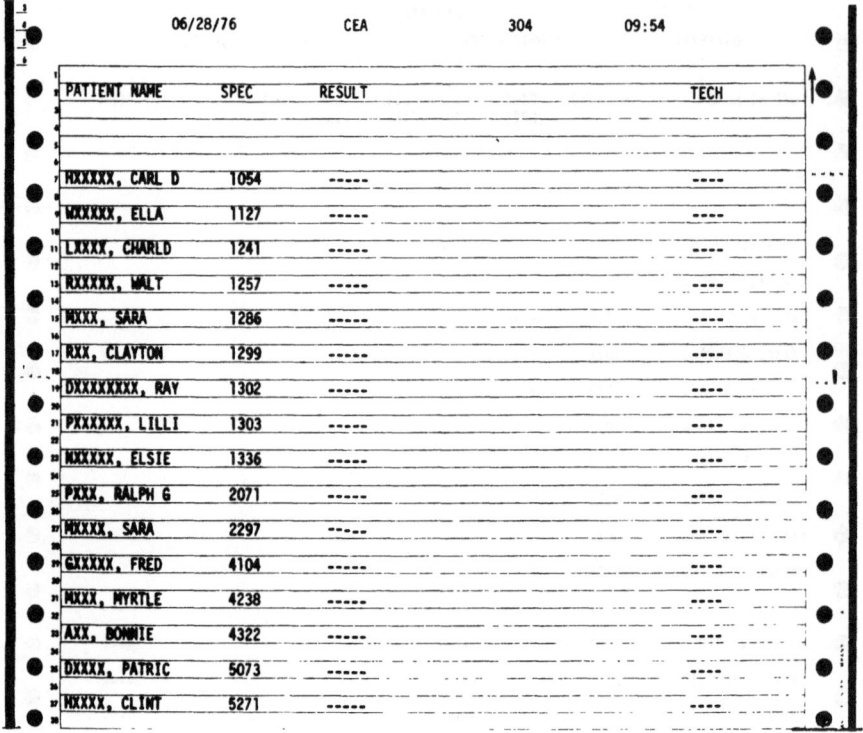

PATIENT NAME	SPEC	RESULT	TECH
RXXXXX, CARL D	1054	-----	----
WXXXXX, ELLA	1127	-----	----
LXXXX, CHARLD	1241	-----	----
RXXXXX, WALT	1257	-----	----
MXXX, SARA	1286	-----	----
RXX, CLAYTON	1299	-----	----
DXXXXXXXX, RAY	1302	-----	----
PXXXXXX, LILLI	1303	-----	----
NXXXXX, ELSIE	1336	-----	----
PXXX, RALPH G	2071	-----	----
MXXXX, SARA	2297	------	----
GXXXXX, FRED	4104	-----	----
MXXX, MYRTLE	4238	-----	----
AXX, BONNIE	4322	-----	----
DXXXX, PATRIC	5073	-----	----
HXXXX, CLINT	5271	-----	----

Date: 06/28/76 CEA 304 09:54

FIG. 28   A CEA worksheet shows the list of patients, their specimen numbers, and a column for results followed by the technologist's signature.

File Maintenance

One time-consuming and demanding job required of any information system is the acute care and handling of the test files. We have delegated this to our chief computer operator, who alone is allowed to make any changes on the system. The protocol has been set up so that the necessary card changes must be made at the same time as the on-line system changes are made. This guarantees continuity of the files and limits the possibilities for inappropriate action being taken without planning and advance notification. Procedures that are added to the system are done so after extensive review by both the laboratory director and the hospital administration. This coordinates appropriate sources and guarantees that the information is sufficient for patient service as well as the mechanical aspects of hospital accounting.

Warning—guard your files! We have had two episodes of file

CHEMISTRY

	03/15/77		ATOMIC ABSOR			110		08:35	

PATIENT NAME	SPEC NO.	CALC (082)	MG (111)	LITH (159)	COP (133)	LEAD (144)	TECH
GXXXXXX, ROLAND	0033	-----					----
AXXXXX, MEREDIT	2321	-----					----
CXXX, BELVA A	2417	-----					----
LXXXX, GLENDA	3040	-----					----
BXXXXXX, SIDNEY	3043	-----					----
CXXXXXXX, PAULA	3047	-----					----
BXXXX, MYRTIE	3074	-----					----
AXXXXXX, CLARA	3075	-----					----
KXXXXXXXXX, WIL	3093	-----					----
HXXXXX, CARL H	3106	-----					----
FXXXX, MARY N	3117	-----					----
MXXXXXXX, GIRL	0004		-----				----
AXXXXX, MEREDIT	2321		-----				--,--
FXXXX, MARY N	3117		-----				----
BXXXXXX, SIDNEY	3043			-----			----

FIG. 29 A chemistry worksheet allows multiple tests to be entered for each of the patients listed in the left hand column.

invasion and only detected this when strange printouts began appearing on all the floors. Instead of saying "Ready," the system started printing "OK Turkey." Calls came in from every area of the hospital asking about the ill-mannered computer. Investigation uncovered a flaw in the program which allowed certain remote terminals access to the files. By playing with the system, someone found out how to get in and change the reference data. A crash program was begun to change this function and now there is software and hardware protection against unauthorized file entry.

7

Admissions

INTRODUCTION

The Admissions area is one of the least appreciated and most demanding areas in the hospital. In this department occur all the critical and essential identification procedures required for patient service. The admission process is one which compels the timely coordination of a number of hospital departments that handle the patients as they arrive. Each step must be efficient yet insist on a quality peculiar to subject identification. Both Admissions and Medical Records require precise patient information so that the old chart or record can be coordinated with the proper individual.

Patients come for admission under four different circumstances, and constitute a unique challenge to master. First, patients arrive who are standard ambulatory admissions in no acute distress and, in most cases, amount to the bulk of admission to a general hospital facility. The general routine admissions process is geared toward this type of patient.

The second category of patients are semiacute admissions who require special handling for proper care. This group utilizes a subsystem

of the general admissions program that often functions suboptimally, since the general routine is broken and additional coordination is required.

The third category of patients arrive in the Emergency Room in acute condition and usually provide minimal information. This group demands the greatest coordination between the emergency facility and admission area for proper identification and subsequent handling. These are the cases that usually cause the greatest problems in the clinical laboratory because the demands are high for immediate service, and, yet, the Admissions process is usually delayed and in limbo because of lack of information.

The fourth category which is rapidly growing is that of outpatient admissions. This can constitute a large bolus of work which has to be handled in addition to stat patients. Special systems and additional people are usually required to execute this properly.

Under adverse admission circumstances, the laboratory is usually faced with the problem of identification and a proper return of information for the chart. Without our admissions module, the standard isolated laboratory system is usually just that—isolated. To solve this problem, one must have access to the source of data and that means a terminal and a system in Admissions, the Emergency Room, and the Outpatient Clinic.

FORMAT

Neither time nor financial resources allowed the development of a total admissions package. Instead, selected key parameters were chosen which are essential to laboratory operation. The design included an interactive software package to support this data set. Our general admission data base includes:

1. A six-digit medical record number which uniquely identifies the patient.
2. Name (21 characters).
3. Sex.
4. Age [with month (m), day (d), or year (y) appended to a two-digit number].
5. A problem consisting of sixteen characters not to be interpreted as a diagnostic statement.
6. A set of doctor numbers not to exceed five per patient.
7. A room, clinic, or Emergency Room designator.

```
**READY
GENRL ADMIT, USER ID:   02,   10:08   06/04/76     STATION   18


   MR# 285801
   NAME: FXXXX, LINDA G   OK?  Y
   SEX:  F   OK?  Y
   AGE:    17Y   OK?  Y
   PROBLEM:  STATUS ASTHMA   OK?  Y
   DR#:  924
   WXXXXX,  H OK?  Y
   ROOM:    A323A  OK? Y
   ADMIS#:  1823879   OK?  Y
   PROT#:   00 OK?   Y
   ENTRY OK?  Y



      -- -- ----
   10:09  ENTRY ACCEPTED
   MR# 011518
   NAME:  WXXXXXXXXX, HAYWOOD  OK?  Y
   SEX:  M   OK?  Y
   AGE:  73Y   OK?  Y
   PROBLEM:  GIL MALIGNOMCY   OK?  Y
   DR#:  537
   MXXXXXX,  T OK?  Y
   ROOM:  H472C  OK?  Y
   ADMIS#:  1832653   OK?  Y
   PROT#:   00 OK?  Y
   ENTRY   OK?  Y
```

FIG. 30   The general admission protocol on our communication system allows the entry of a medical record number, the name, sex, age, problem, doctor number, (not to exceed five physicians), room, admission number (hospital billing number), protocol number (special diagnostic classifications of patients), and finally an entry for verification.

8.   A seven-digit hospital billing code number (admission number) to be used by the hospital IBM accounting system.
9.   A protocol number of two digits for research and retrieval of selected patients on a prospective study basis (Fig. 30).

For the stat admission and those patients who are in need of immediate services without complete identification, the medical record number, name, sex, age, and room location are required before laboratory testing can begin.

The terminal selected for use in the Admissions area was a modernized version of the teletype with a special function keypad along with a standard typewriter keyboard married to a housing allowing direct view of the printer paper. The print mechanism uses a rolled NCR, two-part carbonless paper in which the primary copy is used for patient

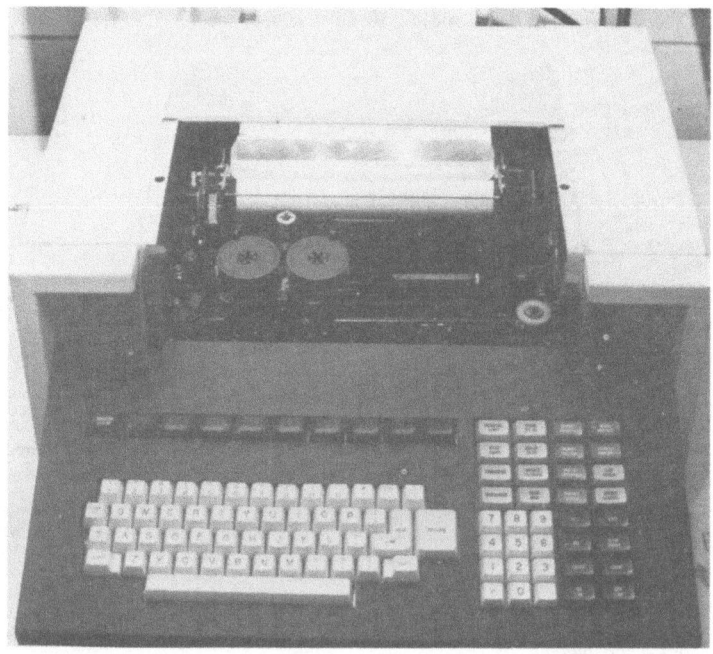

FIG. 31   The original terminal used throughout the communication system was a Model 33 teletype housed in a special cabinet allowing keyboard entry and high volume message keys for control of communication.

purposes and the second copy is used for audit trail. The selection of this terminal for operation was based on the economics of the program, a necessity of having hardcopy audit for normal entry, and the desire to use interactive software for system communication. At the time of the program initiation, no other terminal was available which could provide all of these functions at the cost and convenience of a single teletype. Figure 31 shows this device as it was configured for our communication system.

There is a great misconception about the teletype, and one would have to state at the outset that it certainly is not the most handsome or quiet alternative to data entry. Yet, it certainly has borne the test of time and offers some unique features which, to this date, have not been reproduced by units selling for twice as much. After three years of continuous use of these particular terminals, we are quite convinced that they are a reasonable alternative for low cost operation at a remote site. Subsequent chapters will deal with some of the modernization of this equipment, along with alternative designs for nursing stations, and

areas which require more speed and flexibility in terms of their data handling and retrieval systems.

PROGRAMS REQUIRED

The programs necessary to maintain an on-line admission package as previously described include: the general admissions program, which has an interactive dialog to gather the basic subset of data, a stat admissions package which creates a minimal file for an individual patient, a transfer function in which an individual can be moved from location to location, and a correct patient identification function in which an individual patient's header file can be changed and modified through proper auditable controls.

Through experience we have learned some of the interesting features in these programs which simplify the nature of the design and make it more convenient for operation. When an inpatient is discharged, the patient's data file stays open until all of the results are completed. The handling of the outpatient clinics, emergency room, and the hospital discharge ward are identical and programs can be equated for this function.

By transferring the patient to a discharge ward, one gains the additional flexibility needed to handle readmissions. Frequently, a

3-AWING		LIST CENSUS		06/29/76	08:43	
A312						
306039	GXXXX, FRANK		54Y M REFLUX ESOPH		A312B	
307037	BXXXXXXX, DELL L		63Y M CA RECTUM		A312A	
A314						
307201	MXXXX, GEORGE H		BOY M TIC		A314A	
305955	AXXXX, BENNIE L		26Y M BAL HYPERTEN		A314B	
ZZZZZ						
A316						
A320						
213375	TXXXXX, BEVERLY A		18Y F NONE GIVEN		A320B	
A321						
271635	CXXXXXX, GEORGIA		60Y F CARC BREAST		A321A	
A322						
300965	TXXXXX, MAURICE		36Y M SARC-L AXILLA		A322B	
A323						
244660	GXXXX, SARAH A		43Y F LBP		A323A	
ZZZZZ						

FIG. 32   A census listing by room and by floor shows the patient, medical record number, age, sex, and current problem.

patient is discharged and then subsequently readmitted in a matter of minutes or hours with some medical complication which occurred in the process of leaving the hospital. By simply transferring the patient to a discharge ward in the files, the transfer software allows a direct movement of this patient back into the hospital without additional data handling or programs.

Along with the input programs, output programs are necessary to allow the terminal in the Admissions area to produce selected census reports. Since the printer is not geared for high speeds, complete census documents are prepared in the computer room on a high speed printer. These are subsequently transported to the Admissions area for validation of census and bed board (Fig. 32). Through the use of this same software, it is now feasible to produce the census listings on each individual hospital unit which has a remote terminal and expect ward validation of census.

Nurses may also use this census listing for nursing notes as they handle the patients during their shift. The slow print speed of the peripheral terminal, however, has not encouraged the use of this particular census reporting function on the floors. Its widespread use will probably await a higher-speed printer terminal located in the nursing station area.

ON-LINE OPERATION

Many individuals have questioned the utility of an on-line real-time admission program. It is argued that this particular function could be batched and subsequently distributed to other areas such as the laboratory at a convenient time. Our labs have found this batch approach disastrous, and have suffered from the many shortcomings of this method for years. The only solution to the problem is to go completely to an on-line real-time system and to maintain all of the functions of the active data base using real-time remote terminals.

ADMITS

The admission dialog of our software has saved us over and over again by building into the system checks and balances which eliminate mistakes and maximize the validity of the primary data. In a number of cases, the wrong medical record number has been entered only to have the system reply that this patient is already in the hospital or clinic, and

that a mistake has been made. In other cases, a wrong room was entered and the system would reply: "data error." This kind of minute-by-minute control of the functions and operations of remote facilities makes the data base that much more valuable and accurate; certainly worth every effort put into the establishment of a real time system.

BED CONTROL

One of the critical problems in laboratory operation is the lack of information that usually accompanies a request for subsequent testing. Historically, our lab has spent hundreds of hours annually chasing down lost reports, trying to report information on patients who do not exist, and attempting to find doctors who did not sign their names to the request card, and who then subsequently disappear from the patient care scene to be replaced by other specialists unknown to both the admission area and the clinical laboratory. This patient-data-base merry-go-round kept one to two technologists busy all day trying to sort out the facts and figures. A constant effort was required to provide some effective response to the number of complaints that were raised by the house staff and faculty over lost data, inappropriate results, and the great crisis in the medical records room where the information never seemed really to match the patient's chart and, therefore, had to be discarded. It might seem a bit redundant to emphasize this fact, but our systems study and actual installation and implementation have shown over and over again that the clinical laboratory is an integral part of the hospital and cannot be looked at in terms of an isolated organization to be left on its own and handled as a remote site. The dialog that is active between the clinical labs and the hospital is an incredibly complex real-time equation which must balance if the lab is to service patients and physicians promptly, accurately, and responsively.

UNIQUE PROBLEMS

How to Identify a Patient

The initial classification of a patient by Medical Records requires a unique identifiable number. Here is one of the most crucial steps in the entire admission process. This depends on the successful search and retrieval of previous hospital information regarding files and numbers and the matching and integration of this with the current patient and his

problem. At our particular institution, we use the Soundex system developed by the telephone company. A large rotary file stores cards that contain this information. Any problems that arise using this retrieval mechanism automatically destroy every other hospital system. The domino effect is dramatic and legally devastating. What would be anticipated now and in the future is the integration of an admissions module shown in Chapter 1 with a complete long term on-line archive patient file holding a minimum of identification data with the appropriate, unique number. Before a new number is assigned, the archive patient file should be searched for any possible matches to eliminate duplicates and falsified information. Our system does not currently have this capability and we still rely upon our card files for classification of any single patient. This continues to create problems on a daily basis since it is entirely a manual system dependent on eyesight and proper categorical search for success.

Admission Orders

In most cases, the patient comes to Admissions with written orders from physician which are barely legible. In our hospital, the patient is moved to an outpatient lab facility where initial orders and testing are accomplished. In some cases, a patient is sent directly to the floor and the orders are processed by the nursing service. This has always posed a problem in the past which was only resolved through the use of an order form on which the physician circled or checked his choice of admission orders prior to patient arrival. This places little or no responsibility on the Admissions office to interpret handwriting and puts the obligation in the responsible hands of the nursing clerk and the laboratory staff, who are adequately trained to handle this simplified order document.

Terminal Location

Space is always a problem and is consistently underestimated when architects and designers build hospitals. Our Admissions area was no exception to this rule and initially our Admissions terminal was located in a closet! When a terminal site is selected, time and effort should be spent on human engineering to provide optimal operation. Our initial terminal site had no soundproofing, no ventilation, poor lighting, and created constant problems in day-to-day operation. We have subsequently converted the Admissions area to a high speed cathode ray

tube (CRT) and now have the terminal back in the working area of bed control. With the future addition of the full admissions module, many additional functions and terminals will be added. Until that time, the hospital can take advantage of a real-time census system which is necessary for ancillary service operation.

Hardcopy

Since the Admissions area is the hub of the hospital, it frequently falls within the realm of investigation by various subservices claiming malfunction and inappropriate operation. This means that the Admissions area has to produce documentation to support its activities in terms of patient admission data. The only salvation in this situation is the hardcopy audit which we currently have on our telecommunication terminal. A new design will be described for a remote terminal which accomplishes the function of hardcopy audit and provides the speed and convenience of the CRT. Needless to say, the audit trail in our hands has been shown to be an absolute lifesaver. It should always be available at the outset of any new program, since many months can be anticipated for training and trial-and-error learning by a wide range of employees.

Failure to Transfer

Our initial systems study and practical experience has shown that one of the major problems in locating a patient is the simple failure of the floors promptly to transfer the patient through bed control. Our patients were moved around the hospital from one bed to another, from one clinic to another, with no central control or tracking system. This created utter chaos in the laboratory since we were frequently unable to draw bloods or return reports. To alleviate this problem, the design created a check and balance which would only allow the patient to have his orders recorded if he was on the proper ward. The system can control this process through the terminal matrix, which assigns a terminal to a patient. If orders are attempted through another terminal these can be rejected and the user told that the patient had not been transferred. In the first month of operation, the phone rang about every hour with an irate clerk or nurse insisting that the system was wrong since it had refused to place orders for their patients. On follow-up, the patient had not been transferred by bed control and the system was vindicated. After the first month, the phone calls decreased dramatically and the personnel in the hospital learned they could not beat the system and had to notify

bed control before patient transfer. This process control step plugged a serious breach in our hospital security, and has made the operating systems of the ancillary services that much more successful.

Failure to Discharge

The on-line census has virtually eliminated patient discharge without bed control notification. Prior to the admission package, the lab often sent reports back to the floor many days after discharge. These reports would continue to go to the floors since the census was not a real-time document. By using an on-line control system, this problem can be minimized. If inconsistencies do develop, we have hard copy documentation to indicate that the educational cycle must be activated.

CONSTANT MONITOR

Our ability to control the Admissions data base and to review and validate its content at will, has solved most problems emanating from that area. This monitor and control function is now used by the Admissions Department for their own internal operations and has been requested by other services in the hospital that need timely data. Dietary and Pharmacy currently use the census listing to program their diets and medications so that meals are not sent to the wrong location and medications are not transported to an improper area. Such a system is absolutely essential for the smooth operation of a hospital and truly does require on-line real-time capability.

OUTSIDE DEMANDS

In the development of the Admissions interface, the systems group had the opportunity to study this area and see, on a daily basis, the demands made and the time scales expected for response. In almost every case, the staff in the Admissions area was overused, undersupported, and manipulated 24 hours a day. Many of the assigned ancillary tasks were in addition to the admitting function. For our facility, this has greatly jeopardized the quality and caliber of their work and is one of the key features for investigating a new system. Computers can only accomplish a limited amount when the basic operational demands and expectations

of the department are excessive. A computer system cannot replace good organizational management, and this is often forgotten in the rush to automate.

ADMISSIONS CRITIQUE

If we had an opportunity to reprogram and reconfigure, these are the following areas we would watch and change:

1. Problems have been detected in transferring patients from an outpatient to inpatient status. Our transfer function does not correct a number of parameters, and we are required to reenter these with each transaction. When changing major hospital areas during a transfer, the problem, the doctor number, the room number, and the admission number must be modified. Our current transfer software does not support this one-step data-base update. The same situation exists for emergency room transfers to inpatient status.

2. Our correct patient-ID function does not cover all the parameters of the admission cycle and leaves off room number. The transfer function and the correct patient-ID function should be combined to allow for convenient handling of updates.

3. The terminal selection for the Admission area was appropriate at the time, but has since been shown to be less than optimal. It is very difficult for one terminal to accomplish both bed control and admission functions, since it means that this particular unit had to be split between two different people for daily operations. To service this area adequately, one "silent" terminal with hardcopy audit should be available in the bed control area where phone conversations can be received and files inspected and maintained. The second terminal should be located in the main Admissions area to handle the subset of information for the hospital. Of course, the solution to the whole Admissions problem is to install a complete admissions module. The choice we made at the time of our specification, design, and development was to conquer one system at a time, and then to try to integrate these as time and dollars dictated through a distributed network of processors.

4. Development of the admissions package requires the solid support of the hospital director for proper implementation and training. We were very fortunate to have dedicated people working with us in this area who went through training and later maintained their support and interest in us and the problems which we faced in the clinical laboratories. We, in like manner, supported them totally in their effort

to achieve a better working situation for their personnel. Consequently, our departments have developed a strong working relationship. This is one of the hidden benefits in becoming involved in outside areas, so that problems which are normally interdepartmental stumbling blocks are now areas of active concern on both sides.

Emergency Room

INTRODUCTION

The emergency room (ER) is a miniature hospital. Its normal operations involve admissions, ordering, reporting, processing, therapy, and discharge counseling. Because of this highly integrated collection of services and skills, and the obvious fact that the patients are, in most cases, in severe jeopardy, the emergency room arena becomes a serious challenge and test of systems involved with patient care. As a rule, the people working in emergency rooms are overworked, underpaid, and overutilized. Many physicians do not appreciate being called to the Emergency Room, and therefore are less than hospitable to its working staff. Those that have full-time faculty know that much hostility and antagonism can in fact be defused, and that the operation can be smoothed out to a point where it is a highly successful and rewarding area of work. Nonetheless, the demands are heavy, liabilities are high, and the expectations of patient and family alike are extreme. All of this creates an environment in which systems are tested to their fullest and most certainly fail if there happens to be one slight flaw. Our efforts to work with this department have been extensive and involve a series of

tests during the evaluation of our prototype system. After many changes of hardware and software, we finally are approaching the expectations and requirements of the emergency facility.

FORMS

Every emergency room has some locally-designed paper form used to gather primary information. Physicians use this document to make diagnostic notations and it is subsequently transported to medical records for storage and retrieval. There are heavy demands on this form, since the physician needs adequate space to write and the clerks must have room for essential legal information. In our initial testing phases, we attempted to integrate the emergency room form and admissions dialog in a convenient package so that the clerks would have a smooth system for data entry. This appears to be a highly successful approach and has been utilized without difficulty for over a year.

AUDIT TRAILS

The emergency room is a unit that has high visibility and was initially believed to require an audit trail. Immediate compromises had to be made in this area since the terminal we had available to provide an audit trail was proving too slow under peak loads. During an interim period, we operated with no audit trail of admissions or orders in the emergency room and relied directly on the handwritten form which is the patient's chart in the emergency room. Our final configuration now finds a CRT and high speed printer in tandem. This has proven to be totally satisfactory since hardcopy and speed are now available. The patient paper chart is still kept as the primary medical document and contains the written results of the laboratory tests cited in the physician's notes.

CHART HANDLING AND
DATA RETRIEVAL

Once the initial ER form is completed, it is placed on a clipboard and handed to the physician for physical examination and subsequent testing. During the interview, shorthand notes are made on the record along with appropriate orders so that the nursing staff can become active. Laboratory orders are taken off the sheets by the clerks once

the initial chart has been evaluated, and it is then entered directly into the system using our standard test numbering. Specimen numbers are assigned by the system on the CRT. These numbers are recorded on the chart so that the specimen can be acquired and identified in the laboratory. When the results are completed, the data is transcribed from the CRT to the ER chart, and the physician then makes his final determination. With the addition of the high speed printer, this transcription process can be minimized. This system does use the hardcopy to simplify the work of the physician and the clerk in handling orders and results. This system also supports the single-page chart concept and eliminates the multiple sheets and documents that have proven to be a hazard in handling critical patients.

TERMINAL

Initially, the emergency room started with a teletype terminal and after many complaints regarding speed and noise it was removed. We increased the speed by a factor of 20 and installed a cathode ray tube as

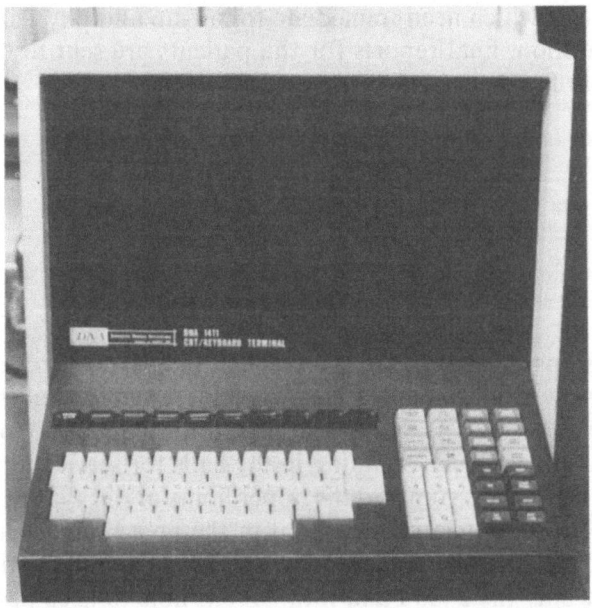

FIG. 33   In certain locations, CRT's are allowed for high speed entry and are primarily utilized for patient inquiry. Medical record documentation is not allowed on CRT entry without hardcopy availability.

shown in Fig. 33. Odd as it may sound, the next complaint was that there was no hardcopy for the doctors to use, and that the terminal did not make any noise so that they never knew when it was printing information. Somewhere between those two extremes is a satisfactory terminal for medicine. The clerks were delighted with the admissions part of the CRT. For data retrieval, it was fast, yet still required a great deal of writing since a hardcopy did not initially exist. With the final addition of our printer, the ER is temporarily satisfied—but for how long?

DAILY REPORTS

Since the emergency room maintains its own record system, it is difficult to use the daily reports that are generated by the computer. Our emergency room likes to keep track of its culture reports and some of its special studies which have to be sent to referral laboratories. The doctors do return to the emergency room to look these up. We currently send charts to this area, and these are sorted by patient name in an accordion file and left for physician review. The nurses review the cultures each day to determine whether there are any positive throat or GC specimens which need immediate follow-up and physician notification. In addition, final reports for the patients are sent to the medical record room for inclusion on the patient's chart.

SPECIAL PROBLEMS

Speed

The admissions element of the emergency room is a fascinating study in itself. Those who work in this area experience two extremes of operation: either the facility is empty and there is nothing to do, or the place is packed and people are standing in the halls for service. In our initial design, we had underestimated the upper limits of this type of operation, and had placed the teletype terminal in the area thinking it would be adequate to handle the admissions cycle. Subsequent investigation has shown that only the 2400-baud-rate CRT is able to keep pace with the admissions process in periods of high utilization. We have had no complaints about maintaining the admissions information using this method.

Personnel

The use of one terminal in an area such as the emergency room becomes a real strain for physicians, nurses, and clerical personnel. Many complaints were initially made about the crowding and the overutilization of the screen since physicians wanted to look up information on their own. The clerks, however, were required to maintain a steady flow of data and believed that the terminal was theirs and not for general use. With the arrival of the CRT, the problem became more acute since the physicians were convinced that this new tool was their personal terminal because it was so fast and simple to use. The situation came nearly to blows one afternoon when the clerical personnel asked that the new CRT terminal be removed. After a brief review of the situation, it was apparent that the problem was real and required attention. As a point of departure, not one extra communication line was available to put in another terminal to decrease the overloading. What was discovered after an hour and half's discussion was that the clerks and nurses were upset with the physicians entering their designated work area and getting into the middle of their traffic patterns. They wanted the physicians to stay on the outside of their work area and get in line to receive the information from them. The house staff and students refused to hear of this plan and insisted that the terminal was there for retrieval of patient results, and that they were therefore required to operate the unit. A brief search of the closets and storage areas of the emergency room turned up the ideal device. A Lazy Susan was made on which the terminal could be placed and allowed to swivel 180 degrees. The CRT was placed on the swivel top with easy access by the clerks. When the clerks were through with their data entry, the physicians could then turn the terminal around and look at it from the outside of the work area to receive their information and proceed. Such a simple physical design solved the problem in the emergency room.

In retrospect, our emergency room does not currently warrant two terminals since the data input and retrieval is only periodically high and often goes through many stages of less than optimal use. The initial installation of two terminals would have been costly and marginal in our particular setting.

9

Ordering Procedure

INTRODUCTION

Two schools of philosophy exist regarding the interfacing of physicians
and communications systems. The first maintains that the physician
must have full-time access to the patients' files and orders, and be able
to manipulate these at a dedicated terminal. The second supports the
physician using a convenient means of interface which requires minimal
medical involvement and training. Arguments and systems exist which
support both alternatives [23, 24]. Historically, each approach has been
successful in the mode in which it operates. Our major difficulty in
dealing with an on-line physician is the cost associated with such high
loading factors. Our staff consists of approximately 800 residents, faculty,
and students. If we failed to intimately reach any one of these individuals, the system would be subjected to severe stress. As a department,
we believed this was an unnecessary risk and well beyond the primary
goals and objectives of the initial hospital's information system program.

ON-LINE VERSUS OFF-LINE

In reviewing the system's documentation, which was originally developed
for our hospital and department, one key element was consistently

found. The lack of direct educational control during the ordering process had created insoluble problems from the floors, clinics, and emergency room areas. The laboratory was always the last to know and the first to be blamed. It was to deal with this experience and dilemma that our ordering process was created. The system had to accomplish direct on-line ordering and had to be smart enough to feed critical information to those entering data so they could make adequate decisions at that time. Cards, multi-part forms, and port-a-punch documents were considered inappropriate to satisfy the requirements established in the ordering cycle.

FORMS

To create a link between the physician and the on-line ordering system, a series of forms were developed to be used by the physicians as they reviewed the patient's chart. No attempt was made to reroute the physician onto the computer terminal for access to the medical record. We feel that this has been an extremely wise decision based on the time and effort that has been spent in training the physicians to use our new order form. Figures 20 and 34–36 show the order forms for all laboratory services. One general form and three specialty forms include everything performed in the separate divisions. The documents are designed to utilize an addressograph plate in the upper left corner. The current problem and the doctors' numbers are recorded on the right. To order, one circles or X's the appropriate test(s) as required. Each of the inpatient order sheets is a single piece of paper which can be printed at minimal cost. No carbons are required. The forms are modified every six months as new procedures are added and corrections or deletions are made. This is a very economical system for handling orders and allows maximum flexibility. Forms can be customized for individual departments that include the procedures most commonly used in a particular area.

An additional form is used for the outpatient clinic in which multipart sheets are available to provide adequate notification for third-party reimbursement by some of the state and federal agencies which require paper documentation for proper payment (Fig. 37).

On each order sheet, the individual procedure is listed with its test code number, its name, a box for expedite, a box for stat, and a special column denoting the type of tube used for collection. A result box is included at the right which can be used in the manual backup system to be described in a later section. Special footnotes are provided for unusual procedures. Expensive procedures require consultation before

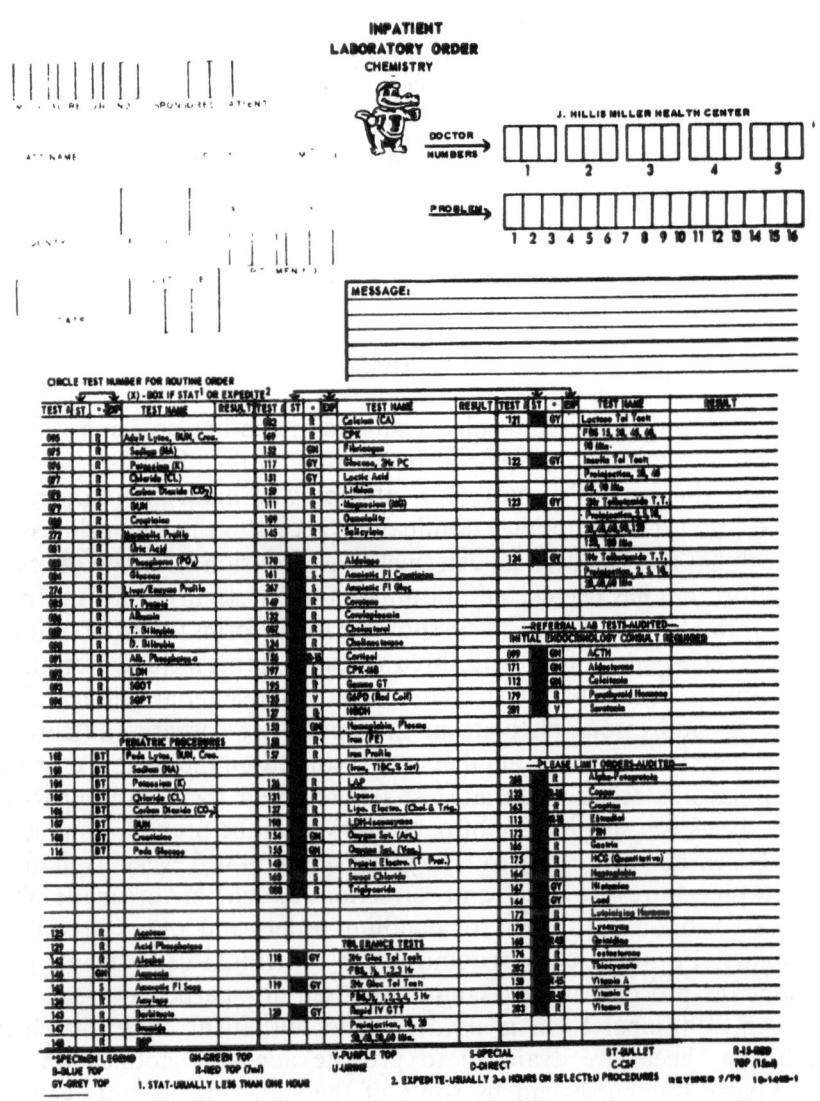

FIG. 34   The chemistry order form allows a sequential list of all chemistry procedures performed in our laboratories. A special section lists referral lab tests. This group is audited and only allowed with initial endocrinology consult.

INPATIENT
LABORATORY ORDER
HEMATOLOGY - BLOOD BANK - MICROSCOPY

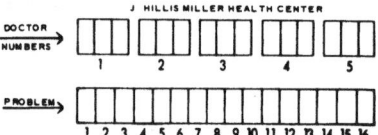

J HILLIS MILLER HEALTH CENTER

DOCTOR →

NUMBERS →   1   2   3   4   5

PROBLEM →

1 2 3 4 5 6 7 8 9 10 11 12 13 14 15 16

MESSAGE

CIRCLE TEST NUMBER FOR ROUTINE ORDER
(X) BOX IF STAT[1] OR EXPEDITE[2]

TEST#	ST	•	EXP	TEST NAME	RESULT	TEST#	ST	EXP	TEST NAME	#UNITS	TEST#	ST	•	TEST NAME	RESULT
				HEMATOLOGY		373	R		WBC Poor Pkd Cells					**RANDOM URINE CHEMISTRY**	
001		V		Hemogram		374	R		Isohemagglutinin		422		U	Amylase	
005		V		WBC		358	R		Prenatal Evaluation		411		U	Chloride (CL)	
002		V		HGB		376	R		Peds Walking Donor		451		U	Myoglobin	
003		V		HCT							478		U	Osmolality	
004		V		RBC					**MICROSCOPY**	RESULT	453		U	Porphyrin Screen	
006		V		Differential (Order Separately)		444		U	Qualitative HCG		409		U	Potassium (K)	
007		B		PT		400		U	Urinalysis		407		U	Sodium (NA)	
008		B		PTT		487		U	Urine Pr Electrophoresis		443		U	Urobilinogen Screen	
009		B		TT							455		U	Amino Acid Screen	
010		V		Platelet Count					**24 HR URINE CHEMISTRY**		413		U	Calcium (CA)	
011		V		ESR		648		U	Addis Count		402		U	Creatinine	
012		V		Retic Count		435		U	Aldosterone		421		U	Glucose, Peds Screen	
022		V		Sickle Screen		656		U	Amino Acid Chrom		454		U	Hemosiderin	
013		V		EOS Count		437		U	Amino Acid Nitrogen		450		U	Homogentisic Acid	
014				Bleeding Time		412		U	Calcium (CA)		452		U	Melanogens	
015				Clotting Time		427		U	Catecholamines		457		U	Phenothiazine	
020		V		HGB Electro		410		U	Chloride (CL)		415		U	Phosphorus (PO₄)	
021		V		Fetal HGB%		402		U	Creatinine		419		U	Protein	
023				Cryoglobulin		438		U	Copper		406		U	Urea	
024				Cryofibrinogen		401		U	Creatinine Clearance		417		U	Uric Acid	
025		V		WBC Alk P'tase		482		U	Delta Amino Lev Acid					**CSF ANALYSIS**	
026				OS Fragility		434		U	Estriol Pregnancy		459		C	CSF Profile (Gluc, Prot, Count & Diff)	
028				Special Stain, Nasal, etc		433		U	Estrogens						
						420		U	Glucose		467		C	CSF Cell Count & Diff	
				BLOOD BANK	#UNITS	432		U	Gonadotropin (HCG)		462		C	CSF Electrolytes (NA K CL)	
350	P			Rhogam		424		U	5 HIAA						
351	R			AHG (Factor VIII)		429		U	Homovanillic Acid		465		C	CSF Chloride	
356	R			ABO Grp Rh Genotype		436		U	Hydroxyproline		461		C	CFS Glucose	
355	R			Antibody Ident		425		U	17 Hydroxysteroids		466		C	CSF LDH	
354	R			Indirect Coombs		426		U	17 Ketosteroids		463		C	CSF Potassium	
375	B			Antibody T ter		479		U	Magnesium (MG)		460		C	CSF Protein	
357	R			Neonatal Eval		449		U	Metals (HG, PB, AS)		464		C	CSF Sodium	
359	R			Elution & ID		428		U	Metanephrines		488		C	CSF Electrophoresis	
360	R			Special Typing		475		U	Oxalate						
364	P			Direct Coombs		414		U	Phosphorus (PO₄)					**BODY FLUIDS**	SOURCE
361				Therapeutic Phlebotomy		641		U	Porphyrin (PBG CP UP)		474		S	Amylase	
362				Therapeutic Plasmaphoresis							477		S	Count & Diff	
363				Therapeutic Leukophoresis		408		U	Potassium (K)		483		S	Electrolytes	
365	R			Whole Blood		430		U	Pregnanediol		472		S	Glucose	
366	R			Fresh Whole Blood		431		U	Pregnanetriol		640		S	LDH	
367	R			Packed Red Cells		418		U	Protein		473		S	Protein	
369	R			Stored Frozen Plasma		406		U	Sodium (NA)						
370	R			Fresh Frozen Plasma		416		U	Uric Acid					**OTHER**	
352	R			Type & Hold		404		U	Urea Clearance		469			Calculi Analysis	
353	R			ABO Grp Rh Type		442		J	Urobilinogen		471		S	Fecal Fat	
371	R			Platelet Concent		423		J	VMA		468		S	Semen Analysis	
372	R			Platelet Rich Fresh Plasma							470			Urobilinogen Fecal	
381	R			Cryoprecipitate							445		UGN	Xylose Absorption	
											446		GN	Xylose Tolerance	

*SPECIMEN LEGEND   GN GREEN TOP   √ PURPLE TOP   S-SPECIAL   BT-BULLET   R-15-RED
B-BLUE TOP   R-RED TOP   , P √F   D-DIRECT   C-CSF   TCP (13 ml)
GY-GREY TOP

1 STAT USUALLY LESS THAN ONE HO •   ····   √ A√ √ / 6 HOURS ON SELECTED PROCEDURES   REVISED 7/76   18-1408/1

FIG. 35 A special Hematology/Blood Bank/Microscopy order sheet encompasses all the tests that are found in our laboratory.

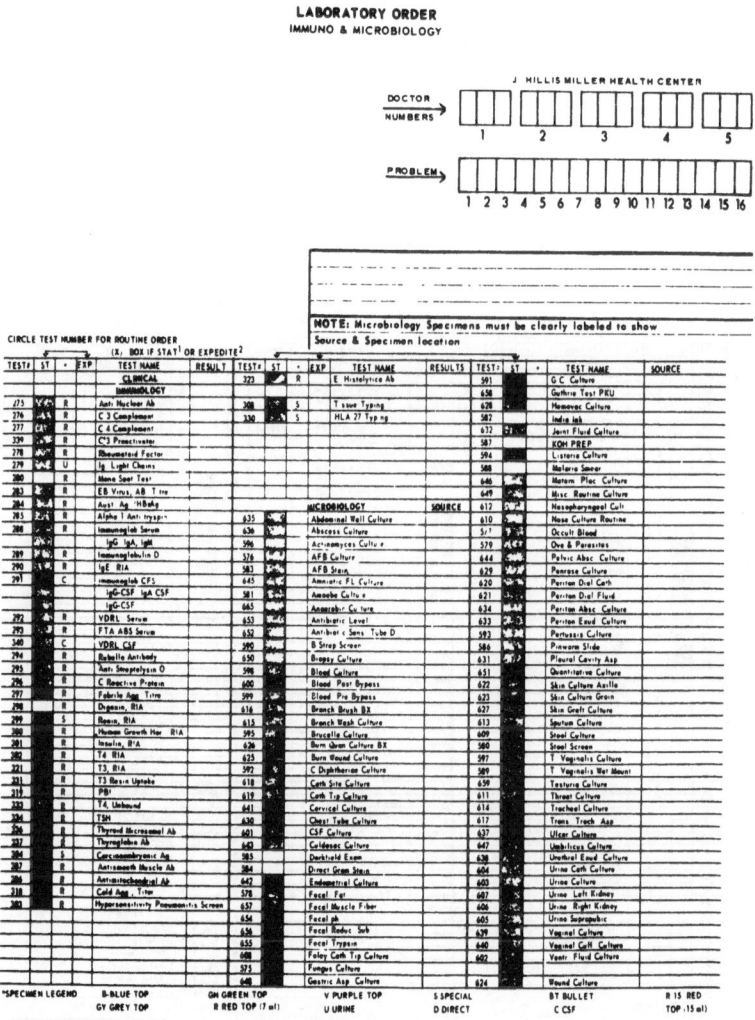

FIG. 36   The Immunology/Microbiology order sheet includes all those procedures which are offered in our laboratory.

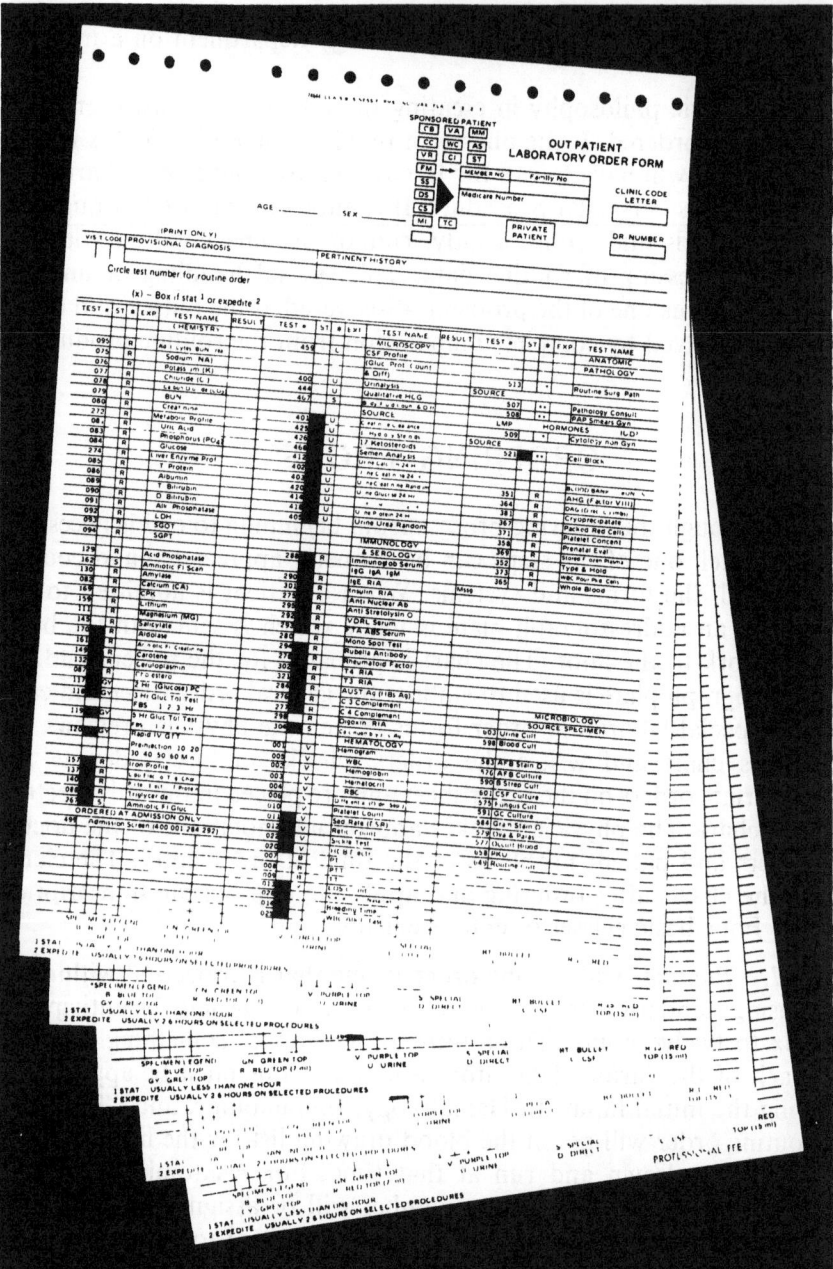

FIG. 37 The outpatient laboratory order form is a multipart document which includes those procedures that are routinely available in the outpatient laboratory. This form uses the same coding and order scheme presented for the inpatient order forms. Additional header information is required for billing and a clinic letter designator specially codes for outpatient laboratory result reporting.

ordering, and are audited by the pathology department on a monthly basis.

The basic philosophy in creating these forms is to list everything that can be ordered. If the physician requires something that is not on the form, he will have to call the laboratory and make special arrangements for this particular procedure. It cannot be submitted through the usual channels and, consequently, cannot become involved with the normal processing of routine data. This special handling of unusual procedures was one of the problems discovered at the outset, and could only be resolved by complete amputation from the routine production process.

ORDERING PROCESS

A trip through the ordering process from beginning to end is necessary so that each one of the steps can be properly appreciated and coordinated with the forms and systems. When a patient is admitted to the hospital, an addressograph plate is made which is sent with the basic paper work to the floor. The chart is prepared for the patient and the addressograph plate is used to emboss the general order sheet and each of the special laboratory order forms. When the physician reviews the patient's chart and writes the orders, checks or circles denote the appropriate orders on the order sheet and are placed in the order section of the chart. The physician makes appropriate notations of the doctor numbers and patient problems at the time of order entry. The clerks take the charts after ordering and apply the appropriate transcription steps. Four basic classes of entries exist.

1. Routine. The routine order is one that is processed within the lab using standard methodologies. The result can usually be anticipated in six to twelve hours. The routine order implies something different in each of the various laboratory areas, and this must be appreciated during the initial input. In Hematology, Immunology, and Chemistry, a routine order will go on the blood drawing list for the next morning and will be drawn and run at that time. For Anatomic Pathology, routine means that a specimen number will be assigned for the order and the Pap smear or biopsy specimen will be sent to the lab with the appropriate specimen number attached. In Microbiology, a routine order will denote the remote printing of a specimen number, and that the appropriate culture material must be acquired and sent to the lab for processing.

2. Expedite. An expedite order allows the physician to acquire a

specimen and bring it to the lab through either personal contact or courier service. The physician is not requesting stat work, but wants the specimen run with the next routine batch. The physician places an expedite order by making a check in the appropriate box.

3. Stat. A stat order is placed by checking the stat column. This, in all cases, means that the floor or physician will draw the blood and transport it to the laboratory. The physician is responsible for the acquisition of the specimen number and the label on that specimen. This, of course, means that the order will not be placed on the morning draw list.

4. Emergency. An emergency specimen indicates a life and death situation in which the laboratory stops everything until the tests are run. This is a very special class of order and is rarely used. All steps involved are manual and the entire information system can be bypassed if necessary.

In the normal setting, the clerk reviews the various orders and begins a dialog with the communications terminal by pressing the lab order button and getting the appropriate date, time, and station notation (Fig. 38). On the initial contact, the system will ask for a medical record number and validate this by providing the name, age, and location of that particular patient. This is confirmed by a touch of the yes

```
T*READY
LAB ORDER, USER ID:  09/22:35  07/09/76, STATION 18


MR#   896413  OK?  Y
NAME:   DXXXX, OTIS G H584A 09 , 22:36  07/09/76 OK? Y
DR#:   751
PROBLEM:   PL EFFUSION OK? Y
T#  095 ADLT LYTS BUN CR   OK?  Y STAT:  N EXP#  N
ENTRY OK?  Y
T#  130  AMYLASE   IU/L  OK?  Y  STAT:  N  EXP#  N
ENTRY OK?  Y
T#  001 HEMOGRAM OK?  Y  STAT:  N  EXP# N
ENTRY OK?  Y
T#
```

FIG. 38   For a lab order that is to be used for morning blood-drawing rounds, the nursing station places the medical record number in the file for verification, then verifies the problem and enters the test number for morning draw. A "no" to stat and a "no" to expedite places this item on the routine blood drawing list for the following morning. Adult electrolytes, BUN, creatinine, amylase, and hemogram are now ordered for morning draw.

button; the system now asks for the test number to be ordered. The clerk merely inputs the three-digit number that has been circled or checked by the physician and is then given a name verification of that particular test or procedure. The system now asks if it is a stat order. If the yes button is pressed, then the appropriate message for a stat order will be printed on the next line along with the specimen number and a "done." The terminal will then ask for verification of that order. If a yes is received, this test will be followed by a system request for another order.

If the order is not a stat, the system will ask if it is an expedite. A yes input will create the appropriate message for specimen handling. With this message also comes a specimen number and a "done." This word is printed to the right of the order so that the nursing station will make a notation when a particular order has been completed.

A routine order is the last alternative that is allowed. If the answer is no to stat and expedite, the appropriate routine message is printed. Certain routine orders are always assigned specimen numbers, such as cultures and urinalysis.

Once the patient's ordering cycle is completed, the physician's order sheet is taken out of the chart and the computer hardcopy order is placed on the patient's record using a page with two adhesive strips (Fig. 39). The order form is verified by the physician with an appropriate signature. When the clerk is working with the chart, the cardex file is updated for the nursing staff by specimen number and test number. The patient's chart is then returned to the rack. The initial ordering form is placed in a basket for 24 hours in case any questions should arise regarding the transcription process. Once the ordering cycle is complete, the information system is ready for business. It has now provided the necessary on-line hardcopy material for informative specimen handling in the hospital complex.

When the nurse or aide prepares to do specimen collection, the cardex file is consulted to reference the patient's order. The detailed instructions of order processing are given on the patient's chart. The "done" statement to the right of the order is initialed and indicates who has "done" the order and what time it was processed. This system provides an audit trail for the physician, so that the physician signing the order sheet knows that the items present have been executed properly by the appropriate personnel. Prior to our on-line control system, it was virtually impossible to produce uniform results since the specimens had such a wide range of processing experience. We know from our own research, and that of others, that the initial specimen handling is critical to the final results produced [25, 26].

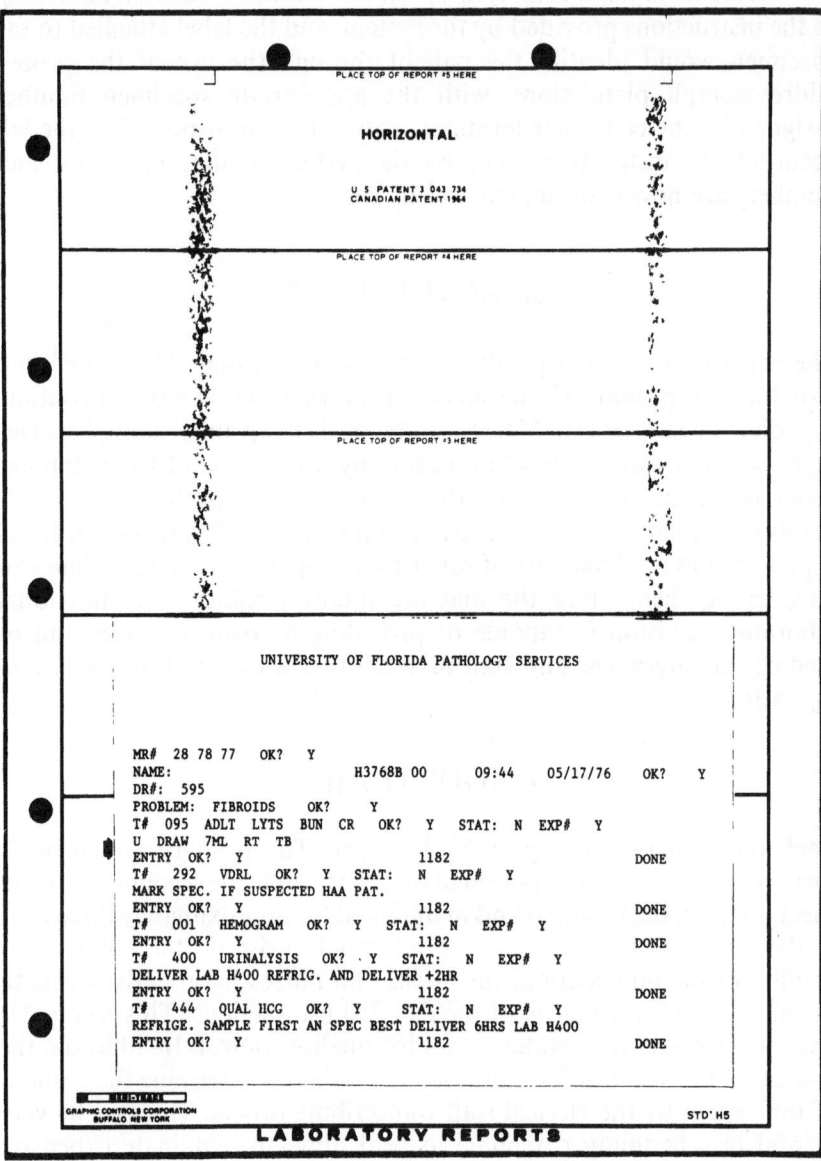

FIG. 39   The transaction of lab ordering is transferred to the patient's chart using vertical gum strips and tacking the hardcopy printout from the terminal directly onto these pages for the chart. These pages are kept with the chart until the time the patient is discharged. At that time, these are destroyed and the final lab records are signed by the physician for verification of order.

As an example, a urinalysis specimen would be handled according to the instructions provided by the system, and the label attached to the specimen would identify the patient through the use of the proper addressograph plate along with the appropriate specimen number assigned by the computer terminal. This is then transported to the lab according to instructions sent by the system. Order, messages, and numbers are now coordinated and uniform.

MESSAGE FILES

The ordering process depends heavily on the message files, which are structured to provide 72 characters of information on either a routine, expedite, or stat order. Messages are broken up into eight-character segments that can be changed on-line by use of one of the computer room terminals. Information about specimen transport media, temperature, patient criteria, extension numbers to call, processing times expected, and a whole host of other patient–physician related data can now be supplied. Since the files are totally flexible, each individual laboratory division is capable of providing its own messages and of feeding the physicians and staff material that is essential for consistent operation.

AUDIT TRAILS

Each terminal uses two-part NCR paper. The primary document is torn from each order and placed in the chart, while the secondary carbon sheet is left on the terminal and maintained for approximately three days at the terminal site. If any questions should arise on the accuracy or validity of the information, the clerks and nurses have ready access to the audit trail for a review of the detailed transactions. This eliminates any guesswork and provides a tool for quality control. In addition, the audit trail can be used for workload recording to determine the amount of time spent by the clerical staff transcribing orders. This can be very helpful in scheduling personnel at peak times to eliminate expensive staffing overlap.

SIGNATURES

The legal demands of the system are satisfied in a number of ways. First, the single-part order sheets are placed on the chart and initialed

by the physician who circles or checks the appropriate items. When the computer order is placed, the hardcopy is attached to the chart and subsequently reviewed and signed by the physician. This allows the doctor a chance to evaluate the nursing service to see that they are performing their functions promptly. In addition, it gives the physician a chance to review the procedures that have been performed and the time frames in which these have been accomplished. As a final step, our state insurance group has agreed to accept signed final computer reports as proof of legal order.

PHYSICIAN INTERFACE

The physician is an integral part of the interface and training required to utilize this method of input. The paper order form we currently use was new to our medical staff. We tried to arrange the forms in convenient groups that relate to high volume areas for quick handling. We alphabetized and categorized the specialty order forms to make it convenient to find some of the exotic tests and procedures offered. The same forms are used in all areas of the health center, so that the individual physician does not have to become acquainted with multiple documents. For the physician wishing personally to perform laboratory work and expedite results, the system does require that the request be input by the clerk before leaving the floor. This guarantees that an order and appropriate document is found on the patient's chart, and that duplicate testing is not encouraged. Prior to the installation of the system, many duplicates were ordered by medical students, residents, and interns without any means of control or audit.

Every order that is placed and every result that is generated must correlate on a one-to-one basis. Any audit of the charts will find appropriate orders with instructions and specimen numbers assigned, along with the associated answers. This eliminates the possibility of "lost" results for procedures that were not "ordered".

NURSING STATION OPERATION

The discussion of a nursing station is a complex subject. Here we find no single category of individual on which to focus. Clerks, aides, nurses, administrators, physicians, students, and inspectors all interface with the nursing station on a minute-by-minute basis and affect its normal daily operations—what they do and what they expect. Our system

changed the operation of the nursing station somewhat and placed an increased demand on clerical support. This was not done to burden the staff, but to expedite the care of the patients.

The laboratory has traditionally been given the job of ironing out the ordering mistakes that arrive after a nursing station has misidentified the patient or provided the wrong documents for transmittal. A busy laboratory is the last and poorest place to make these corrections and changes, and many of them are not done properly. The only person that suffers is the patient. We believe that it is exceedingly important that the nursing station be given the necessary personnel, and quality of personnel, to sustain a consistent effort. Because of this, we have advocated the upgrading of clerical lines on the nursing stations to the category of computer operator. This would provide rewards appropriate to the skills that are required. Without exception, most nursing station clerical personnel are the lowest paid and most abused employees in the hospital. Tremendous expectations are levied on this group without adequate justification or reward.

In our hospital, the clerks and nurses who work with the information system receive special training regarding the proper handling of specimens. This in-service program on the system is essential. Coordination of the program falls within the confines of our systems team and the laboratory/floor coordinator.

CRITIQUE

Our original specifications called for only two categories of orders: routine and stat. After the initial study, we immediately discovered a giant hole—the expedite category. In this case, a physician or nurse would draw the specimen and transport it to the lab. They did not expect stat handling, yet wanted it in the next batch for results. We were fortunate enough to have the programming done to deal with this situation before the system was implemented.

If we were to redesign the ordering system again, we would strongly consider the option of a fourth category of on-line order: emergency. This would provide for the rare exception in which a specimen is so critical it must take total precedence over all other stats. In our institution, the word stat means one hour or less. Since stats come from every area of the hospital all day long, it becomes a bit difficult to differentiate those patients who are critical or terminal from those who just routinely need the results back in one to two hours. This would be the rationale for having a fourth on-line order category.

We are not totally satisfied with the shingling process of lab orders for the patient's chart, and hope to make some progress in this area by looking at some other type of paper system. It is quite difficult to modify this step since the medical record is such a conservative document at this time, with little latitude for change.

Another area of critical concern is the actual specimen numbers that are assigned by the system. The specimen numbers are divided numerically for convenience. Any number less than 1000 is a stat specimen number and is recycled daily following successful completion of results. The specimen number stays outstanding for a patient until such time as all results assigned to that number have been completed. At the end of that time, the number goes back into the pool to be utilized for someone else. For routine or expedite specimen numbers, the system starts at 1000 and goes up to 8000, incrementing 1000 each day of the week. This means that Sunday is 1000 to 1999, Monday goes from 2000 to 2999, and so on. This provides a very convenient log within the laboratory to determine the day the specimen was ordered. We have found some interesting problems in handling the specimen number system and have required additional software changes for clarification.

A doctor can order one test stat, one expedite, and the other one routine. This is done in a random fashion on the form. The software will take each one of these in order to determine whether it needs a specimen number for each individual test.

Initially, Chemistry, Hematology, and Immunology all obtained separate specimen numbers for every individual test. This meant that on one sample at check-in, multiple specimen numbers were entered and required additional time for processing. After becoming dissatisfied with the approach, the numbering system was changed so that one specific number was assigned to each patient. This meant that all the routine orders for hematology, chemistry, and immunology tests would be given exactly the same number. This turned out to be successful, with one additional drawback. If the individual orders were input in the order in which they were created on the form, a specimen number would be assigned for a routine order. Following that would be a stat order, and the specimen number would come back with a number less than 1000. In returning to a routine order on the same patient, the system would not recognize that it had already assigned a number, and give another new number. This process again resulted in tubes of blood arriving in the laboratory with eight to ten specimen numbers attached, all of which had to be confirmed and subsequently handled. This created an immense problem for the laboratory in trying to split specimens and allocate work for various divisions. Multiple specimen numbers were residing in

the system for the same patient which required extensive bookkeeping to follow.

To solve this problem, the specimen number assignment was made a bit more sophisticated. In the first place, each individual terminal must have a buffer assigned which contains the specimen number assigned for stat, expedite, and routine orders. When the specimen number program assigns a number, it must remember what it has done. An alteration of category should not change the basic minimum group of numbers. The final result is that the maximum of specimen numbers per tube which can be received is two; a number for stats and a number for expedite/routine. This is an extremely convenient and practical numbering scheme. We have only been able to develop and implement such a technique by retrospectively looking at our internal problems within each selected division.

Another simple basic parameter which was forgotten during the initial design requires the terminal to forget the specimen numbers that have been assigned and clear the buffers when the terminal stops or advances to another patient. Our initial system did not provide this step, and programming changes were made to eliminate the possibility of having specimen numbers assigned inappropriately to the same patient.

As an example, a patient is on the floor and has several orders entered at one time. The blood is sent to the laboratory and is verified against the system stored specimen numbers. That ordering terminal is put in a stand-by mode and about 15 minutes later another set of orders arrives for the same patient. Our initial system was not smart enough to reload its buffers with zeros and assign new specimen numbers. It made the mistake of assuming that this was part of the original order and again assigned the original specimen numbers. The problem occurred only three or four times in the first six months of operation and usually happened on weekends or holidays when the hospital was at low census and the area load was light. The likelihood of ordering on the same patient twice becomes much higher at that point. This is one logical error to be avoided.

10

Laboratory/Nursing Station Interface

INTRODUCTION

Placing any medical system within the operating confines of the nursing station is the ultimate challenge. In a busy nursing station environment employees are usually conservative and show a great reluctance to change anything. Only when a situation becomes a crisis will there come a cry for change. This philosophy is a direct result of the highly skilled and detailed schedule which exists in this environment, and the extreme expectations and demands of the physicians who manipulate and control the staff for their patients. The hospital is always pressed between the demands of the physicians and the requirements of reasonable administrative control. If a new system does not provide some concrete, useful material for the nursing station and its personnel, it will be promptly rejected by the users. The nursing personnel have a close allegiance to practicing physicians and can mobilize their strength and power to inhibit anything that impinges on their personal ideas of success. All it takes is one nurse saying that the system has compromised

patient care: one such statement made to a single physician can jeopardize a whole project. For this reason the coordination of any system with the nursing station personnel and clerks is a very highly sensitive task that deserves the undivided attention of any group attempting to interface with them to create such a working relationship.

TERMINAL

The terminal that is placed on the nursing station should be extremely reliable, sturdy, and reasonably quiet. We used our telecommunication terminal, shown in Fig. 31, on all of our nursing station installations no matter what their size or capacity. In some areas, the noise created by the terminal was not even noticed because of the din of respirators, pumps, and patient-support equipment. In other stations, the terminal racket became a major problem and required insulation and sound-proofing to achieve a measure of success. A special terminal cover had to be designed for the unit to decrease the noise level to an acceptable point (Fig. 40).

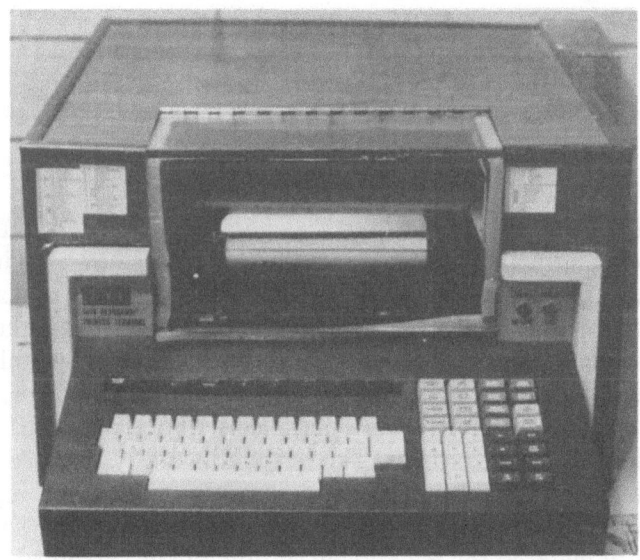

FIG. 40   Although the initial terminal appeared to be satisfactory, the noise level created by the teletype was beyond what the nursing station could tolerate. Therefore, sound-proof covers were constructed to increase visibility and to decrease noise. Unfortunately, the vendor refused to make such adjustments in their terminals and we were forced to do this in-house.

It was quite apparent that the large, busy nursing station requires more terminal power than can be provided by one single unit. In these cases, high-speed printing capability is a necessity. In other areas, the teletype is more than adequate since it provides an effective terminal for both hardcopy, audit, and interactive dialogue. Although the current range of options is not large, it would be advantageous to match the type of terminal to the demand and select a reasonably priced unit to meet expectations. We continue, to this day, to use our teletype communication terminals, and at this point have found few flaws other than their speed and noise to justify their replacement.

ORDERS

The orders that are placed at the nursing station are entered by the clerical staff. Only after midnight, when clerks are unavailable, is the nursing staff intimately involved with the terminal. We initially had a great many problems establishing the ownership of the terminals on the floor because the clerks and the medical students tended to seek the unit at the same time. Clerks, house staff, and students all maintained that the terminal was for their exclusive benefit. Major disputes were fought over what was primary—an order or an inquiry. We settled the issue by proclamation: the students could use the terminal only when the clerks were not busy with data input or retrieval. We had never anticipated such a competitive spirit over the use of the terminal.

CHART OPERATION

Our current charting operation uses carts and carousels to hold notebooks. This varies depending on the ward and physician who manages the unit. It makes no difference what kind of chart format is used as long as the clerks are acquainted with the approach for handling the orders and properly manipulate the paper work. The charting operation works quite smoothly using the mounting sheets for orders and has been integrated with the medical record room without much difficulty.

BLUE CROSS APPROVAL

Our communication system was presented to Blue Cross of Florida and was approved for operation under the following guidelines. *1.* Doctors

would initial all order sheets. *2.* Doctors would initial all hardcopy orders on mounting sheets. *3.* Doctors would sign all seven-day chart reports. *4.* Mounting sheets would be discarded by medical records at discharge. *5.* All initialed order sheets could be destroyed after patient discharge.

REPORTS

A large series of reports can be obtained on the nursing station terminal by the use of our interactive software. Short reports are quite conveniently printed using the teletype, and others that are more extensive do not make optimal use of this terminal. The large volume reports that are required can be minimized by the use of documents printed by the computer room and distributed daily. The capability exists, however, of creating the charts and additional documents at the peripheral station, and this does provide a great deal of flexibility for future system development.

Ward Reports

The ward report displays all the information which has been entered into the system since the last daily chart report was printed. The worst case could include 23 hours of information, since the chart reports are printed daily. Figure 41 shows this document. The ward report can also be called up on the peripheral terminals by doctor number and ward.

Daily Charts

Daily charts are delivered to the floors and nursing station areas at approximately 5 PM each day, seven days a week. They summarize the activity for each of the patients who has had work performed in the previous 24 hours. Daily charts use a cumulative format. In most cases, the date and time is the header and the laboratory work performed is listed on the side of the page with the appropriate results in the proper column. In areas such as Microbiology, a paragraph or horizontal format is used for the narrative information. The daily charts are printed on green striped paper and require approximately 45 minutes of printing time running at 300 lines per minute (Fig. 42).

```
5-A WING              WARD REPORT           09/25/76      12:26      PAGE 1


A507B  EXXXXX, DELORES*                    MEDICAL RECORD # 485736

   URINE CULTURE         REQUEST RECEIVED              09/25/76  09:00
   URINE CULTURE         REQUEST RECEIVED              09/23/76  00:00
   URINALYSIS            REQUEST RECEIVED              09/23/76  00:00


A507A  AXXXXXX, MARSHA A                   MEDICAL RECORD # 847365

   DIFF                  REQUEST RECEIVED              09/25/76  00:00
   HEMOGRAM              REQUEST RECEIVED              09/25/76  00:00
   MISC ROUTINE CUL      REQUEST RECEIVED              09/21/76  20:45
   MISC ROUTINE CUL      REQUEST RECEIVED              09/21/76  20:45


A514B  GXXXX, JEFF E                       MEDICAL RECORD # 495836

   HBS  AG (AUST. AG    NEG                            09/23/76  17:15


A515B  SXXXXXX, RICKY E                    MEDICAL RECORD # 4837560

   URINE CULTURE         URINE-CLEAN CAT   NO GROWTH      09/24/76  09:15
   URINE CULTURE         TEST COMPLETE                   09/24/76  09:15


A516A  CXXXX, JOHN                         MEDICAL RECORD # 573655

   URINE CULTURE         REQUEST RECEIVED              09/28/76  16:30
   CATH TIP CULTURE      REQUEST RECEIVED              09/24/76  11:00
   BLOOD CULTURE         REQUEST RECEIVED              09/20/76  07:45


A517B  TXXXXX, MARK A                      MEDICAL RECORD # 583758

   MISC ROUTINE CUL      REQUEST RECEIVED              09/23/76  14:15


A518B  NXXX, PAMELA C                      MEDICAL RECORD # 843791

   CATH TIP CULTURE      FOLEY CATH TIP    IN SUBCULTURE          ECOL 1
   CATH TIP CULTURE      FOLEY CATH TIP       ECOL1  S        TETRACYCLINE  09/22/76
   CATH TIP CULTURE      FOLEY CATH TIP       ECOL1  S        AMPICILLIN    09/22/76
   CATH TIP CULTURE      FOLEY CATH TIP       ECOL1  S        KANAMYCIN     09/22/76
   CATH TIP CULTURE      FOLEY CATH TIP       ECOL1  S        CARBENCILLIN  09/22/76
```

FIG. 41 A ward report by floor shows each patient, tests requested or received, and results currently pending. The ward report runs on a clock basis starting from the last daily chart report.

Seven-Day/Final Charts

Figure 43 shows a seven-day/final chart for a patient. The chart is identical in format to the daily chart, but is printed on blue barred paper. Medical records and the floor personnel know they must save this final copy. The files in the system are limited, and each seven-day period results in the purging of the patient's results from the files and the printing of a seven-day/final chart report. This final chart report can also be triggered by an excess of result reporting—anything that exceeds 165 results per patient. At that point, a final chart is produced and the patient's files are cleared for additional work. Both the seven-day and

```
SHANDS TEACHING*HOSPITAL/CLINICS                    LABORATORY CHART REPORT


WARD:  7TH PEDS              DAILY        CHART REPORT              PAGE 2

NAME:  XXXXXXXX, JONATHAN D                       MEDICAL RECORD #305867

ROOM:  H749D    04M   M   00    DR:  GXXXX, I H               16:50  17/27/76

PROBLEM:  ECD


TEST              LIMITS          07/27
                                  09/30

CHEMISTRY
CALCIUM MG/DL      8.5-10.5        10.0
PED LYTE.BUN.CRE
  NA MEQ/L         135-145         137
   K MEQ/L         3.1-5.3         5.0
  CL MEQ/L         98-109          100
  CO2 MEQ/L        24-30           28
  BUN MG/DL        8-18            8
CREATININE MG/DL   0.6-1.2         0.5*
```

FIG. 42   The daily laboratory chart report is printed on green bar paper. Most laboratories use the column type presentation headed by date and time.

daily charts are produced by the high-speed line printer located in the computer room.

Although result files are closed every seven days, the data is still available on the system for 28 days. The seven-day/final chart program

```
SHANDS TEACHING HOSPITAL*HOSPITAL/CLINICS           LABORATORY CHART REPORT


WARD:  7th PEDS              FINAL  --   CHART REPORT              PAGE 1

NAME:  JXXXX, MELISSA                    MEDICAL RECORD  395837

ROOM:  H394B    05Y   F   00   DR:  FXXX, R         07:54       07/26/76

PROBLEM:  ILL


TEST              LIMITS          07/25
                                  14:15

CHEMISTRY
CL      MEQ/L      95-105          107*
CO2     MEQ/L      24-32           32
BUN     MG/DL      10/20           21*
CREA    MG/DL      0.7-1.4         1.4
URIC AC MG/DL      2.5-8           6.8
```

FIG. 43   The final charts are printed on blue bar paper and are the final copy to be kept on the medical record. Both the floor clerks and the medical record staff make sure that there are no green charts on the pages of the patient's chart. Only blue copies should be in the patient's chart when completed.

```
MEDICAL           LIST CENSUS           07/02/76        10:51

WF07

A406
299384    HXXX, RAYMOND S       32Y M REJECT-TR-KIDNEY    A406A

A409
309584    SXXXXXX, GERTRUDE C    54Y F NONE GIVEN          A409A

A417
013847    SXXXX, ROOSEVELT*      62Y M CHEST PAIN          A417B

ZZZZZ

A418
302937    BXXXXX, FRANCES E      54Y F HORNES SYNDROME     A418B
307284    SXXXX, VELMA M         40Y F NOT GIVEN           A418A

MEDICAL           LIST CENSUS           07/02/76        10:51

A419
004837    GXXXX, DORIS L         48Y F HYPERPARATHY        A419A

A421
302947    RXXXXXXX, KAREN M      32Y F SUBARO HEMMORAGE    A421B
304837    MXXXXX, ELNORA U       39Y F CHF                 A421A

H435
306281    SXXXX, PATRICIA A      29Y F RETINAL EMBOLUS     H435B
306154    WXXXXXX, HELEN J       53Y F REFLUX EXOPH        H435A

H439
305483    MXXXX, WILLIE*         69Y PLEURAL EFFUSION      H439D
304958    MXXXXXX, LEROY R       69Y M MALABSO             H439C
307903    HXXXX, VINCENT E       70Y MS.O.E.               H439B

ZZZZZ

H441
304851    NXXX, JOHNNIE MAE      59Y F OBS JDCE            H441A
091393    WXXXXXXX, ESTEL. M     76Y F DEHYDRATION         H441B
```

FIG. 44 A census list can be called by room, by floor, or by area. On this list is shown the medical record number, the name, the age, the sex, the current problem, and the specific bed location.

takes care of file housekeeping and distributes the paper handling requirements.

Census

The nursing station has access to the census system through the peripheral terminal. Here one can inquire into current bed locations or can search the entire ward for a list of all patients. Figure 44 shows a census listing in a selected area. On this listing is the name, age, sex, problem, and medical record number associated with each patient. The same type of document, in an expanded form, is used by the admissions area for bed control.

Inquiry

The nursing terminal allows the floor and physicians to inquire into every aspect of the patient's laboratory-data base.

1. The physician may want to obtain a current census listing for himself. By inquiring under doctor number, the system will deliver a personal physician's list of patients in the clinics, emergency room, and hospital area. This can be used for rounds or to assign individual billing (Fig. 45).

2. The patients' files can be individually reviewed. During the patient inquiry, the system will ask for the medical record number and verify the patient name. Data can be received in three categories (Fig. 46).

```
**READY
INQUIRY-DOCTOR  , USER ID:  22,  14:46  09/03/76 , STATION  12


DR#:  001.
A XXXX%  S C  OK?  Y

        312515    GXXXXXXXX LXXXXX          ILL          H441B
REPORT COMPLETE

        --------
DR#:
```

FIG. 45 An inquiry by physician is accomplished by entering the doctor number (001) followed by a period. The doctor name is then verified and the list census for that individual physician is printed along with the current problem, medical record number, and patient location. This function is extremely helpful to the staff in the hospital so they can locate their patients and make rounds.

INQUIRY-PATIENT , USER ID: 22, 10:47   12/13/77 , STATION   1

MR# 345502 OK? Y CXXXXXXXXX, MARY H661D OK? Y
TYPE: 095 ADLT LYTS BUN CR OK? Y
LIF/FIF? 1 05 OK? Y

NA MEQ/L	143 MEQ/L	12/13	08:30
NA MEQ/L	144 MEQ/L	12/13	05:00
NA MEQ/L	144 MEQ/L	12/12	06·45
NA MEQ/L	141 MEQ/L	12/11	22:15
NA MEQ/L	142 MEQ/L	12/11	14:30
K MEQ/L	3.6 MEQ/L	12/13	08:30
K MEQ/L	3.5 MEQ/L	12/13	05:00
K MEQ/L	3.5 MEQ/L	12/12	22:30
K MEQ/L	3.4* MEQ/L	12/12	12:45
K MEQ/L	3.4* MEQ/L	12/12	06:45
CL MEQ/L	104 MEQ/L	12/13	08:30
CL MEQ/L	104 MEQ/L	12/13	05:00
CL MEQ/L	102 MEQ/L	12/12	06:45
CL MEQ/L	102 MEQ/L	12/11	22:15
CL MEQ/L	103 MEQ/L	12/11	14:30
CO2 MEQ/L	33* MEQ/L	12/11	14:30
CO2 MEQ/L	35* MEQ/L	12/13	05:00
CO2 MEQ/L	35* MEQ/L	12/12	06:45
CO2 MEQ/L	34* MEQ/L	12/11	22:15
CO2 MEQ/L	34* MEQ/L	12/11	14:30
BUN MG/DL	21* MG/DL	12/13	08:30
BUN MG/DL	23* MG/DL	12/13	05:00
BUN MG/DL	25* MG/DL	12/12	06:45
BUN MG/DL	25* MG/DL	12/11	22:15
BUN MG/DL	24* MG/DL	12/11	14:30
CREATININE MG/DL	0.8 MG/DL	12/13	08:30
CREATININE MG/DL	0.9 MG/DL	12/13	05:00
CREATININE MG/DL	0.9 MG/DL	12/12	06:45
CREATININE MG/DL	1.0 MG/DL	12/11	22:15
CREATININE MG/DL	1.0 MG/DL	12/11	14:30

REPORT COMPLETE
TYPE:
**READY

FIG. 46 The inquiry procedure begins with the entry of the medical record number followed by the validation of the patient. "Type" is then asked for, and all the unfinished work, all the work since the last ward report, and all the laboratory data stored by specific test can be called. In each of these cases, the system allows a LIFO or FIFO presentation (last in–first out; first in–first out) and up to 99 items called by specific test category. As an example, if the physician would like to see the last five sodiums, he would enter "L 05". With this entry he would receive the last five sodiums displayed in sequence.

INQUIRY-PATIENT , USER ID: 22, 10:53 12/13/77 , STATION   1

MR# 345502 OK? Y CXXXXXXXX, MARY H661D OK? Y
TYPE: 001 HEMOGRAM OK? Y
LIF/FIF? F o5 OK? Y

HGB	GM	11.0*	GM	12/10	07:00
HGB	GM	10.9*	GM	12/11	06:45
HGB	GM	11.3*	GM	12/11	18:15
HGB	GM	11.2*	GM	12/12	06:45
HGB	GM	12.6	GM	12/12	22:30
HCT	%	32.9*	PERCENT	12/10	07:00
HCT	%	32.6*	PERCENT	12/11	06:45
HCT	%	33.4*	PERCENT	12/11	18:15
HCT	%	33.4*	PERCENT	12/11	22:15
HCT	%	33.5*	PERCENT	12/12	04:15
RBC	10X6/CMM	3.62*	10X6/CMM	12/10	07:00
RBC	10X6/CMM	3.55*	10X6/CMM	12/11	06:45
RBC	10X6/CMM	3.60*	10X6/CMM	12/11	18:15
RBC	10X6/CMM	3.62*	10X6/CMM	12/12	06:45
RBC	10X6/CMM	4.17*	10X6/CMM	12/12	22:30
WBC	10X3/CMM	11.3*	10X3/CMM	12/10	07:00
WBC	10X3/CMM	11.4*	10X3/CMM	12/11	06:45
WBC	10X3/CMM	12.1*	10X3/CMM	12/11	18:15
WBC	10X3/CMM	10.9	10X3/CMM	12/12	06:45
WBC	10X3/CMM	9.9	10X3/CMM	12/12	22:30

REPORT COMPLETE

FIG. 47   Inquiry for hemograms creates the output of the last five basic data sets from the hemogram profile.

a.   One can ask for all the uncompleted test requests on the patient's file. The system will display specimen number, test number, and name along with the date of order and the time of specimen arrival.

b.   An individual can inquire about a specific test result by entering the test number (Fig. 47). As an added feature, the system is programmed to access the patient files as a first-in first-out (FIFO) or last-in first-out (LIFO) function. An additional code of 0–99 brings up the specified number of test results required. An L 02 will execute a LIFO search for the last two tests on file for a specific test item.

c.   The third option available is the printing of the ward report for that individual patient. This will list all the information, both

```
WARD REPORT , USER ID:  22, 14:31  09/03/76 , STATION  12


TYPE:  001.
A XXXXXX S C  OK?  Y


MEDICAL          WARD REPORT            09/03/76    14:32  PAGE   1
DOCTOR: AXXXXX S C


H44IB    G XXXXXXX LXXXXX          MEDICAL RECORD # 312515

 HEMOGRAM                         09/03/76   00:00
      HGB  GM            10.8*  GM             09/03/76    00:00
      HCT  %             34.1*  PERCENT        09/03/76    00:00
      RBC  10X6/CMM       3.68*  10X6/CMM      09/03/76    00:00
      WBC  10X3/CMM      12.4*  10X3/CMM       09/03/76    00:00
      MCV  CUB MIC         93   CUB MIC        09/03/76    00:00
      MCH MC MC GM       29.3   MC MC GM       09/03/76    00:00
      MCHC  %            31.7*  PERCENT        09/03/76    00:00
   PT CONTROL SEC        1C.8   SEC            09/03/76    13:00
   PT SEC                13.8   SEC            09/03/76    13:00
   PTT CONTRL SEC          30   SEC            09/03/76    13:00
   PTT SEC                 32   SEC            09/03/76    13:00
   SGPT    IU/L        REQUEST RECEIVED        09/03/76    00:00
   VDRL                REQUEST RECEIVED        09/03/76    00:00
   HBS AG (AUST AG)    REQUEST RECEIVED        09/03/76    00:00
   RETIC CT            REQUEST RECEIVED        09/03/76    00:00
   ESR                 REQUEST RECEIVED        09/03/76    00:00
   PLAT CT 10X3 CUM    REQUEST RECEIVED        09/03/76    00:00
   DIFF                REQUEST RECEIVED        09/03/76    00:00
   MG      MG/DL       REQUEST RECEIVED        09/03/76    00:00
   CPK     MIU/ML      REQUEST RECEIVED        09/03/76    00:00
   AMYLASE  IU/L       REQUEST RECEIVED        09/03/76    00:00
   SGOT    IU/L        REQUEST RECEIVED        09/03/76    00:00
   ALK PHOS    IU/L    REQUEST RECEIVED        09/03/76    00:00
   D BIL   MG/DL       REQUEST RECEIVED        09/03/76    00:00
   T BIL   MG/DL       REQUEST RECEIVED        09/03/76    00:00
   ALBUMIN GM/DL       REQUEST RECEIVED        09/03/76    00:00
   T PROT  GM/DL       REQUEST RECEIVED        09/03/76    00:00
   CALCIUM MG/DL       REQUEST RECEIVED        09/03/76    00:00
   GLUCOSE MG/DL       REQUEST RECEIVED        09/03/76    00:00
   ADLT LYTS BUN CR    REQUEST RECEIVED        09/03/76    13:00
   HEMOGRAM            REQUEST RECEIVED        09/03/76    13:00
 REPORT COMPLETE
```

FIG. 48 A ward report called by a physician will produce all the data since the last chart report for that physician. This document will show both complete and incomplete work at the time of printing.

complete and incomplete, that has been processed since the last chart report was generated (Fig. 48).

3. An additional inquiry can be made through the use of the specimen number. In this case, the floor personnel can track a specimen number that has been misplaced or questioned. The system will present the patient's name assigned to that specimen number and list all the associated laboratory work that is currently ordered for that patient in addition to the individual specimen number requested. This gives maximum utilization of the test file data (Fig. 49).

```
**READY
INQUIRY-SPECIMEN, USER ID: 22, 13:41  09/02/76 , STATION 12



ACQ#:  2166  MXXXXX, ARTHUR J   OK? Y  BURN H541B  941
       BXXXXXX, HG


    4320 603   URINE CULTURE                        09/02  00:00
    4289 625   BURN WOUND CULT                       09/02  12:45
    4283 625   BURN WOUND CULT                       09/02  12:45
    3396 619   CATH TIP CULTURE                      09/01  21:00
    3141 426   17-KETOSTERO-24U                      09/01  10:30
    3141 425   17-OH 24U                             09/01  10:30
    2166 427   CATECHOL-24U                          08/31  09:45



    REPORT COMPLETE
```

FIG. 49   An inquiry by specimen number begins by the validation of the name of the patient. Following verification of name, the system then produces all tests pending on that patient and allows the reviewer to see the specimen number, the test number, the test name, the date and time of order or check-in. This allows a convenient means of cross checking any specimens which may have questions raised regarding their validity on the floor or in the laboratory.

Archive

The archive system was designed to meet the needs of the medical staff and ultimately to offer a solution to the mass storage requirements of the laboratory. At each of the peripheral terminals, the archive system can be activated at the depression of a button and the input of the patient medical record number. The system will then respond with the appropriate identification for that particular record number. Following verification, the terminal will present the following information: date of service, problem, age, sex, "I" for inpatient or "O" for outpatient, and microfilm page and cassette number associated with that particular collection of patient information. Each line of information represents one admission or treatment cycle. The presentation is problem-oriented, as is shown in Fig. 50. All data is routinely microfilmed on a daily basis and entered into this retrieval system for long term storage. Currently, it is possible for the physicians to have access to their patients' laboratory information by seeking the index in the archive file and retrieving the specific data by microfilm reader/printers at locations outside the laboratory. This is a cost-effective approach to mass storage and re-

MR#:   016467

RXXXXX, DONALD I   MALE

DATE	AGE	PROBLEM	CART	PAGE	I/O
06/31/76	49	MICARDIAL	0002	0045	I
08/15/76	49	ANXIETY	0005	0123	I
09/22/76	49	CHEST PAIN	0006	0003	I

FIG. 50   A search under the archive entry button allows the reviewer to see the patient name, sex, dates of service, age, problem, microfilm cartridge and page number, and an inpatient or outpatient status code. This then acts as a reference source for physicians to access the specific laboratory data on a low cost storage media such as microfilm or microfiche.

trieval, and offers a very convenient alternative to the medical record room and its inherent problems.

SPECIMEN HANDLING

Specimen handling on the nursing station is always a tenuous situation. The policing and 24-hour enforcement of specimen requirements is difficult. Through the use of our communications system and the appropriate messages printed on the patient's chart, we developed a painless method of handling the specimen control process which satisfies the nursing requirements for information. Before the development of our files, procedure manuals were located on the floors which listed hundreds of items and the appropriate steps to be taken for each test. As anyone will testify who has worked on a busy nursing station, the book was hardly ever opened, and when it was needed, it wasn't to be found. With our current system, adequate documentation and management material is always provided to ensure that the patient receives the greatest benefit. Because of the high cost of procedures and manpower, the precise execution of each order is very important. This is just one more potent argument establishing that it is both prudent and cost-effective to have floor terminals to eliminate this possibility of error.

PROBLEMS

Crowding

Our initial configuration was limited to 32 peripheral terminals. This amounts to approximately one terminal per nursing station, which

immediately creates the problem of crowding. If two clerks wanted to order at the same time, they had either to wait in line or to schedule their work. This does not become too serious a problem as long as the workload is light. If one were trying to handle several areas, such as Pharmacy and X-ray, the burden would become extremely heavy. In some areas, a single terminal devoted to the laboratory may be necessary because of high demand and great utilization.

Overutilization

The students versus the staff. Our overutilization problem is still with us and will only be resolved when we have enough money for communication lines and terminals to satisfy everyone. Fortunately, the student demand on the system is sporadic and highly teaching-oriented; it therefore becomes very difficult to cost justify within a routine hospital environment. Plans are being made to provide additional lines of communication and a new type of terminal for the student and staff which will more than adequately meet their needs.

Sabotage

One must be very cautious when multi-user systems are installed to be sure there cannot be a systematic, well-planned effort of sabotage. One employee or individual can do great damage to the system if any of the loopholes are not anticipated beforehand. The use of the audit trail has discouraged a great many of the initial pranks since one would need to destroy it, and this would be quite visible. Less destructive attacks have occurred, which makes one believe that possibly some of the designers of vending machines ought to be consulted when looking at nursing station terminals. We have had terminals fail because of paper clips, gum wrappers, pencils, hairpins, lipstick containers, and all sorts of unusual objects being dropped into the electronics and mechanical mechanisms. In addition, the terminal often serves as a support for soda, coffee, sandwiches, and peanuts, which eventually end up being tipped or spilled. When this happens, there is a great cry on the floor about terminal failure. We have established a very simple policy which states that if the individual floor is responsible for damage to the terminal, the necessary repair and replacement comes out of their budget. This has helped to foster responsible action regarding the actual use and abuse of the terminal.

Audit Trail

When the system was started, four to five times a day a concerned physician would arrive in my office seeking retribution on the "imbecile" in the laboratory. Mistakes were obviously made, and it was our fault. We initiated a policy of immediately following up on all complaints. For about one month, every incident was investigated. The audit trails on the individual floors were absolutely invaluable in demonstrating that the physician and the nursing staff had actually created the problem. There is no doubt that without these documents we would have been shut down and turned off by popular demand. Even after seven to eight months of operation, I still find physicians who complain and are only satisfied after a review of the facts determines that the true source of malfunction was the nursing personnel, or residents, or house staff, or students. This easy delineation of responsibility and authority creates an environment within the hospital for proper patient management and administration. With this tool, one can document individual failures and provide appropriate retraining or discipline. Prior to the implementation of our system, everything was hearsay and innuendo, which never resulted in any meaningful direct action ever being taken. Now there is direct delineation of responsibility, and we can deal with real issues to ultimately solve problems.

Space

There is currently a great need for an architectural systems approach to the nursing station and its physical structure in light of communication system problems and requirements. The charting function must be convenient to the terminal and in many of our stations, this was not possible. In the case of counter-top terminal break down, we have a spare terminal on a cart which can be wheeled to the area of need. There are, however, additional problems in handling these terminals because of their weight and size. Each terminal weighs about a hundred pounds, and it is impractical for our female operators to lift the terminal off the cart, onto the counter top, move the malfunctioning unit to the cart, and return the terminal for repair. It is also impractical to leave the cart with the replacement terminal at the station since this clogs up working space. The countertop unit in our hospital is not the answer for a nursing station or a standard peripheral terminal. Benchtop models require such careful integration into the long-range architectural planning of the floor that it becomes very difficult to coordinate as changes are made and requirements modified.

Sound

Documentation regarding the sound levels and noise problems associated with our current teletype printers has been published [27, 28]. The obvious source of all this noise is the printing mechanism. Vendors in the computer industry have never been asked nor required to recognize this problem. We hope to press for changes in this area.

As a practical consideration, a nursing terminal cannot create more than 55 decibels (dB) of noise before it begins interfering with speech and normal activity at the station. Above 55 dB, the terminal becomes a hazard to the extent that personnel find it difficult to talk on the phone, take orders from physicians, and communicate about serious problems. In some cases, the personnel working in the noisy environment did not really understand why they felt irritable and upset. When the terminal was turned off, there was a great sigh of relief, and people just felt better.

DESIGN CRITERIA FOR A NURSING STATION TERMINAL

We personally looked at many communication terminals and have had a chance to review systems in operation. After experiencing our situation and working with our personnel and system, we have come to some definite conclusions about what is needed in the nursing station area to support and satisfy some of the basic activities.

As a beginning, one must look at the cost of a communication system, and break it down into line costs and the number of lines it takes to support each terminal. One can directly correlate costs of communication systems and number of lines required for the system. The cost not only relates to the line itself but also the terminal to which it connects.

Being both practical and expedient, the communication terminal offered by most vendors is probably a duplicate of those used in other data processing centers and has not been customized for a medical environment. This is where we get into serious problems regarding noise and reliability. It may be convenient to use a noisy printer in a computer center, but such a device on a nursing station is impractical. In addition, the nursing terminal must be seriously looked at since on-site service is expensive. The hospital's 24-hour operation requires repairs within five to ten minutes in almost all cases. It is too expensive to have service people on call 24 hours a day; therefore, a redundant series of terminals must be available on a cart system.

IDEAL TERMINAL

Our ideal terminal must integrate a line printer, cathode ray tube (CRT), broad function keyboard, communications controller, and transport and storage device that is compatible with the following specifications.

Printer

1. The unit must support "multipart" printing of at least one original and four carbon copies.

2. Sound level of the terminal at the user's ear must be at or below 55 decibels in all directions.

3. The printing must be visible to the user as it is processed by the machine.

4. Paper and ribbon changing must be simple and easily accessible.

5. On the average, the printer must operate at least two months without repair or service.

6. The printer must operate at a minimum of 2400 baud.

7. Edge-perforated/fan-fold multipart paper should be supported to permit high speed printer and high speed page ejections, as well as accurate registration of preprinted forms.

8. Form feed must be selectable so that it can match the application area.

9. The printer must offer the full 64 character monocase character set—including all alphanumerics and symbolics.

10. Printed characters must be impact formed in full-font, rather than dot-matrix character approximations.

11. The printer unit must include provisions for automatic "turn-off" during periods of inactivity—with automatic "turn on" when data printing is required.

12. The printer must be able to print at least 80 columns width at standard spacing of 10 characters per inch (horizontal) and the standard line spacing of six lines per inch (vertical).

Cathode Ray Tube (CRT)

1. The screen should allow at least 80 character columns by at least 24 lines.

2. The screen should offer minimal distortion characteristics at the edges.

3. The terminal should include both "brightness" (separate) and "contrast" (separate) controls exposed for easy access and adjustment by the user.

4. Both white on black and black on white presentation should be available.

5. The terminal should operate at a minimum of 2400 baud and allow expansion up to 19.2 kilobaud.

6. The CRT display module should be "tilt" adjustable from the horizontal to suit the individual user's requirements.

7. The terminal should be modular and flexible enough to permit easy future expansion into a colored CRT display.

8. The terminal should be flexible enough to allow easy future expansion for incorporation of a "light pen" input selection device.

9. The terminal should have cursor control via the keyboard.

Keyboard

1. The keyboard should offer a standard typewriter array.

2. The keyboard should offer an adding machine keyboard for numerical entry.

3. The keyboard should offer a variety of function keys for ease of selection.

4. The keyboard should offer a series of action keys for interactive software control.

5. The keyboard should have local command keys for control of the CRT, printer, and microprocessor.

6. The keyboard should include at least two "status" indicators to permit operator observation of the terminal microprocessor hardware.

7. The keyboard should include programmable lighted indicators to provide operator indication of the various applications states of the terminal programs (firmware).

Communications

1. The communications port of the terminal must include provision for connection to a standard asynchronous modem, via the RS232C standard interface and connector.

2. The communications portion of the terminal must allow for full duplex operation over a direct connection 20 milliamp "loop." Connection to the "loop" circuit should be via a connector with pro-

visions for a separate "transmit" twisted pair, and a separate "receiver" twisted pair.

3. The communications portion of this terminal must allow for direct connection to a four-wire, full-duplex, bidirectional circuit to provide for transmission/reception at baud rates greater than 2400.

4. The terminal must include internal capability for asynchronous (10 unit code) transmission/reception of data at baud rates up to 19,200.

5. A standard communications code for the terminal should be USASCII (ANSI X3.4). All alphanumeric, symbolic, and most standard control codes should be supported.

Terminal Design

1. The operation of the printer, CRT, and keyboard should be under the direct control of the microprocessor in the terminal.

2. Add on modules should be possible to allow: (*a*) local mass storage such as a floppy disc, (*b*) local expansion of memory such as additional ROMs and RAMs, (*c*) local expansion of additional microprocessors, (*d*) local entry and processing of microprocessors remote from the terminal, (*e*) the manipulation of fixed format keyboards designed for special purpose applications, and (*f*) a badge reader option.

3. Internal design should permit redundancy so that either the printer of the CRT could be used if the other fails.

4. The packaging should be as small and compact as possible to stay within the requirements of the noise specifications as listed above.

5. Spare logic bays should be available for the expansion of both memory and microprocessor.

6. Units should offer heavy duty power and communication cable with at least 8–10 feet of spare line for service.

7. The terminal should be easy to repair and allow for internal diagnostics to be performed as a test mode.

Cart or Mounting Media

1. The support base for the terminal should be adjustable from a sitting to a standing height.

2. The cart or support media should hold the paper in a convenient location and allow for proper paper feed.

3. If a second copy is used for audit, the terminal base should store the second page in a convenient location.

4. The support or transport device should have wide 4-inch diameter rubber wheels that roll easily and lock.

5. The terminal should support a knee space in the front direction to allow for easy access on an average nursing station.

Figure 51 shows our idealized terminal, which is self-contained, mobile, and meets the criteria we have established through months of operation and working with our personnel and system constraints. We would propose to use this same terminal for physician inquiry since we have noted that they, in most cases, are dissatisfied by the use of the CRT only, and continue to demand hard copy. They appreciate the speed of the CRT, yet want to take a printed page with them. This places us right back in the same conceptual design we are using for the

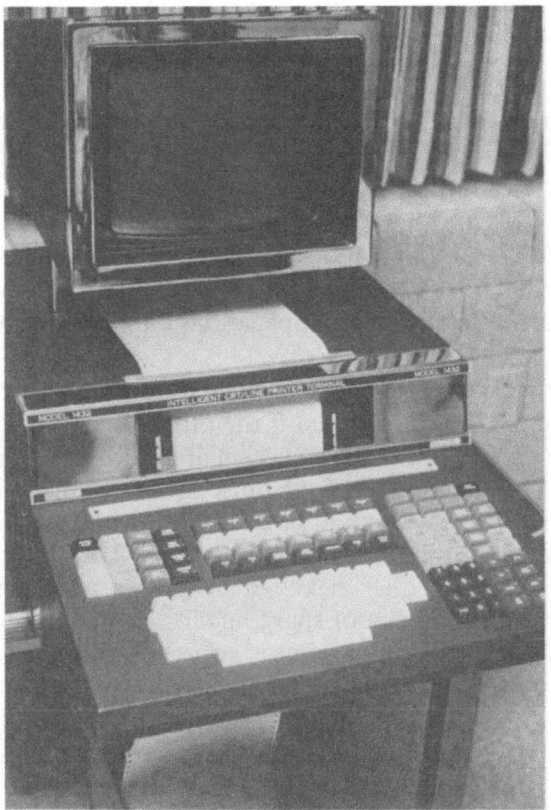

FIG. 51   The nursing station is an extremely difficult environment to accommodate, and a special terminal was built to reach the speed requirements as well as the hardcopy demands in this challenging area.

nursing station. By standardizing on one unit, it would seem that we can service all areas and drastically simplify our maintenance problems. This approach also puts us in a position of having a unit that has volume potential, so that we can begin decreasing the cost of a single terminal.

This particular design and function allows virtually every nursing station to create an open space in which a chair can be approximated to the terminal. The terminal can be brought up against a counter or other existing structure for use. With this design, there are no holes being cut in countertops, no special knee space required, no special chair, none of the customary physical plant changes that are required with most countertop units. Our design also creates a unit that is easy for the laboratory to handle on a daily basis and eliminates many of the human engineering problems experienced with current modules.

11

Outpatient Operation

INTRODUCTION

Our Outpatient Clinic had been a constant problem for the hospital laboratories. Since all clinics ran autonomously and synchronously, specimens would arrive in shoe boxes, snuff cans, and soda bottles with very little identifying information. This was the legacy of the outpatient laboratory services inherited as part of the original systems design.

To make a major change in this service required a dialog between the clinics and the laboratory to coordinate efforts. One of the first criteria was to insist that all outpatient specimens be brought to the outpatient lab. Prior to system installation, outpatient specimens were sporadically delivered to the main hospital laboratory, and usually mixed with inpatient specimens with no way of untangling the mess. A sharp delineation was made between these two sources of specimens, and this has been maintained by the system.

OUTPATIENT ADMISSIONS

Each outpatient requires admission to the communication system. This function is performed in the outpatient laboratory. One full-time

technical person handles demographic data entry and ordering through a remote CRT terminal. This guarantees that we have the proper data in our files for reporting and the right number of specimens for evaluation. Unfortunately, there are not enough communication lines currently available to provide individual clinic terminals. Despite this current limitation, it is very convenient to have a central outpatient lab station for specimen evaluation and data control.

ORDER FORMS

The form used is very similar to the inpatient ordering form, except that additional information is required for outpatient billing (Fig. 37). An outpatient designation is the key for reporting. This letter code sorts the reports coming to the Outpatient Clinic and solved the problem of lost reports.

RESULT ENTRY

Once the specimens have been ordered and the proper admission data has been collected, they can be transported to the main lab for testing and reporting. The results for an outpatient are now in the communication system and are available to any doctor within the hospital as soon as they are entered and verified. A few basic tests are still performed in the outpatient lab, and until additional communication lines are available, these cannot be added to the real-time data base.

CHART REPORTING

Daily charts are run with outpatient results at about 4 PM each day. The clinic designator helps the outpatient lab to distribute the proper forms and reports to the appropriate area. Daily charts are placed in accordion files by the clinic clerks for the doctors to review on a later visit. In some clinics, the patient charts are saved and the appropriate reports are placed in the patient's chart before they are returned to medical records. This drastically reduces clerical effort when accomplished.

PROBLEMS

Terminals

Without enough peripheral terminals in the Outpatient Clinics, specimen collection still remains uncontrolled. In some cases, the wrong tube is drawn. This is usually detected too late and the courier has to be sent back and the patient redrawn. The obvious solution is simple—install more hardware.

Transport

Since our clinics are widespread and include pediatrics, specimens are often drawn in the clinic. Transporting the specimen between the clinic and outpatient lab can be complicated. Courier service cannot always be depended upon for expeditious transits. Only architectural assistance will resolve this issue by providing adequate horizontal and vertical conveyance for outpatient laboratory material.

Data Accuracy

After two years of indoctrination, we are still receiving requests from the outpatient area for which the primary identifying data is incomplete. This creates additional problems in trying to retrieve information to notify the appropriate person. One must still rely on a constant program of education to handle this procedural area.

Remote Operation

The configuration of our current system and the number of communication lines available makes it impossible to run an outpatient laboratory in a true remote sense. We continue to use the central lab as the major source of testing and data entry. Soon, we will be expanding to a full outpatient laboratory and have equipment on order to enlarge the size of our current information system to handle additional laboratory communication lines.

12

Specimen Handling

KEY SYSTEM

Probably the most significant design challenge for a laboratory system is to devise a method by which the specimens can be transported to and from the laboratory and coordinated with the proper results and retrieval of information. There are not many choices available when approaching this type of work, and most of the information we have gathered has been by trial and error, using the actual environment of the hospital laboratory facilities as a test medium. In fact, virtually every combination and permutation of specimen problem has been run against our current configuration; so far there are no known failures to report.

PROTOCOLS

Stats

The stat specimen is assigned a unique number less than 1000 at the site of ordering along with the appropriate handling information. It is anticipated that this order will go on the chart at that time, and that

119

subsequent persons reviewing the chart will not reorder or duplicate that particular procedure.

Expedites

The expedite category of order requires a different type of specimen number which begins with 1000 and increases in intervals of 1000 for each day of the week. This scheme rotates all numbers each week and is automatically initialized every midnight. Such an order process allows the physicians individually to handle their own routine specimens without activating the stat mechanism of the laboratory. The system provides a message for the expedite orders using the same basic data we provide for routine orders, since these tests are going to be handled identically in the laboratory.

Routines

Routine orders, in some cases, will be assigned a routine specimen number, and in other cases are merely put in a holding file for blood drawing the next morning. These differences are uniquely coded in the individual test files established for the laboratory at the time of system initialization. For a routine order such as urinalysis, a special message is printed that tells the floor exactly how to process the specimen and handle it from the time they contact the patient until the time it is delivered to the lab.

SPECIMEN SCREENING

Once the specimen is transported to the laboratory, there is a central window for receiving. At that time, the specimen number and patient identification are checked. For coagulation studies, the tube is inspected for volume to ensure the proper amount of anticoagulant. For timed procedures and tolerance tests, a check is made to insure that both time and necessary specimens are available. Before acceptance, an additional verification of the order is done using the unfinished test file via CRT. This pinpoints duplicates, identification errors, and incomplete orders. If there are any problems related to the screening process, they are immediately phoned back to the floor for resolution before the specimen is accepted. Any errors verified at this stage are entered on-line into the patient result file for PSRO audit and floor physician education [29] (Fig. 52).

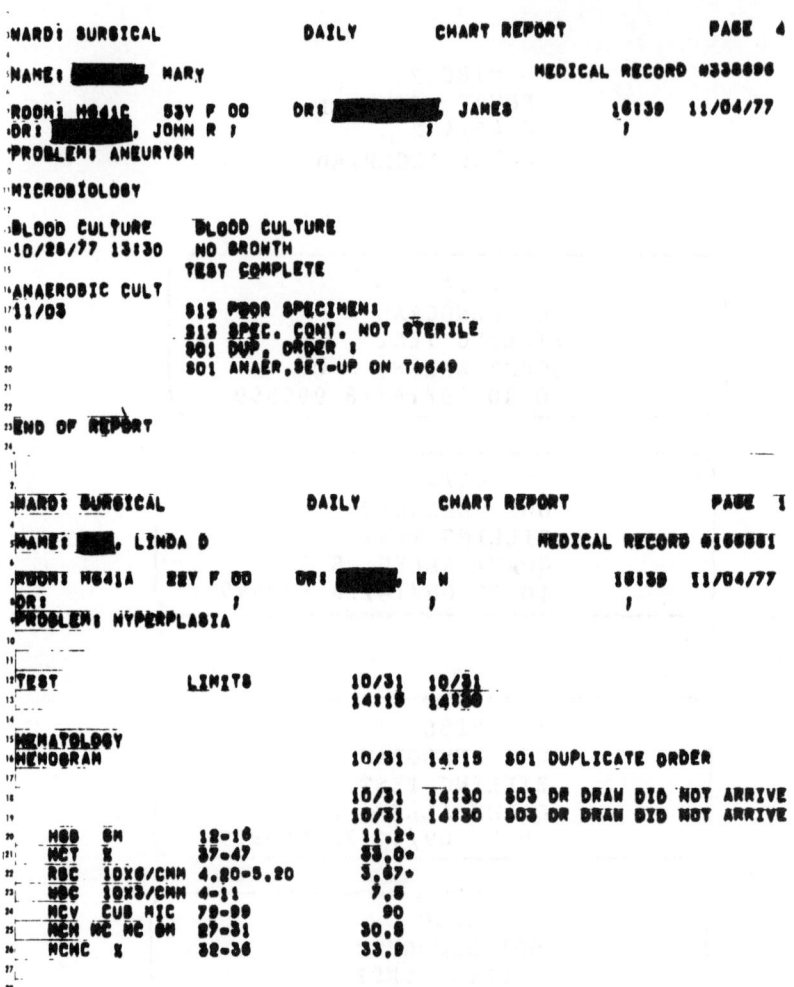

FIG. 52 The patient chart report shows the errors. This PSRO audit is carried on by the laboratory following each specimen inspection and handling. Each mistake is coded with a specific number and given an English interpretation. This data is then tabulated and maintained by physician, by service, and by floor so that areas of difficulty can be identified and corrective measures taken.

CHECK-IN AND TIMING

Once the specimen is accepted at the front window of the laboratory, it is finally checked into the system by the use of a dedicated CRT. The terminal allows the specimen number entry, followed by the selection

```
U  0180 2
ENTRY  ACCEPTED
U  4574 2
ENTRY  ACCEPTED
```

```
          4574
001 HEMOGRAM
BILLING TEST
QCRMX ALLEN, S C
10:30 09/14/78 999999
```

```
          4574
001 HEMOGRAM
BILLING TEST
QCRMX ALLEN, S C
10:30 09/14/78 999999
```

```
          0180
001 HEMOGRAM
BILLING TEST
QCRMX ALLEN, S C
10:30 09/14/78 999999
```

```
          0180
001 HEMOGRAM
BILLING TEST
QCRMX ALLEN, S C
10:30 09/14/78 999999
```

FIG. 53   The input of the specimen number during the check-in process begins with an identification code "u," specimen number, followed by the number of labels required for subsequent processing. If a date or a time change is required, this is entered along with the standard format and allows the update of the files for this corrected information. After receiving an entry accepted, the system then prints the specific labels required for those procedures and allows this information to be passed on for laboratory testing.

of the number of labels required by the individual laboratories. Figure 53 shows the label produced by the high speed label printer in the normal check-in procedure. There are built-in overrides in the check-in process to allow the specimen's time and date to be modified for the individual requirements of the specimen. The check-in process also allows up to nine labels to be generated for each individual specimen number verified. This permits one to customize the number of label-generating steps for each laboratory.

One of the major problems in handling stats and expedites in the laboratory is that they are sporadic and inconvenient for work sheets. To solve this problem, our labels are attached directly to a blank work sheet on which the answers are written. Using this technique, there are no transcription steps involved in stat and expedite work-sheet generation. The technologists are free to perform only the testing and entry functions.

SPECIMEN AUDIT

The specimen audit trail is one area in which our specifications were quite detailed as a direct result of the initial systems study. Some means was necessary to determine when the specimen was ordered, how the specimen was drawn, if the laboratory was properly contacted, and whether the specimen ever arrived in the laboratory. Prior to computer logging, it was a nightmare to unravel some of the complex problems associated with locating specimens and missing results.

Our current system requires timing inputs when a test is ordered, when a test is checked in at the laboratory, and when the test is reported. The initial time assigned is 00:00. This means that the order has been placed, but no specimen has arrived in the laboratory. When a specimen number greater than zero is assigned, this indicates that there is active work being done on that specimen. A specimen number of 0000 indicates that the individual specimen is pending on the blood drawing list and has had no formal action taken yet.

When the specimen arrives in the laboratory, it is checked in and a time is assigned on a 2400-hour military clock. This is incremented in 15-minute intervals through the real-time computer-clock system. In most cases, specimens ordered arrive the same day and, therefore, we have an accurate correlation between specimen order data and date of arrival in the laboratory. A secondary assumption made is that there is not more than a half hour delay between the time the specimen is ordered from the floor and the time it arrives in the laboratory. In most

cases, we assign the date and time of check-in at the laboratory as the time of specimen acquisition from the patient. For more than 90% of the cases, this is true. In the other cases, urines are held or tests are delayed and a different date and time are required. This calls for a special branch of the software which allows us to insert a new date and a new time appropriate for that particular order. This is done at the time of check-in when labels are being printed.

By the use of the time and dating function, it is very easy for the house staff and clinical personnel to determine the status of their orders at any point and decipher whether the order is still in the hands of the floor or has been transferred to the laboratory for subsequent performance.

SPECIMEN NUMBER ASSIGNMENT

Microbiology, Blood Bank, Microscopy, and Anatomic Pathology all require unique specimen numbers for each individual order. This occurs because these areas very rarely have split specimens headed to different parts of the laboratory. These stand in contradistinction to Chemistry, Hematology, and Immunology, which need common numbers to minimize their logging function. This common number simplifies ordering, confirmation, and the bookwork that is necessary for reporting.

LABEL PRODUCTION

Before the routine AM blood drawing, labels are printed which contain the necessary information for sample identification. This is acquired, along with a draw sheet which itemizes the patients to be visited for venipuncture and lists the procedures for each of those particular patients (Fig. 54). Technologists are then free to make the rounds, acquire the appropriate tubes, and later return to the laboratory for check-in. Individual phlebotomists use the check-in CRT terminal and input the appropriate specimen number for the work they have performed. This places the specimen time and date function in proper sequence so that the faculty and staff know the lab has performed its job. As for procedures which are not accomplished, these are not checked in and are left for subsequent follow-up using a "doctor draw" routine.

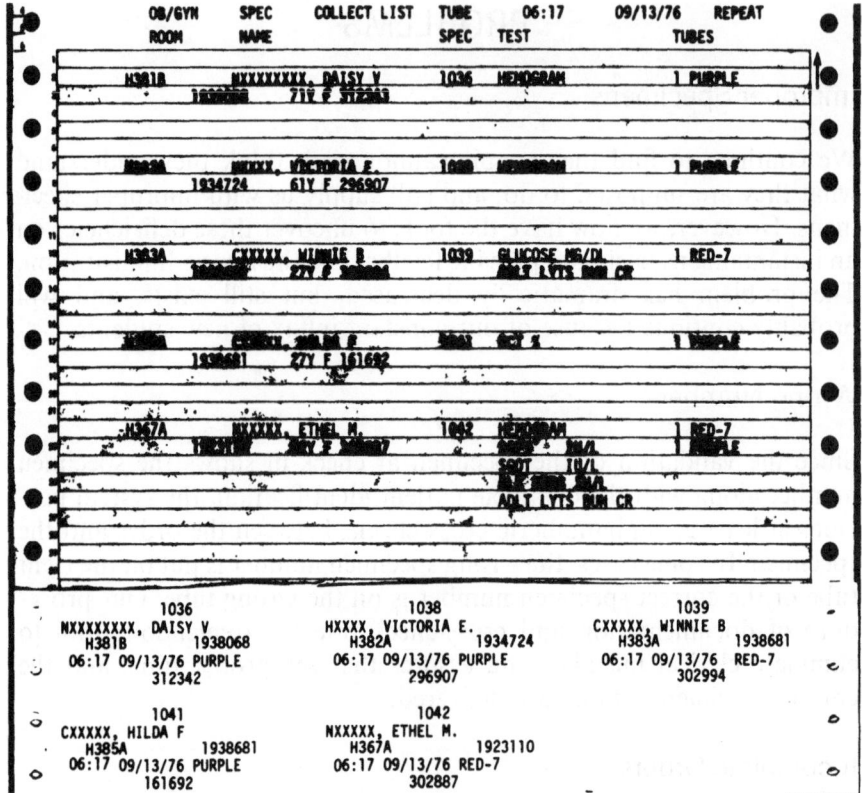

FIG. 54   The morning collection list for specimen pick-up is printed just before the blood drawing team leaves. A hardcopy is generated, along with appropriate labels defining what type of tests are to be performed and what kind of tube is required.

TRAINING ARENA

The sample check-in desk and master console operation for the computer system turns out to be an ideal training arena for medical technologists, medical students, and pathology residents. This is truly the crossroads of the lab, at which all of the acute problems encountered by the staff reach the system at its highest state of activity. There is no question that the training and experience gained by handling the daily specimens is essential for the proper orientation and appreciation of students to the dynamic field of clinical pathology.

PROBLEMS

Improper Specimens

We continue to find that people cannot read, think they understand what they are supposed to do, and still supply us with improper specimens. However, we now have the tools to uncover these deficiencies on an instantaneous basis and provide feedback to the floor administration. The problem has dramatically decreased, but still exists, and will probably continue because of our constant influx of new students.

Wrong Numbers

Since the validation of the specimen at check-in shows the specimen number along with the complete patient identification, the system provides at least 25 alphanumeric cross-checks between the order and the specimen. In some cases, the wrong specimen number is put on the right tube or the correct specimen number is on the wrong tube. Our procedure of documentation and cross-check offers a tremendous tool to eliminate clerical mistakes and assures that the proper tube, and the correct specimen number are delivered.

Incomplete Orders

Using the specimen numbering system as described, there is a potential inconsistency that relates to incomplete orders. If someone should deliver two tubes with the appropriate specimen number, and yet leave a third tube behind which is still part of the original order, we usually did not detect the error until the tubes were back in the laboratory. It requires a very careful inspection at the front window to make sure the tubes are appropriate for the tests ordered. If they are not, the tubes are held for floor correction. To solve this problem, we now use the CRT to list the complete order set before specimen check-in. A very quick calculation by the computer operator will detect inadequate specimens and result in an immediate correction.

"IDEAL" SPECIMEN NUMBER PROGRAM

An ideal specimen number system would require numbers to be placed in a terminal buffer for each individual patient order sequence. A single

number would be assigned for routine, stat, and expedite orders. This would eliminate the possibility of getting multiple specimen numbers on one tube. After several months of programming, we are happy to say that we now have this function and it works.

LABEL SPEED

In our initial configuration we used a modified teletype for a label printer. This particular device proved totally unsatisfactory in the first week of operation because the unit was just too slow. To keep pace with the number of stat and expedite specimens brought to the check-in window required a unit three to four times faster. Our miscalculation was almost fatal. We quickly replaced our original unit with one that was six times faster and have been very satisfied with the results. One must very accurately judge the number of stat and expedite specimens and the amount of time spent in handling these to stipulate the speed of the label printer required for daily operation.

COORDINATION WITH A CENTRAL PROCESSING UNIT

The people who maintain and operate the computer on a 24-hour basis also handle all the specimens and do the routine check-ins. This requires a level of skill in a new category within the clinical labs. We have found it quite difficult to train individuals who come from outside the hospital environment for this new position. Those who were trained at large data centers find it exceedingly difficult to work within the hospital laboratory environment, since they are placed under a constant level of stress owing to the demands of the faculty and the expectations of the technologists. As a high volume area, it requires knowledgeable, well-oriented, cool-thinking operators. Many of the clerks and secretaries who were originally taken from the laboratory and retrained in computer operation found this job too stressful and demanding, and have subsequently taken jobs elsewhere within the Health Center. We found the greatest personnel resource to be the clerks and secretaries on the floors in the hospital. These people possess the needed background, knowledge, and familiarity with the terminology used within the laboratory, and have a genuine feeling for the problems related to floor operation. They can talk knowledgeably with floor personnel, and usually have a good liaison with the physicians in the hospital. It is a natural promotion for them in this new area of training.

CENTRAL COMMUNICATIONS FOR THE LAB

Centralizing the check-in process and the data control system centralizes laboratory communication. Adequate resource staff and personnel are required to maintain the necessary functions of the individual laboratory facilities as they process the daily problems. A pathologist will find great utility in becoming very familiar with this operation since many of the problems resolved in this area require medical decisions related to patient therapy and ultimate disposition.

SPECIMEN ACQUISITION

Blood Drawing

Blood drawing in our facility amounts to morning draws, Monday through Friday, and a reliance on the house staff and faculty for acquisition of the remaining specimens. As a result of both economics and logistics, the laboratory is unable to provide a blood-drawing team substantial enough to service the entire Health Center complex. Our morning team does receive specific blood-draw instructions each morning at about 07:00, which are generated only moments before they proceed on rounds.

Previously, lists were generated at midnight, causing many serious problems. Delayed orders and missing patients were common. Somewhere between 20 and 30% of all reports regarding patient location were wrong. An additional hour or two each morning was spent tracking down patients who could not be found. Our on-line real-time blood-drawing list and label production has totally eliminated this problem.

Specimen Check-In

When the blood-drawing team completes its rounds, the tubes are brought to the laboratory for check-in. The technologists enter a zero when specifying labels since these are not required. This particular function takes just a matter of seconds and places the proper dates and times in the patient record for audit and review.

Doctor Draws

For those patients who are not in their beds or who are extremely difficult to draw, the tubes and labels are left on the floor for the appro-

priate doctor to draw. When the technologists check the specimens into the lab, they do not check in the doctor draws. The physician then draws the tubes, brings them to the lab, and the appropriate labels are checked in by the computer operators and passed on to the various laboratories for handling.

CREDITS

Billing credits for laboratory work can only be executed by the individual laboratories on signed credit forms. They can be entered directly through on-line communications by our remote laboratory terminal. The actual credit is logged in a book in each one of the lab areas, along with an explanation for the credit to make certain these orders are canceled accurately. This allows no recriminations by a physician on the floor insisting that the cancellation or credit was inappropriate (Fig. 55).

```
MR#          121212          OK? Y  GXXXX, RALPH R        ERMA  OK? Y



        0000  002    HGB              02/03  00:00
        0011  018    G6PD U/GHB/MIN   02/03  12:30
        2011  598    BLOOD CULTURE    02/03  12.15
        0008  298    DIGOXIN RIA      02/03  12:15
        0007  002    HGB              02/03  12:15
        0006  001    HEMOGRAM         02/03  12·15


    REPORT COMPLETE
    CANC T#·  002  HGB      OK?  Y

    CANC T#   018  G6PD SCREEN    OK?  Y

    CANC T#   001  HEMOGRAM  OK?  Y
```

FIG. 55   In order to cancel a test, one enters the medical record number and validates the name. From this is produced the list of unfinished tests along with their specimen, test number, and date of check-in. One then enters the test number, validates the test name, and then enters specimen number for appropriate cancellation. This process can only be done in the central computer room.

STAT SPECIMENS

Stat specimens flow through the lab with a specimen number of less than 1000. They are transported directly to the lab area of interest and are handled preferentially. Our computer check-in label is transferred to a stat worksheet and the necessary work is performed. Expedite and routine orders are handled in a similar manner and are batched for normal testing.

SPECIAL ORDERS

There are always those cases that do not fit any of the above situations or systems. These usually occur for a doctor's wife, office nurse, or medical student who wants special care and handling. These very special, rare requests do not go through the system, but use a notebook in each lab for reporting. This is reviewed weekly to process billing information. These results are only reported by phone to a specific individual. We find that this escape valve system is used once or twice a week in special cases, and is certainly not to be advocated or encouraged in any circumstance.

OUTPATIENT SPECIMENS

Outpatient specimens are initially preprocessed in the outpatient area and the appropriate specimen numbers are acquired. An outpatient terminal gathers admission data and places the order. The specimens are then brought to the main lab area for check-in, labeling, and distribution to the individual divisions.

13

Chemistry System

INTRODUCTION

Chemistry was the most dynamic division in the installation of the information system, since the number of stat and expedite specimens arriving after morning blood drawing exceeded the total AM pickups. This volume implied a huge workload, which was unscheduled yet expected to be completed in less than two hours. Solving this problem required the integration of chemistry instrumentation and working schedules to put together a new package sufficient to meet the demands for service. Our chemistry operation utilizes a SMAC, ACA, GEMSAEC, 4 + 2 Autoanalyzer, 4 dual Autoanalyzers, and atomic absorption equipment, along with some special stat single-item testing devices that are maintained around the clock. Through the coordination of these devices, the computer, and chemistry staff, it is possible to create a tremendously responsive unit with very high through-put. Using this approach, however, requires a very high dependency on technology. Training and coordination must be maintained at a very high level to keep mechanical up-time on a day-to-day basis acceptable.

FORMS

The chemistry order form shown in Fig. 34 provides those data the faculty and staff need to decide what should be done stat and what may be considered routine. If the test or procedure is not done by the lab, they will not find it on the form, and it must then be requested through one of the pathologists. This single step has eliminated many of the problems associated with the ordering of outlandish procedures, unknown to anyone in the lab, and the former lack of communication and coordination is now minimized since the problem is dealt with directly through a physician/pathologist interface.

SPECIMEN PREPARATION

When the tubes and labels reach the splitting section or specimen-preparation area in Chemistry, they are centrifuged and the appropriate label is placed on the work sheet and subsequent splitting tube for sample allocation. Two people are assigned on a rotating basis to the front desk of clinical chemistry each day to guarantee the continuity of this process and to follow through on any special splits that are required to feed Immunology and Microscopy. Stat orders are, of course, processed expeditiously and the results are entered as soon as they are finished.

SPECIAL ORDERS

Special tests requiring a referral laboratory are monitored at the specimen check-in desk, and are subsequently spun and processed for shipping. This process is very time-consuming, and will ultimately require the services of one full-time individual. There are many special-handling procedures and instructions required for the exotic tests, and they must be done with exactitude or the whole procedure is a waste of time. Some difficulty has been experienced in coordinating this process, and we are now working with the area specialty groups, medicine and pediatrics (endocrinology and gastroenterology), to coordinate the consultation mechanism with the ordering of referral tests. Our current test files ask the individual clinician who orders a test such as an ACTH to contact one of the endocrinologists prior to placing this order. The consultants are well aware of the procedures involved in these tests, and

can therefore act as monitors of the procedure and guarantee that the lab will have adequate specimen control and follow-through when the test is initiated.

WORK SHEETS

The laboratory enters its initial volume of work on work sheets generated by the system once blood drawing is completed. These work sheets are quite flexible, as shown in Figs. 56–58, and provide different options for display. Results are transcribed onto these sheets for subsequent data entry by the medical technologist performing the work.

PATIENT NAME	SPEC NO.	NA (075)	K (076)	CL (077)	CO2 (078)	BUN (079)	CREAT (080)	UR AC (081)	TECH
						96		08:37	
MXXXX, NANCY P	1081	-----							----
BXXXXXX, BETTY	1111	-----							----
FXXXXXX, ELMER	7174	-----							----
MXXXX, NANCY P	1081		-----						----
TXXXXX, SAM	1101		-----						----
BXXXXXX, BETTY	1111		-----						----
MXXXX, NANCY P	1081			-----					----
BXXXXXX, BETTY	1111			-----					----
MXXXX, NANCY P	1081				-----				----
BXXXXXX, BETTY	1111				-----				----
PXXXXX, THOMAS	0008					-----			----
AXXXX, ROBERT	1057					-----			----
AXXXXX, THOMAS	1097					-----			----
BXXXXXX, BETTY	1111					-----			----
PXXXXX, THOMAS	0008						-----		----
BXXXX, MAGGIE	1051						-----		----
AXXXX, ROBERT	1057						-----		----
EXXXXXX, VERNO	1059						-----		----
AXXXXX, THOMAS	1097						-----		----
WXXXXXX, NANCY	1159							-----	----

Date: 03/06/77   SMAC GROUP 1

FIG. 56   Special worksheets are prepared for group tests, such as the SMAC and Coulter Counter, in which dotted lines indicate those patients who have specific tests to be run.

| | | 05/16/77 | ACA TESTS | 128 | 08:40 | | | | |

PATIENT NAME	SPEC NO.	AC PHOS (129)	CPK (169)	SAL (145)	HBDH (127)	L-LDH (126)	LAC AC (151)	ALC (142)	TECH
WXXXXX, ROBERT*	2050	-----							----
PXXXXX, COLLIE	2079	-----							----
MXXXXXXXXX, BER	0036		-----						----
LXXXXXX, AUSTIN	2030		-----						----
PXXXXXX, ETHEL	2075		-----						----
LXXXXXX, AUSTIN	0105		-----						----
JXXXXX, ANNA	2099		-----						----
BXXXXXXX, AMLIN	2121		-----						----
MXXXXXXXXX, BER	2151				-----				----

FIG. 57   A worksheet for the ACA Chemical Analyzer shows the patient name, specimen number, and appropriate tests to be performed.

| | 09/01/76 | OSMOLALITY | 109 | 8:38 | |

PATIENT NAME	SPEC	RESULT	TECH
PXXXXXXX, ANGE	0097	-----	----
HXXXX, SYBLE	0102	-----	----
CXXXXX, CHERYL	0160	-----	----

FIG. 58   For singular tests a standard one-column report is provided, along with space for technologists' verification.

INPUT TERMINALS

Four modes of entry are available for clinical chemistry results. Using special function keyboards, high volume special messages are used along with the numerical result for the bulk of routine entry. This method provides a hardcopy audit and verification of each entry as the technologist enters data from the work sheet. The second mode of entry is the mark-sense card on which the technologist can mark in the appropriate answer and submit these as a batch for subsequent verification. A third mode of entry uses the free-format CRT keyboard on which one can enter information in a dialog fashion. It is interesting to note

that, having these three options available, the technologists uniformly enjoy the use of the fixed-format keyboard with the special buttons. This is by far the most commonly used and most popular terminal in the lab. A fourth mode of entry is via computer-readable media such as that employed for the SMAC.

SMAC INTERFACE

A special technique of interface has been designed for the Sequential Multiple Analyzer plus Computer (SMAC) using punch paper tape. Previous information has been published on the technical aspects of this interface [30]. It is sufficient to state that the SMAC is a complicated instrument utilizing a computer system for storage and retrieval of its internal information. It can produce a tremendous amount of data in a single hour, and should anything happen to that information during a run, a serious problem would be created in the laboratory, requiring manual entry. The laboratory initially elected to interface the SMAC through punch paper tape generated by a teletype terminal. As of this date, the technologists are extremely happy with the choice and have had no real desire to move to an on-line system.

The normal procedure in creating a SMAC paper tape is simple. Specimens are brought to the SMAC unit with the appropriate specimen number attached. The operator places the specimen number in the SMAC header field in place of name and identifying information. All procedures are ordered for all specimens. This requires minimum input via the SMAC CRT. SMAC subsequently generates all the answers for each one of the specimens and punches this out on paper tape on the teletype. The tape can be monitored by watching the print-out on the paper to guarantee it is accomplishing the proper information transfer. Once the tape is completed, it is transported to the computer room, loaded on a high-speed paper-tape reader, and entered into the patient's files. The programs initially used simulated the manual input terminal through the use of the paper-tape system. This is a highly unsatisfactory approach and was rewritten for a more convenient mode of data handling. Using our current software, the SMAC tape is quickly read into a buffer. A second program pass checks the orders for the individual specimen numbers. One can then print out, using the high-speed printer, a summary of those orders requested against the various specimen numbers. A validation of that matrix before and after file entry is all that is necessary. This involves a minimum number of steps and a maximum amount of data through-put.

UNFINISHED TEST REPORT

Throughout the day, it is necessary for the laboratory to audit its books and determine specimen–result continuity. This information can be called up at any time during the working cycle as the "unfinished test report." We currently print this report twice a day and have a medical

```
UNFINISHED TEST REPORT   CHEMISTRY          06/28/77   13:10    PAGE 1

PATIENT NAME          PATIENT NUM      SPEC. TEST  IDENTIFICATION      REQ DATE


PXXX, BARBARA *       H225A  101483     1221   180 PARATHY-PC      09:15 06/20/77



GXXXXXX, EDMUND       A320B  342702     1037   923 LIPO-INTERPRET  08:15 06/27/77
                                        1037   922   EL ALB GM/D   08:15 06/27/77
                                        1037   921   ALPHA-1 GM/   08:15 06/27/77
                                        1037   920   ALPHA-2 GM/   08:15 06/27/77
                                        1037   919   BETA    GM/   08:15 06/27/77
                                        1037   918   GAMMA   GM/   08:15 06/27/77
                                        1037   917   PROT ELP IN   08:15 06/27/77
                                        2184   119 5-HOUR-GTT      00:00 06/28/77

MXXXXX, VIRGINIA *    A322B  319480     2183   119 5-HOUR-GTT      00:00 06/28/77


BXXXXX, WAUNA         A327B  303306     3367   099 ACTH            16:30 06/22/77



HXXXXXX, VIOLA        A328A  340633     2207   274 LIVER/ENZY. PR  11:30 06/28/77
                                        2207   095 ADLT LYTS BUN   11:30 06/28/77


SXXXXXXXXX, JOHN      A329B  265850     2213   081 URIC AC MG/DL   11:30 06/28/77
                                        2213   095 ADLT LYTS BUN   11:30 06/28/77
                                        2213   084 GLUCOSE MG/DL   11:30 06/28/77


FXXXXXX, JACK P       A332A  329327     2029   129 ACID PHOS IU/L  12:45 06/28/77
                                        2029   084 GLUCOSE MG/DL   12:45 06/28/77
```

FIG. 59 For each laboratory an unfinished test report is produced at any time during the day to validate what specimens have not been processed and what the current information shows regarding specimen handling. On this report is shown the patient's name, medical record number, the specimen number, and test number requested, and also the requisition date and time. If the time is 00:00, the specimen has not been checked into the laboratory.

technologist assigned to evaluate it and to point out problems. In essence, this is the bookkeeping system which keeps the clinical labs honest and clears up the problems which have arisen during each shift. Figure 59 shows this document as an integral part of the quality control function of the laboratory.

The use of the unfinished test report minimizes the number of clerical hours and mistakes, and at the same time provides absolute control of each laboratory. Our initial experience with this document was quite frustrating since many of the technologists and laboratory directors were accustomed to accounting for procedural mistakes through manual systems. However, the report now has a great deal of credibility because of the absolute accuracy and its instantaneous availability.

ABNORMAL TEST REPORT

An abnormal test report can be called up at any time and used for system audit, teaching, or patient rounds. The abnormal test report will produce

6-A WING		ABNORMAL RESULTS		09/04/76	PAGE 1	
H360A	35Y F	OODXXXXXX, JUDY M		ILL	MEDICAL RECOR	451783
	ALBUMIN GM/DL		3.5 GM/DL			
	ALBUMIN GM/DL		3.5 GM/DL			
	ALK PHOS IU/L		40 IU/L			
	TOT LDH IU/L		85 MIU/ML			
	SGOT IU/L		51 IU/L			
A618A	15Y M	OOBXXXXXX, BARNEY JR.		ORT	MEDICAL RECOR	476931
	BUN MG/DL		36 MG/DL			
	SGPT IU/L		140 IU/L			
	CPK MIU/ML		86 MIU/ML			
H359C	03D M	OO BOY		NEWBORN	MEDICAL RECOR	621893
	BUN MG/DL		92 MG/DL			
	CREA MG/DL		9.3 MG/DL			
H655A	69Y F	OOFXXXXXX, JULIA, M		ORT	MEDICAL RECOR	402861
	BUN MG/DL		8 MG/DL			
	URIC AC MG/DL		1.6 MG/DL			
H658B	52Y M	OOBXXXXXX, HOWARD C		ILL	MEDICAL RECOR	692714
	NA MEQ/L		128 MEQ/L			

FIG. 60   Abnormal test reports can be produced by the system and show those tests which are outside the age and sex corrected limits stored on the files. An additional package allows the system to check for a certain percentage change in the patient's results since last testing.

the listing of all abnormal tests created in the system since the last daily chart reports were printed. Figure 60 shows this particular document. Along with any abnormal tests which are outside normal limits, it is possible to set in delta check limits to allow for changes between results on a daily basis. This delta checking mechanism, however, has become very difficult for us to use since we have so many patients with abnormal results. In our hospital, too many patients are receiving variable changing therapy, making the calculation difficult to interpret.

SHANDS TEACHING*HOSPITAL/CLINICS   LABORATORY CHART REPORT

WARD: 7TH PEDS   DAILY   CHART REPORT   PAGE 2

NAME: RXXXXX, NICOLE M   MEDICAL RECORD #305813

ROOM: H777B   01Y F 00   DR: GXXXXXXXX, A D   20:02 11/17/76

PROBLEM: REYES SYND

TEST		LIMITS	11/14 00:15	11/14 16:45	11/14 19:00	11/15 13:45	11/16 15:30
CHEMISTRY							
CALCIUM MG/DL		8.5-10.5	8.3*	8.7*			
PO4	MG/DL	2.5-4.5	2.2*	1.2*			
T PROT	GM/DL	6-8		5.5*			
ALBUMIN GM/DL		3-5.5		4.0			
ALK PHOS	IU/L	30-115	117*				
SGOT	IU/L	7-40	170*	183*			
SGPT	IU/L	6-53	106*	102*			
PED LYTE, BUN CRE							
NA	MEQ/L	135-145	135	137 CONFIR	139	147	
K	MEQ/L	3.1-5.3	2.6*	2.4* CONFIR	3.8 MDHEM	5.2	
CL	MEQ/L	98-109	100	95*	95*	107	
CO2	MEQ/L	24-30	17*	28	33*	22*	
BUN	MG/DL	8-18	14	6*	2*	5*	
CREATININE MG/DL		0.6-1.2	1.1	0.6	0.5*	0.3*	
PEDGLUC	MG/DL	65-110	220*				
L-LDH	PERCENT	0-10	11/14 00:15 QNS REORDER LDH ISOENZYMES. 11/14 19:00 QNS				
AMYLASE IU/L		60-180	229* 11/14 16:45 QNS 11/14 19:00 QNS				
L AMIN PEP IU/L		8-22	15				
ASLICY	MG/DL		41.9	14.5	1.1		
AMMONIA	MCG/DL	18-48	51*				
FIBRIND	MG/DL	200-500	339				
CPK	MUI/ML	2-75	1425*				

FIG. 61   The daily chart report for chemistry shows the vertical array of time and date with the appropriate messages appended to the actual test value. Comments are inserted by time and date on a horizontal format—QNS (quantity not sufficient) along with specific instructions for the physicians to review and act upon. Asterisks indicate abnormal values with age and sex corrections internal to the system.

CHART REPORTS

Chart reports are reviewed in Chemistry each day to determine the actual output of information, to look for duplicate entries, and to uncover problems with terminals and technologists. It is easy to identify an employee who does not understand the system by looking at the chart

```
SHANDS TEACHING*HOSPITAL/CLINICS                        LABORATORY CHART REPORT

WARD: 3-AWING                    DAILY        CHART REPORT          PAGE 2
NAME: WXXXXX, ALVA J                               MEDICAL RECORD #308555
ROOM: A324A    37Y M 00   DR: WXXXXX, E R               17:35  07/15/76
PROBLEM: MORBID OBESITY


TEST             LIMITS        07/12    07/13   07/14   07/15
                               12:15    10:00   21:15   09:15

CHEMISTRY
  NA   MEQ/L     135-145        141
  K    MEQ/L     3.5-5          4.1
  CL   MEQ/L     95-105         101
  CO2  MEQ/L     24-32          30
  BUN  MG/DL     10-20          18
  CREATININE MG/DL  0.7-1.4     1.1
  URIC AC MG/DL  2.5-8          7.9
  CALCIUM MG/DL  2.5-10.5                9.8
  PO4  MG/DL     2.5-4.5                 2.8
  GLUCOSE MG/DL  65-110         105
  T PROT  GM/DL  6-8                     7.4
  ALBUMIN GM/DL  3-5.5                   4.9
  T BIL  MG/DL   0.1-1                   0.8
  D BIL  MG/DL   0-0.3                   0.2
  ALK PHOS  IU/L 30-115                  85
  SGOT   IU/L    7-40           20
  SGPT   IU/L    6-53                    26
  MG     MG/DL   1.8-2.8                 2.0
  5-HOUR-GTT
    FBS  MG/DL   65-110                          100
    30MIN MG/DL                                  163
    1 HR  MG/DL                                  127
    2 HR  MG/DL                                  138
    3 HR  MG/DL                                  112
    4 HR  MG/DL                                  86
    5 HR  MG/DL                                  95
  RAPID IV GTT
    PREINJ MG/DL 65-110                                          95
    10 MIN MG/DL                                                190
    20 MIN MG/DL                                                170
    30 MIN MG/DL                                                154
    40 MIN MG/DL                                                141
    50 MIN MG/DL                                                129
    60 MIN MG/DL                                                119
  LIPO-ELETROPHOR
    CHOL  MG/DL                          158
    TRIG  MG/DL                          308
  PROTEIN-ELECTRO
    T PROT  GM/DL  6-8                    7.4
```

FIG. 62 Special formats can be arranged for group tests, such as the 5-h glucose tolerance test, in which the format allows indentation of the subset for ease of reading.

```
SHANDS TEACHING*HOSPITAL/CLINICS                    LABORATORY CHART REPORT


WARD:  OB/GYN                  DAILY        CHART REPORT              PAGE 2

NAME:  DXXXXX, ANN M                        MEDICAL RECORD #278982

ROOM:  H347A    29Y F 00    DR: CXXXXX, B                  16:19  07/10/76

PROBLEM:  IUP


TEST                LIMITS      07/08  07/09  07/09  07/09  07/09  07/09
                                20:45  07:15  13:45  16:15  17:00  18:15

CHEMISTRY
NA    MEQ/L         135-145                                 134*
K     MEQ/L         3.5-5                                   4.2
CL    MEQ/L         95-105                                  107*
CO2   MEQ/L         24-32                                   23*
GLUCOSE  MG/DL      65-110        67    292*   459*         314*   261*
ACETONE  MG/DL      0-1          NEG                  40*    10*   NEG


TEST                LIMITS      07/09  07/09  07/09  07/10  07/10  07/10
                                19:00  21:30  22:30  04:00  07:00  10:30

CHEMISTRY
NA    MEQ/L         135-145             135
K     MEQ/L         3.5-5               4.4
CL    MEQ/L         95-105              107*
CO2   MEQ/L         24-32               23*
GLUCOSE  MG/DL      65-110       287*   143*   148*   39*    96
                                                     CONFIR
2HR-PC   MG/DL      70-120                                          222*
ACETONE  MG/DL      0-1          NEG    NEG    NEG


TEST                LIMITS      07/10


CHEMISTRY
2-HR-PC  MG/DL      70-120       249*


END OF REPORT
```

FIG. 63 To minimize paper loss, it is possible to double-format a single page if the number of tests ordered does not exceed the vertical limit for one individual.

reports, since any data that is improperly entered will stand out quite clearly. Figures 61–63 show some of the characteristic chemistry reports generated by the system.

STAFFING AND ORGANIZATION

To accommodate our change in technology, we now group our technologists in teams of two. It seems that each one of our major functions in the lab requires two people to operate properly: SMAC, specimen check-in desk, and stats. The pairs work together on a preset schedule, and this has allowed us to stretch the staff pool and provide coverage on Saturday and Sunday.

QUALITY CONTROL

There is nothing specific in the laboratory information system which supports quality control. We found that this was such a difficult and individualized task that it would be most appropriately implemented through a separate comprehensive program. Quality control is instrument-specific and laboratory-specific, and requires many different processes to define adequately. Currently, we are creating an on-line SMAC control sera-result pool to be kept by the system. This is extracted from the daily charts and used for statistical analysis of the instrument. Many special programs have been written for a batch computer so that our on-line system can optimize its time.

REFERRAL LABS

Specimens sent to referral laboratories are a constant problem for chemistry and, of course, require special handling, shipping, and follow-through to guarantee reasonably prompt results. It is certainly uneconomical for us to consider performing these special procedures even though the laboratory expends a great deal of money and effort in the initial acquisition and transportation of the specimen. Even cost-conscious physicians who routinely compare the basic prices of tests sent to outside labs generally overlook these hidden costs. Our processing instructions, which are sent by the system to the floor or the physician, have greatly improved our current performance in this area.

MARK-SENSE CARDS

Each terminal within Chemistry is backed up by mark-sense cards which can be used to input all the data in case a terminal goes down for any length of time. This reserve mechanism is always available to the lab, and is exercised on a training basis for potential emergencies. A full description of the backup system will be given in a later chapter. Figure 64 shows the mark-sense cards used by Chemistry.

CRITIQUE

The chemistry operation initially suffered two types of difficulty, both of which have since been totally eliminated. First, the SMAC program

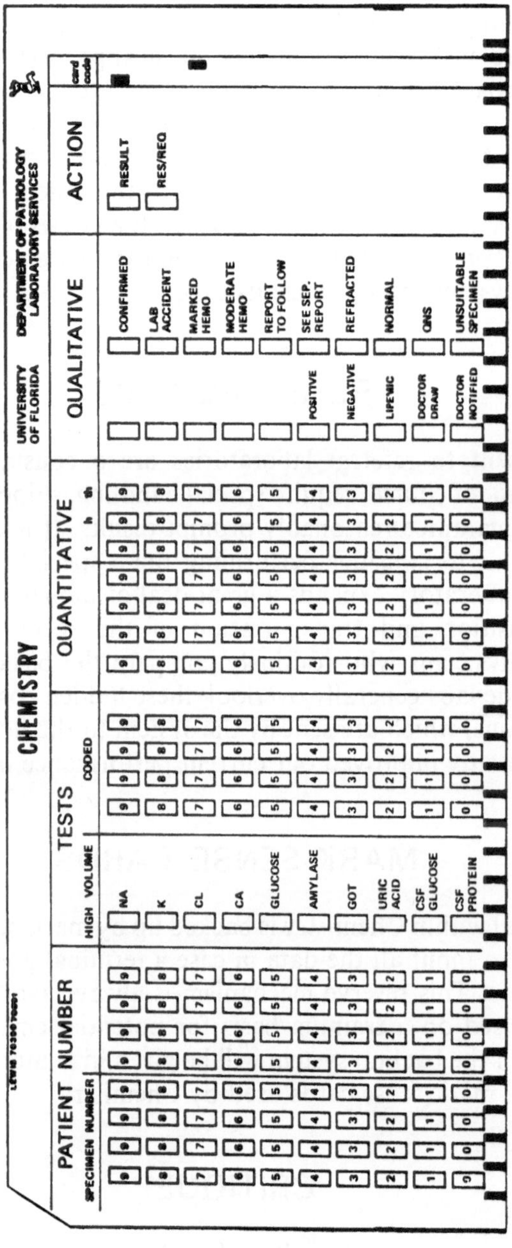

FIG. 64. The chemistry mark-sense order form allows high volume tests to be entered with a single pencil stroke, along with qualitative messages for result reporting.

we used was unsatisfactory for day-to-day operation. Secondly, our specimen numbering system for stat and expedites caused great difficulty because of the excess numbers per tube. With the two programs now appropriately corrected, the rapid flow of material and reports is routine.

14

Hematology

INTRODUCTION

Hematology offers a special challenge for information systems since there is a diversity of procedures and equipment which require direct human interface using visual interpretation before data input. In our hematology laboratory we use the Coulter S, Coagulizer, Honeywell ACS 1000, and associated microscopes for cell counts.

FORMS

The primary form for Hematology shown in Fig. 35 represents a convenient mode of communication with the physician. The structure of the form gives an idea of what is within a major test battery such as a Coulter S, and allows the physician to order subtests when that is all that is required. In most cases, the price rewards judicious ordering.

SPECIMEN PREPARATION

Special precautions must be exercised in specimen preparation for coagulation studies to be sure they are properly anticoagulated before acceptance at the laboratory. This has created some problems, and requires constant vigilance to minimize the amount of personnel time involved when errors occur. During a normal day, routine and expedite specimens are brought directly to the hematology area with the appropriate labels and work sheets. These are processed on an immediate basis. Very little hematology work is batched and much of it is done as it arrives. Only such things as alkaline phosphatase and hemoglobin electrophoresis are held over for the following day for batch processing.

SPECIAL ORDERS

Certain tests require that a message be sent to the laboratory for proper patient/procedure coordination. This is accomplished through the test file by setting up a code in which a particular procedure is given a logical terminal number on which a copy of the order is to be printed. As an example, a bleeding time requested on the floor will be immediately sent to the hematology lab area as soon as the order is complete. This notifies the responsible lab about the work to be done. At the same time, the message generated on the floor terminal tells the clerks to call the lab and schedule this procedure. With this double notification mechanism we are assured that the order is processed properly. This special laboratory print-out can be executed for any of the orders if the files are properly coded (Fig. 65).

```
REQUEST            311732          RXXXXX, JOHN          H449A    08/31/76
        2380   BLEED TIME
```

FIG. 65   Certain orders are sent on-line to the appropriate laboratory so that coordination can be achieved and a rapid response anticipated.

WORK SHEETS

Work sheets are not a major problem for hematology since much of its work is stat oriented and is processed continually. We do provide work sheets in the morning after blood drawing, as seen in Figs. 66 and 67.

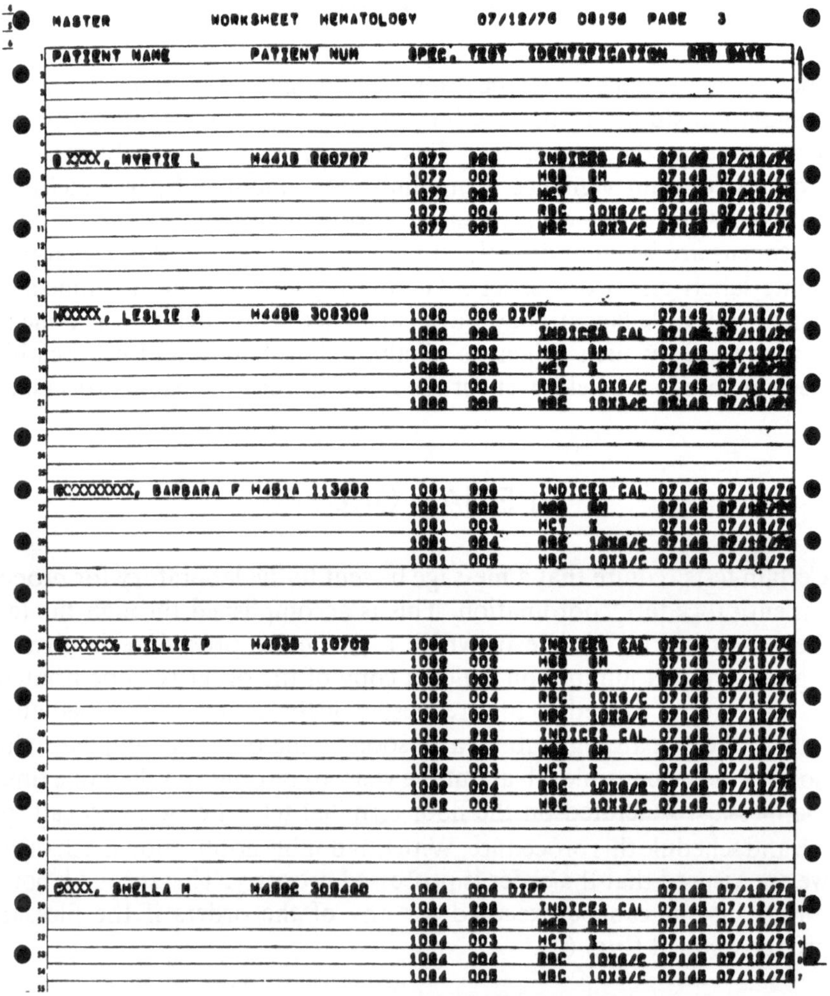

MASTER WORKSHEET HEMATOLOGY 07/12/76 08156 PAGE 3

PATIENT NAME	PATIENT NUM	SPEC.	TEST	IDENTIFICATION		REQ	DATE
XXXX, MYRTIE L	H441B 880707	1077	001	INDICES CAL		07148	07/12/76
		1077	002	HGB	GM	07148	07/12/76
		1077	003	HCT	%	07148	07/12/76
		1077	004	RBC	10X6/C	07148	07/12/76
		1077	005	WBC	10X3/C	07148	07/12/76
XXXXX, LESLIE B	H448B 308308	1080	006 DIFF			07148	07/12/76
		1080	001	INDICES CAL		07148	07/12/76
		1080	002	HGB	GM	07148	07/12/76
		1080	003	HCT	%	07148	07/12/76
		1080	004	RBC	10X6/C	07148	07/12/76
		1080	005	WBC	10X3/C	07148	07/12/76
XXXXXXXXX, BARBARA F	H451A 113602	1081	001	INDICES CAL		07148	07/12/76
		1081	002	HGB	GM	07148	07/12/76
		1081	003	HCT	%	07148	07/12/76
		1081	004	RBC	10X6/C	07148	07/12/76
		1081	005	WBC	10X3/C	07148	07/12/76
XXXXXX, LILLIE P	H453B 110762	1082	001	INDICES CAL		07148	07/12/76
		1082	002	HGB	GM	07148	07/12/76
		1082	003	HCT	%	07148	07/12/76
		1082	004	RBC	10X6/C	07148	07/12/76
		1082	005	WBC	10X3/C	07148	07/12/76
		1082	001	INDICES CAL		07148	07/12/76
		1082	002	HGB	GM	07148	07/12/76
		1082	003	HCT	%	07148	07/12/76
		1082	004	RBC	10X6/C	07148	07/12/76
		1082	005	WBC	10X3/C	07148	07/12/76
XXXX, SHELLA M	H488C 308480	1084	006 DIFF			07148	07/12/76
		1084	001	INDICES CAL		07148	07/12/76
		1084	002	HGB	GM	07148	07/12/76
		1084	003	HCT	%	07148	07/12/76
		1084	004	RBC	10X6/C	07148	07/12/76
		1084	005	WBC	10X3/C	07148	07/12/76

FIG. 66 Master worksheets display the totality of tests ordered for each individual patient by subsections of the laboratory.

INPUT TERMINALS

The Coulter S produces a high volume of information in a short period of time and certainly justifies on-line connection. A special control terminal plus a logging printer keeps track of the Coulter information and guarantees that it is properly placed in the files of the appropriate patient.

A special subsystem was designed for input of differential blood counts. This involves the use of a microprocessor connected to special

HEMATOLOGY

	06/03/77		RETIC CT	12	09:01	

PATIENT NAME	SPEC	RESULT	TECH
RXXXX, RICHARD	3068	-----	----
CXXX, SHELLA M	3080	-----	----
HXXXX, MAC S	3082	-----	----
BXXXXXX, ANNIE	2087	-----	----
BXXXXXX, VERA M	2089	-----	----

FIG. 67 A standard hematology worksheet allows the singular entry of one test result for a series of patients.

key pads by individual technologists at their microscopes. It provides an input of the morphologic characteristics of cells, and automatically keeps a tally of total cells, sounding off when 100 have been counted. A special numerical code closes out the result file, and the appropriate information is then sent to the main computer for file insertion (Fig. 68).

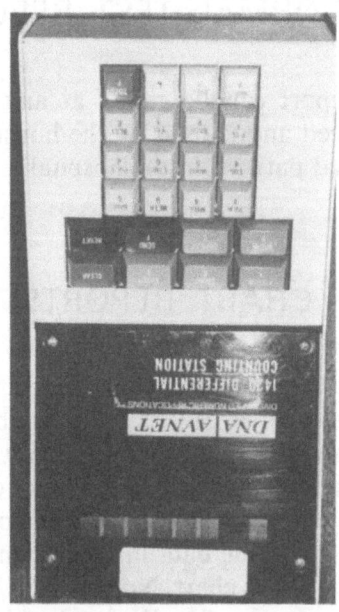

FIG. 68 A special diff pad is provided by the system to allow entry of differential counts on either peripheral smears or bone marrows. Appropriate comments are allowed for chart insertion.

The Honeywell differential cell counter (ACS 1000) provides a similar function yet requires an interface to accept the information provided by its terminal. The morphologic codes sent from that unit are not as extensive as those contained in our current library on the diff-pads, and this provides some difficulty in coordinating the two systems. We currently use a diff-pad located next to the Honeywell unit to input the data required and have not yet interfaced this instrument.

UNFINISHED TEST REPORT

An unfinished test report is the primary bookkeeping document for hematology and is evaluated twice a day to make sure that all reports have been completed and all patient work has been accomplished. It is an essential document and one of the substantive advantages of a laboratory system.

ABNORMAL TEST REPORT

An abnormal test report can be called at any time. The format is patient-room sequenced and is used by the house staff and laboratory for detecting abnormal patients in the hospital.

CHART REPORTS

Figures 69–71 show the standard chart reports generated from the programs for Hematology. Because of the flexibility of the software, double entries are possible. This occurs when a set of morphologic codes are expected for a differential and the files are not closed. The unfinished test report will show that this test has not been completed, and another individual may place the same data in the system. This then puts two sets of results on the patient's chart. No harm has been done, but it does result in redundant work (Fig. 72). We are looking into ways to eliminate this possibility through procedural changes in the use of the unfinished test report, and the possibility of software protection.

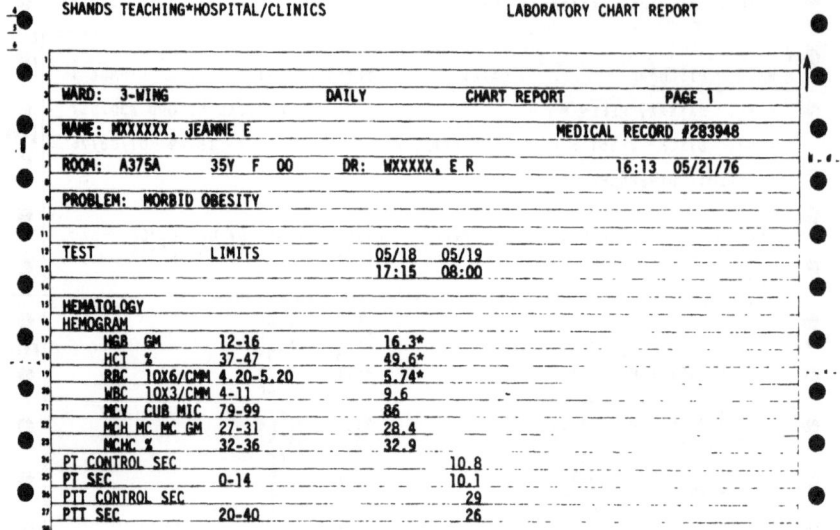

FIG. 69 The daily chart report for hematology uses the same vertical array and indentation formatting for convenient user review.

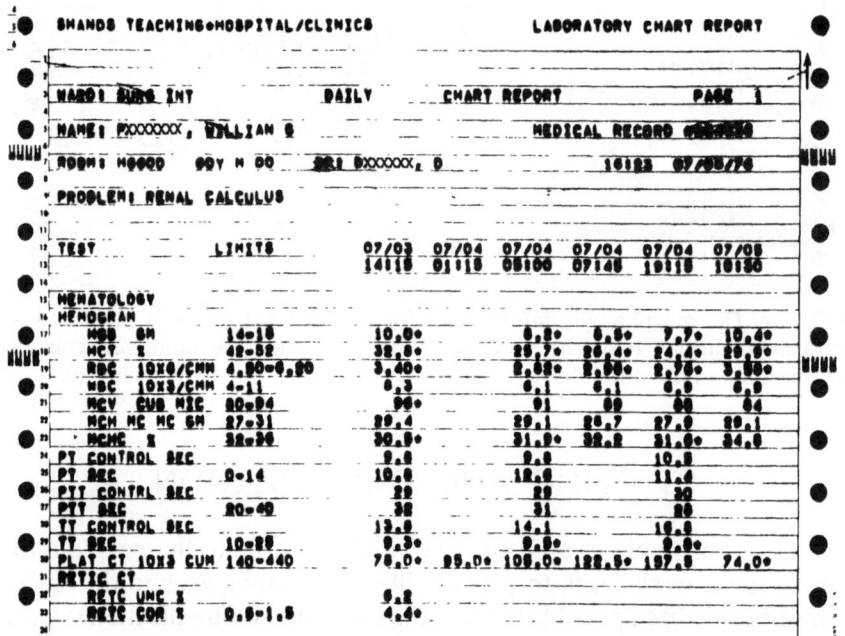

FIG. 70 For more complicated cases in which sequential data is essential, the system allows indentation of the chart report for physician review.

SHANDS TEACHING*HOSPITAL/CLINICS   LABORATORY CHART REPORT

WARD: DISCHARG   DAILY   CHART REPORT   PAGE 1
NAME: SXXXXX, HELEN M   MEDICAL RECORD #307937
ROOM: DISCH   55Y F 00   DR: GXXXXX, M   18:49 07/08/76
PROBLEM: HYPERNEPHROMA

TEST	LIMITS	07/05 00:00	07/05 12:15	07/06 07:45	07/06 12:45	07/06 20:15
HEMATOLOGY						
HEMOGRAM						
HGB GM	12-16		9.5*	7.6*		
HCT %	37-47		28.6*	22.9*		
RBC 10X6/CMN	4.20-5.20		3.03*	2.33*		
WBC 10X3/CMN	4-11		45.1*	56.3*		
				CR WBC		
MCV CUB MIC	79-99		94	98		
MCH MC MC GM	27-31		31.4*	32.6*		
MCHC X	32-36		33.2	33.2		
DIFF-POLY	50-75		84	82		
BANDS %	0-7		7	8		
LYMPHS %	25-45		1	4		
MONOS %	0-10		1	4		
EOS %	0-6		1			
META %			4	1		
MYEL %			2	1		
NRBC %				11		
MORPHOLOGY		07/05	12:15	PLAT DEC		
		07/05	12:15	RBC NORM		
		07/05	12:15	ATYPICAL LYMPHS		
		07/06	07:45	MOD ANISO		
		07/06	07:45	MOD POIK		
		07/06	07:45	SPHEROCYTES		
		07/06	07:45	MOD POLY		
		07/06	07:45	MOD MACRO		
		07/06	07:45	SCHISTOCYTES		
PT CONTROL SEC			9.5	10.5		
PT SEC	0-14		16.5*	90.0*		
PTT CONTROL SEC			29	30	29	
PTT SEC	20-40		90*	90*	90*	
TT CONTROL SEC				13.3	13.3	
TT SEC	10-25		20.3	23.3		
PLAT CT 10X3 CUM	140-440		24.5	11.0*		
ESR						
ESRU MM/HH			8			
ESRC MM/HH	0-20		0			
RETIC CT						
RETC UNC %				8.5		
RETC COR %	0.5-1.5			4.7*		

FIG. 71 The morphologic information for a peripheral smear is presented in horizontal display based on date and time. This could be more conveniently arranged in a horizontal display with paragraph formatting by date and time.

STAFFING AND ORGANIZATION

We have been able to split our staff and redistribute the people on a seven-day a week basis to provide liberal coverage around-the-clock. This has only been possible because the use of the communication system has eliminated most phone calls and a massive share of the data entry problems.

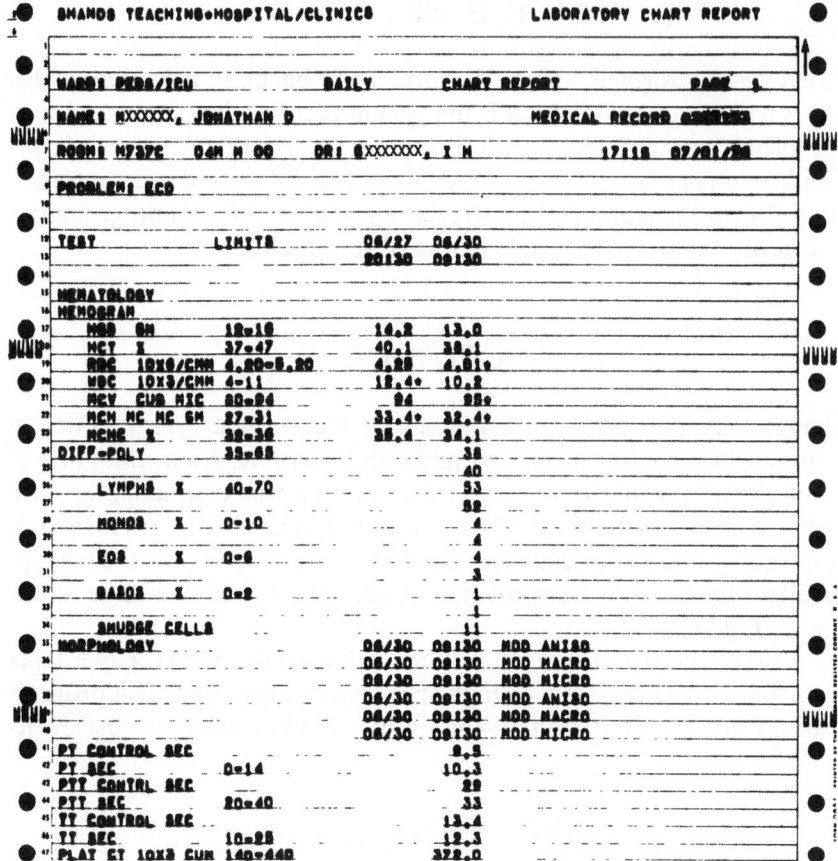

FIG. 72 It is possible to fool the system because of the flexibility of the peripheral input stations and to obtain two results for the same patient. This must be watched very carefully by the technologist since the option of closing out an individual test for complicated items such as peripheral smears is at the discretion of the technologist. Charts are reviewed daily by the laboratory director and the chief technologist, and corrected at the earliest possible time.

QUALITY CONTROL

The laboratory communication system does not support any specific quality control program for Hematology. We use alternative computers, other programs, or special log books. Quality control has been too volatile an area to make specific plans for centralization. Our system strives for response time and communication speed, and relies on a number of support procedures for accuracy and precision.

MARK-SENSE CARDS

Every test performed within Hematology is backed up by mark-sense cards which can be filled out if the system becomes inoperative. One of the problems with these cards in our system is that seven cards per Coulter run per patient are required to include all the necessary information. This will eventually be corrected through additional programming and proper design of a single new card for Coulter entry.

CRITIQUE

Hematology has performed well using the on-line system, but has required two major changes to make this possible. First, the noise of printers and logging terminals in the lab area was distracting to technologists attempting to study a peripheral smear. This problem was resolved by using a special ventilated, soundproof box over the teletype printer. Our box was not provided by the vendor and had to be home-made (Fig. 73).

A second area of concern was created when the SMAC paper tapes were first fed to the system by high-speed paper-tape input. This program used so much CPU time that the on-line Coulter data was lost or de-

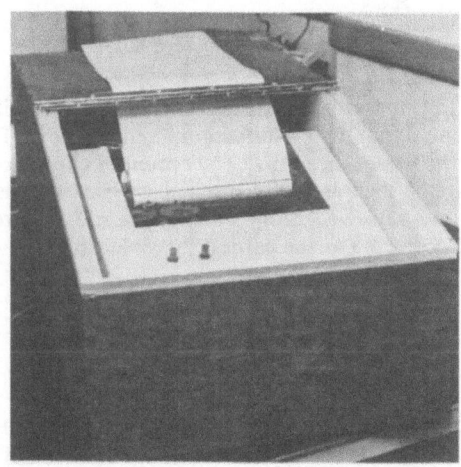

FIG. 73   The logging printers located in the laboratory were constant sources of irritation. The only solution to this problem was the installation of a plexiglass-wood box to decrease the noise level.

stroyed during parallel operation. Hand entry of the Coulter results is tedious, and if persistent, creates a serious morale problem. For seven to eight months we suffered from the Coulter/SMAC malady. This led to psychological warfare between Chemistry and Hematology—Hematology believing that the Chemistry equipment was out to destroy them. After a long period of agony, the program was finally modified so that each could operate independently. This loading problem usually becomes more serious as on-line devices are added and through-puts are increased.

15

Microbiology

INTRODUCTION

Microbiology stands as the ultimate challenge for a laboratory system since it incorporates a vast array of names, dates, places, organisms, and cultures. This primary reference material is far in excess of that of any other laboratory data base. It also represents an area in which flexibility is crucial, since many of the specimens require special handling and individualized testing procedures. Initially, we looked at the log of sources available for cultures and came to the conclusion that it was infinite. We were faced with designing a system which incorporated the advantages of nursing station ordering along with the flexibility of free-format English.

REQUEST AND SOURCE FILE

A request for a microbiology order automatically requires that the individual doctor, nurse, or clinic obtain a specimen for the laboratory. Each order is assigned a unique specimen number at the time of entry at

```
LAB ORDER , USER ID:  2, 13:45   09/11/76   ,    STATION 12


MR#  295130  OK?  Y
NAME:  MXXXXX, PAULA   WF02   22    , 13:45     09/11/76    OK?  Y
DR#  250 260 231 241
PROBLEM:  LOW FEVER  OK?  Y
T#  649  MISC ROUTINE CUL   OK?  Y STAT:  N  EXP#  Y
 EXPEDITE TRANSPORT--ONLY FOR UNLISTED SOURCE-LABEL SOURCE+TYPE MSG
MSG:  LEFT EAR
ENTRY OK?  Y                              2250         DONE
T#
**READY
```

FIG. 74   The laboratory order for microbiology begins with the medical record number entry and verification of name and problem. Following this, the test number is entered and the message is requested from the user specifying the source of culture. Upon the completion of that message, a specimen number is assigned along with a "Done" statement for nursing verification. At the okay of that order, a copy of the exact order is teleprocessed to the microbiology logging terminal so that the laboratory is able to monitor cultures and sources at the time of entry.

the terminal. There are only five or six items in Microbiology that are allowed on an expedite or stat basis. The major share of the requests are set up for routine specimen numbers. Figures 20 and 36 show request forms used for microbiology which ask for both a specific type of culture and an anatomical source of culture. For orders which are general in nature, such as a routine culture, the system files seek a source message input by the clerk ordering the culture. Figure 74 demonstrates this dialog. The message allows input of 32 (alphanumeric) characters, which is then followed by the assignment of the appropriate specimen number and a "done" statement. The test files are coded immediately to transmit this entire order, including message, to a logging printer located in Microbiology. As soon as the order is completed, the printer displays this data and allows complete prospective communication regarding every culture and specimen.

SPECIMEN PREPARATION

With each one of the orders that are entered, special instructions have been put in the computer files to direct the floor personnel to the proper type of media, timing, and sequencing to allow for optimal culture results. This has greatly improved the quality of specimens arriving in

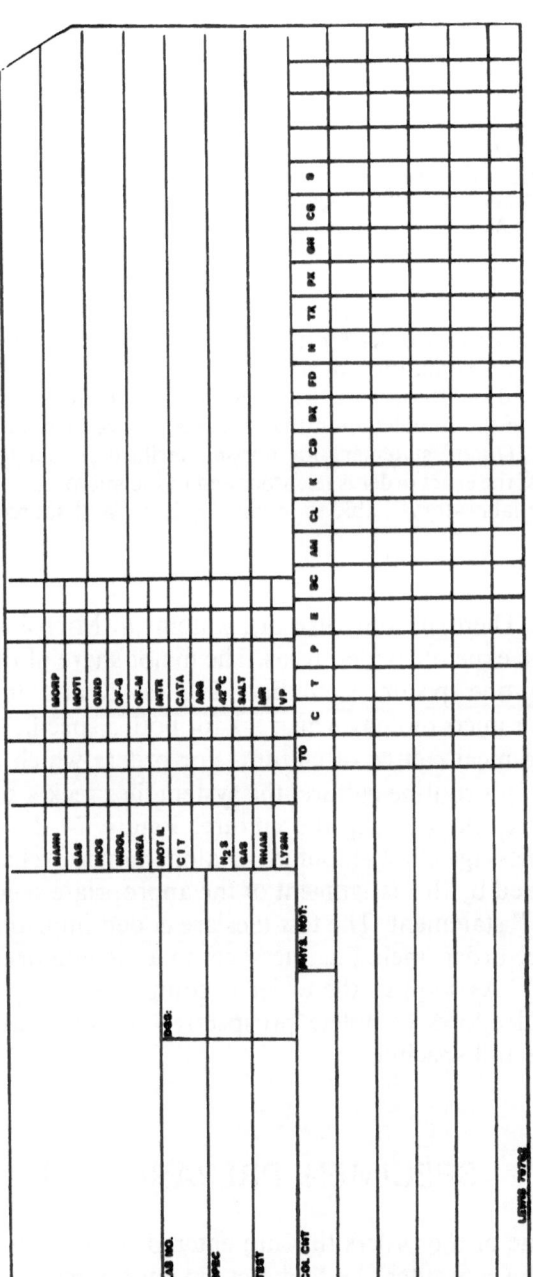

FIG. 75   The microbiology reporting card allows the application of a computer-printed label in the left upper corner. The coding of specific culture and sensitivity information along with biochemical data by the technologist is accomplished while they work with each of the culture plates and media.

the lab, and is a constant source of educational reinforcement since people rarely appreciate the necessity of proper specimen handling for consistent microbiological results.

Once the specimen has been acquired and properly labeled, the sample is transported to the laboratory. The number is checked in at the front window and given computer labels which are carried back with the specimen to the microbiology area. One label is assigned to a work card (Fig. 75), and the other is assigned to the culture plate. Our culture work card requires no transcription and is used for complete evaluation of all organisms. The work card includes categories for sensitivity data and the biochemicals necessary for identification. In addition to making up a work card, individual specimens are manually logged into a source log book. This allows easy reference to culture site-related inquiries.

For special requests, the individual technologist can go to the microbiology logging printer and determine the appropriate information which has been sent by the floor terminal. This minimizes the need for the phone calls and dialog between clerk and lab that previously led to inconsistent results.

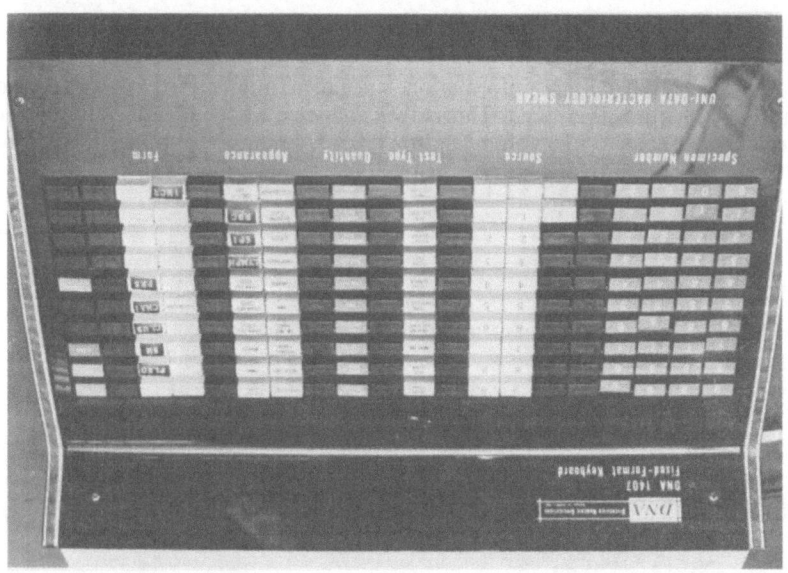

FIG. 76   The fixed-format keyboard for microbiology allows the entry of smear information by the depression of specimen number, source, code of culture, type of test, quantity visualized on the smear, and the form of the organism seen. This is entered and then verified by CRT.

INPUT TERMINALS

A special terminal (fixed-format type) is used for entering information related to smears (Fig. 76). A second fixed-format terminal is used for data on cultures and sensitivities (Fig. 77). A third alphanumeric key-

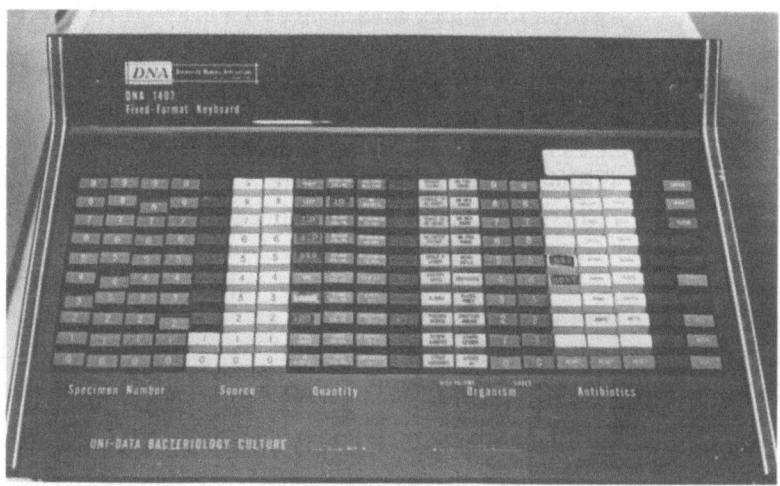

FIG. 77   For the culture information, specimen number, source code, and quantity of organism is entered. This is then followed by the identification of the organism, by either the high volume button or coded number, and then the appropriate selection of antibiotics for sensitivity or resistance reporting.

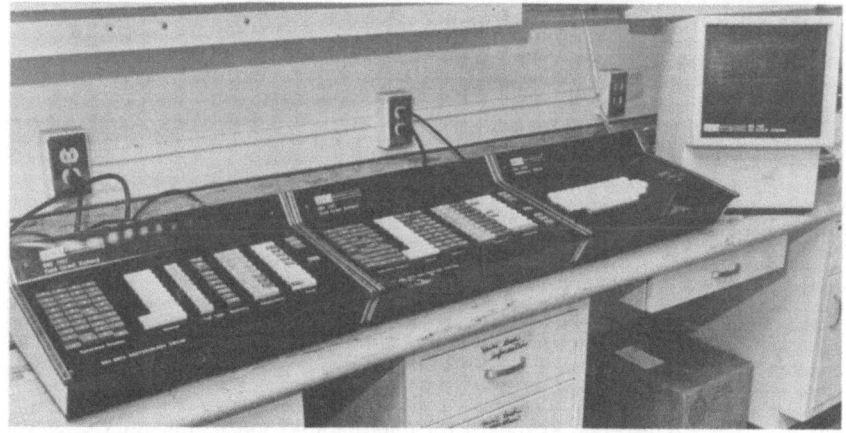

FIG. 78   For those cases in which the fixed-format keyboard is insufficient, a free-text alphanumeric keyboard is used and verified by CRT.

board allows free text entry (Fig. 78). The entry of culture information is considered part of the technologist's responsibility, since the data must be carefully reviewed and scrutinized before it is released to the physician on the floor. Using these standard terminals, we are able to handle the entire gambit of microbiology and meet the great diversity of requests received for this area.

UNFINISHED TEST REPORT

Microbiology receives the longest unfinished test report in the entire laboratory. Incomplete culture data accounts for most pending work and the greatest backlog of information in terms of retrieval and recovery. We have set up a screening process which scans one week's work to determine whether we have been negligent with certain cultures or selected procedures. This has worked well in eliminating the problems of lost specimens and missing results. Such things as fungus and AFB cultures are handled in a separate mode and reported out to the physician as: "report to follow if the culture is positive." This is necessary to avoid having an excessive number of patients with open data files awaiting results. Our files currently are not large enough to handle this backlog of information. Positive cultures found in a year's time do not justify an unlimited file capacity. The positives that are detected are referred to infectious disease for follow-up and require extensive medical input outside the communication system. A manual report is sent to medical records for all positive fungus or AFB cultures for patient report continuity.

CHART REPORTS

Microbiology chart reports are unique (Figs. 79–81). They were designed to maximize the information content and display the material in a readable fashion. The primary smear or organism data is in paragraph format. Information appears in short statements without excessive verbiage. For a culture, the source and quantities of the organism form a matrix in which the organisms are arranged across the top of the page and the antibiotics are printed down the left column of the page. "S" or "R" are used to delineate sensitivity or resistance. For smears, the quantity and descriptive material are presented in paragraph format

```
SHANDS TEACHING*HOSPITAL/CLINICS                    LABORATORY CHART REPORT


WARD:  OB/GYN                    DAILY    CHART REPORT              PAGE 1

NAME:  KXXX, GLENDA JEAN                         MEDICAL RECORD #204967

ROOM: H386C    48Y  F  00    DR:  BXXXXX, D S              16:15  07/13/76

PROBLEM:  CA/CERVIX

MICROBIOLOGY

URINE CULTURE     URINE-CLEAN CAT
07/11/76  22:45   ENTEROBACTER  CLO  100,000 COL/ML
                  TEST COMPLETE


                  ENTEROBACTER

TOBRAMYCIN        S
CEPHALOTHIN       R
TMP/SXT           S
GENTA             S
AMPICILLIN        R
KANAMYCIN         S
CARBENICILLIN     R
NITROFURADANTIN   R
TETRACYCLINE      R


END OF REPORT
```

FIG. 79 A daily chart for microbiology identifies the type of culture ordered, the date and time, along with the organism and quantity. A matrix of antibiotics is used for sensitivity testing along with a column header for the organism being tested. The S and R stands for sensitive or resistant.

```
SHANDS TEACHING*HOSPITAL/CLINICS                    LABORATORY CHART REPORT


WARD: MEDICAL                    DAILY    CHART REPORT              PAGE 2

NAME: RXXXXXXXXX, THOMAS O                       MEDICAL RECORD #304100

ROOM: H464A    62Y  M  00    DR: BXXXXX, E R               17:40  07/08/76

PROBLEM: R/O OBE

MICROBIOLOGY

BLOOD CULTURE     BLOOD CULTURE
06/30/76  09:15   NO GROWTH
                  TEST COMPLETE

BLOOD CULTURE     BLOOD CULTURE
06/30/76  21:15   NO GROWTH
                  TEST COMPLETE

ANTIBIOTIC SENS
06/11             GENTAMICIN: MIC=0.15 UG/ML
                  GENTAMICIN: MBC=0.30 UG/ML
                  PENICILLIN: MIC=0.3 U/ML
                  PENICILLIN: MBC=0.3 U/ML

END OF REPORT
```

FIG. 80 For certain microbiology orders, free-text entry is necessary to delimit the minimum inhibitory concentration for gentamicin and penicillin.

```
SHANDS TEACHING-HOSPITAL/CLINICS            LABORATORY CHART REPORT

    WARD: SURGICAL              DAILY       CHART REPORT           PAGE  3
    NAME: Xxxxxxxxx, CATHERINA A                MEDICAL RECORD #306658
    ROOM: H641C    82Y F 00    DR: Rxxxxxxxx, R          16114  07/18/76
    PROBLEM: NONE GIVEN

    MICROBIOLOGY

    BLOOD CULTURE       BLOOD CULTURE
    07/07/76 16119      NO GROWTH
                        TEST COMPLETE

    BLOOD CULTURE       BLOOD CULTURE
    07/07/76 16130      NO GROWTH
                        TEST COMPLETE

    MISC ROUTINE CUL WOUND
    07/18/76 09145      PSEUDO AERUGIN LIGHT (1+)
                        ENTEROCOCCI FEW (+/-)
                        BACTEROIDES FRAG MODERATE (2+)
                        PROTEUS MIRABILI IN SUBCULTURE
                        TEST COMPLETE


                        PSEUDO AERUGI ENTEROCOCCI   BACTEROIDES F PROTEUS MIRAB

    TOBRAMYCIN              S            R                        S
    DOXYCYCLINE                                      R
    CEPHALOTHIN            R            R            R            S
    GENTA                 S            R                        S
    AMPICILLIN            R            S            R            S
    KANAMYCIN            R            R                        S
    CARBENICILLIN        S            R                        S
    CHLORAMPHENICOL      R            S            S            S
    ERYTH                                           S
    PENICILLIN                                      R
    TETRACYCLINE        R            R            R            R

    END OF REPORT
```

FIG. 81 For more complex cultures, the system allows a matrix entry of organisms in which these organisms can be displayed along with the appropriate antibiotic-sensitivity testing result. This allows the physician quickly to scan the page and select the antibiotic with uniform sensitivity.

sufficient to communicate with the physician. Special statements regarding the organism or culture can be entered using the comment function available on the free-format microbiology terminal.

STAFFING

Microbiology, by its nature, must be staffed seven days a week since the organisms will not stop growing. This lab has shown the least effect since the installation of the system, inasmuch as their clerical effort was high before and now continues to be high because of the direct use of technologists for data interpretation. The flexibility and complexity

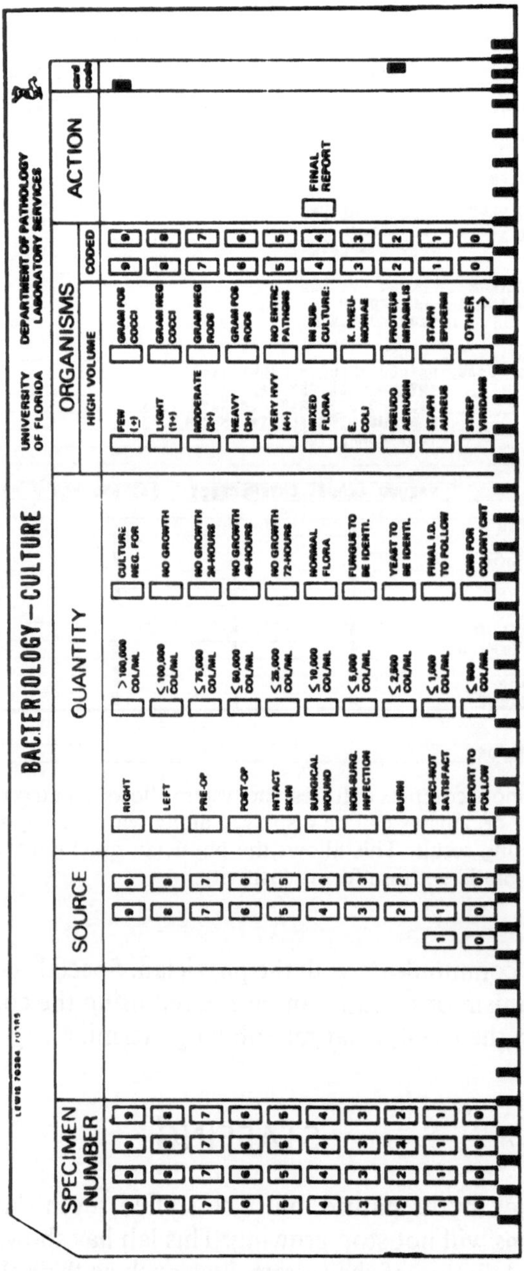

FIG. 82   As back-up, bacteriology has a mark-sense card which allows entry of the specimen number, source, quantity, and organism.

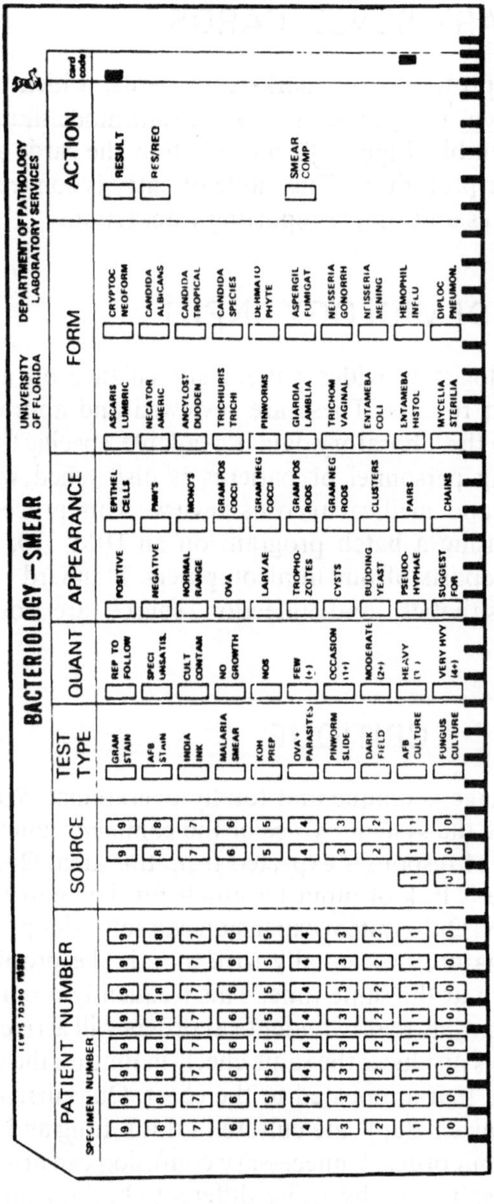

FIG. 83 The bacteriology smear card is a duplicate of the fixed-format keyboard, and allows the technologist to enter their results through mark-sense forms in case of terminal failure.

of microbiological work demands qualified data-handling personnel, and this cannot be delegated to inexperienced clerical staff.

MARK-SENSE CARDS

Microbiology is fully protected by mark-sense cards, which allows entry of organism and sensitivity patterns in an off-line mode should the terminals become inoperable. Figures 82 and 83 show the cards associated with this particular procedure. This mode of entry is conveniently used for negative cultures and simple-reporting transactions.

EPIDEMIOLOGY INPUT

The hospital epidemiologist provides patient surveillance on a daily basis through our chart reports. These are reviewed and appropriate action is taken. Since all the laboratory data is available, specific therapy or procedures regarding personnel or patients is dispatched without extensive chart search and medical records review. This process has now been automated using a batch program on an IBM 370, which audits the daily chart reports of our minicomputers. Standard reports about organisms, sensitivities, and infection source are routinely available.

CRITIQUE

Our microbiology package is unique and totally operational. We have been able to manipulate the system by use of the comment function to provide the wide range of responses expected from this area. Our most serious problem to date is lack of input terminals for data entry in the microbiology laboratory. Only system expansion can solve this problem.

Of a less serious nature, yet equally irritating, is the problem of duplicate cultures drawn at the same time. This frequently occurs with blood or sputums, and means that two identical orders will arrive in the lab at the same time. This produces the same check-in time on the system and confuses the results that are posted to the chart. Our current software is unable to recognize a duplicate culture in this setting and places results in a first-in-first-out order. Unnecessary confusion can arise from this situation, and we solve this by using different check-in times for duplicate requests on the same patient. This problem eventually should be resolved by software modifications.

16

___

Immunology

INTRODUCTION

Our Immunology laboratory is very similar to Chemistry on a procedural basis. However, in its daily operation it employs some of the newer techniques that are quite expensive and, therefore, can only be done in batches during the week. This makes the use of work sheets quite helpful since these can be called for each batch and run once or twice a week.

REQUEST FORMS

The immunology request forms shown in Figs. 20 and 36 present a collection of information necessary for the ordering physician. We have had some problems with thyroid function tests since many of the specialized tests are not that familiar to the house staff. We produced a series of educational materials for the physicians to help them understand the differences, and have grouped them together for convenience and continuity on the order form.

SPECIMEN PREPARATION

Very few tests are ordered stat since all immunological tests are time-consuming special projects that are usually run in batches. The major share of our specimen splitting occurs at the check-in area in central chemistry, where the appropriate tubes are placed in a basket for refrigeration. This does pose a procedural problem and is a possible area for confusion.

WORK SHEETS

Immunology receives a set of specialized work sheets which allows it to process information in a convenient fashion. Figures 84 and 85 illustrate examples of these particular items.

			FAST	10MIN	20MIN	30MIN	40MIN	50MIN	60MIN		TECH
06/26/77		INSULIN RIA			301		08:45				
PATIENT NAME	SPEC NO.		FAST 120MN	10MIN 180MN	20MIN 240MN	30MIN 300MN	40MIN 360MN	50MIN	60MIN		TECH
KXXXXXX, MICHAEL	2266		----- -----	----- -----	----- -----	----- -----	----- -----	-----	-----		----
TXXXXXXX, PATRIC	8371		----- -----	----- -----	----- -----	----- -----	----- -----	-----	-----		----
SXXXX, JAMES	4413		----- -----	----- -----	----- -----	----- -----	----- -----	-----	-----		----
GXXXXXXXXXX, ROB	6239		----- -----	----- -----	----- -----	----- -----	----- -----	-----	-----		----

FIG. 84   Special types of worksheets are provided for areas such as immunology, which have many specimens per test such as the insulin tolerance procedure.

INPUT TERMINALS

Immunology has designed its own special purpose input terminal and uses an alphanumeric keyboard for textual input of special information present in many of its results. This combination of terminals plus logging printer serves the function of Immunology well and allows for adequate data collection. Figure 86 shows the associated input terminal.

| 09/13/76 | | HBS | AG (AUGT AG) | 284 | 09:02 |
PATIENT NAME	SPEC	RESULT			TECH
FXXXXXX, FRAN	1045	-----			----
AXXXX, ROBERT	1057	-----			----
EXXXXXX, VERNO	1059	-----			----
WXXXXX, NANCY	1159	-----			----
AXXXX, LEWIS H	5284	-----			----
RXXXX, FLORENC	5351	-----			----
WXXXXXX, JANIS L	7058	-----			----
RXXXXXXX, TYNIE	7062	-----			----
RXXXXXXXX, LAURA	7063	-----			----
NXXX, GUY G	7111	-----			----
HXXXXXX, VELMA	7112	-----			----
HXXXXX, CLARIS	7116	-----			----
BXXXX, HERBERT	7120	-----			----

FIG. 85 Immunology also uses the single test worksheet for convenience of data gathering.

FIG. 86 Immunology has a fixed-format keyboard specifically designed to handle their unique requirements. This peripheral allows entry of high-volume immunology tests, in which are used such things as titers and the special qualitative messages unique to that laboratory discipline.

UNFINISHED TEST REPORT

Immunology receives an individualized unfinished-test report, which is used for audit of procedures. Since many of its tests are performed at a preset time, this report must be scrutinized closely to insure that tests are not in an upcoming batch. Initially, there was some difficulty in establishing daily use of the unfinished test reports, but through an educational process these timing problems were resolved.

ABNORMAL TEST REPORT

An abnormal test report can be called up on individual patients to review atypical immunologic data. The report is less useful in this area since many of the results from immunology do not have absolute limits, but are qualitative verbal responses with yes–no limits.

CHART REPORTS

Figures 87 and 88 show the actual chart reports available from Immunology. These are very similar to Chemistry and employ the cumulative record system with dates and times as column headers.

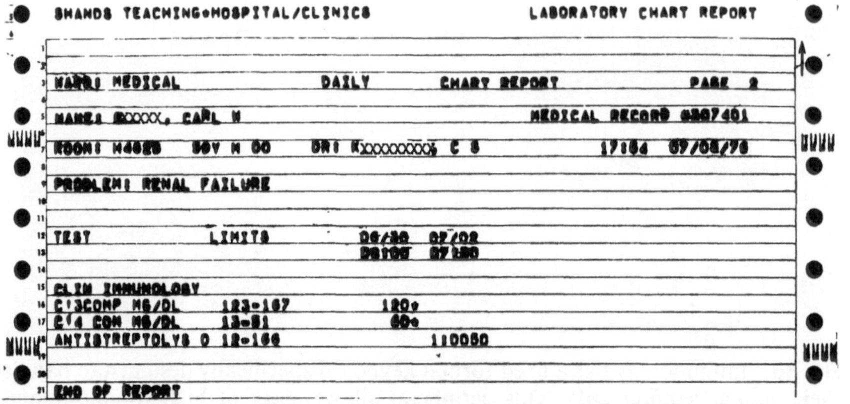

SHANDS TEACHING•HOSPITAL/CLINICS LABORATORY CHART REPORT

WARD: MEDICAL DAILY CHART REPORT PAGE 2
NAME: BXXXXX, CARL H MEDICAL RECORD #307401
ROOM: H4025 56Y M 00 DR: KXXXXXXXXX C S 17:54 07/05/76
PROBLEM: RENAL FAILURE

TEST	LIMITS	06/30 08:00	07/02 07:30
CLIN IMMUNOLOGY			
C'3COMP MG/DL	123-167	120+	
C'4 COM MG/DL	13-51	60+	
ANTISTREPTOLYS O	12-166		1:0050

END OF REPORT

FIG. 87 The immunology laboratory report is a standard vertical array but also offers the option of reporting horizontal titer information in selected areas.

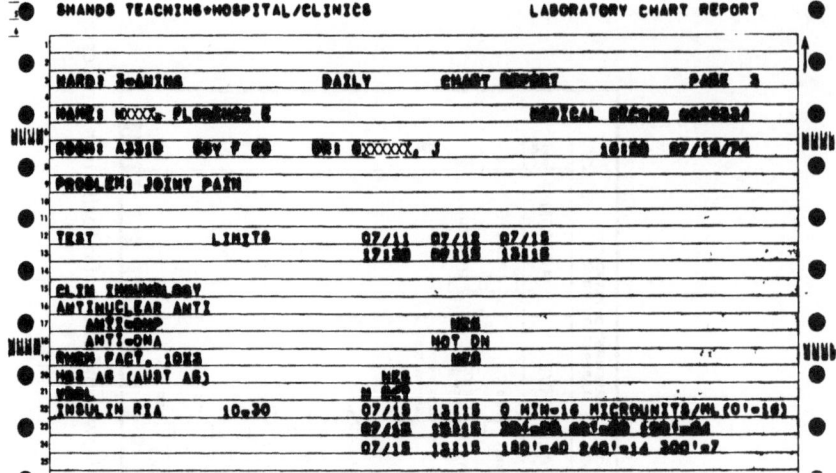

FIG. 88   In certain cases, only free-text entry will allow adequate reporting of results. In this case the insulin tolerance procedure is reported by the horizontal array of information, with time and date noted so that the physician can adequately review the information.

STAFFING AND ORGANIZATION

Our immunology lab currently operates 18 hours a day, five days a week and maintains a skeleton call-in crew on weekends. The major demand is for Australia Antigen testing and an occasional digoxin level requested on a stat basis. Other procedures are conveniently handled on a weekly schedule because of their cost and the frequency of demand.

QUALITY CONTROL

Our laboratory system provides no on-line quality control system for the immunology area. The current program uses modular units and many different techniques to decide the range of acceptance and quality of performance.

MARK-SENSE CARDS

Mark-sense cards are maintained as backup for all the procedures that are performed in immunology. These exactly match the manual-entry special-function keyboard (Fig. 89).

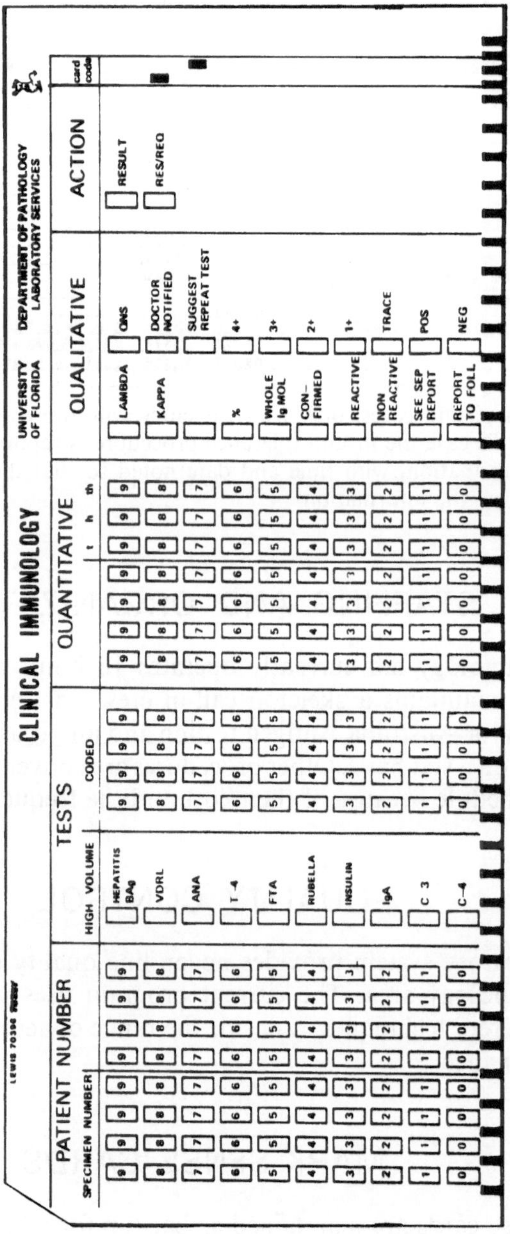

FIG. 89   The immunology mark-sense card is used in case of system failure, and can allow rapid entry of information if necessary.

CRITIQUE

The most demanding problems we faced in Immunology were the timed procedures, such as insulin tolerance tests and other serial RIA measures. No matter what times we specified, they were always drawn differently. This meant that subtests with preset times were impossible, and we finally settled for a single test number which was answered in the laboratory by comment. This allows total flexibility as long as the times are properly written on the submitted specimen collection tubes.

17

Blood Bank

INTRODUCTION

The establishment of an information system for blood banking confronts a hospital with the need to incorporate an almost endless series of forms and documents, all of which are very tightly controlled by the American Association of Blood Banks and require certification. The attempt to encompass all of the individual donor cards, patient recipient records, and associated cross-reference files becomes an extremely expansive project. In looking at a fully operational blood bank, it becomes clear that the physician really is involved with only a small section daily. Our system study showed that the major share of difficulties arose from the frequent calls for information regarding the status of blood products. Another primary concern to the physician is the order that is placed and the ability of the Blood Bank to respond promptly with the particular item required. In developing information for the blood-bank package, our initial choice was to optimize the potential of the communications mode and minimize the data involvement with the basic record system in the Blood Bank proper. We anticipate that a separate blood-bank system will be required to handle the full recordkeeping capability expected of this area.

REQUEST FORM

Blood-bank request items can be seen on both the general and the specific order forms (Figs. 20 and 35). They are somewhat different from other items since these requests allow a quantity to be ordered. When an order is placed for this area on the floor, the message file for that particular test is set so that it will ask for a specific comment from the clerk regarding the number of units or number of products to be available. This is then transmitted directly through the communications system onto a logging terminal in the Blood Bank and made available on an immediate basis. The requestor is also asked to call to deal with any problems that might have arisen in the procurement of these products.

SPECIMEN HANDLING

The Blood Bank has been designed to be operated peripherally with its own specimen check-in functions. It was found that all blood-bank tubes brought to the central labs had to be subsequently transmitted to the Blood Bank on a stat basis. Most of the type and crossmatch tubes and the emergency tubes sent to the bank needed immediate attention and could not go through a secondary source. At that time, it was decided that the specimen had to be diverted directly to the check-in desk at the bank where they could be directly inspected for the proper signatures and patient identification by Blood Bank personnel.

For those elements that require results such as titers and antibody identification, a free-format keyboard is provided that allows users to type specific comments in English that are then transmitted to the patient's chart. Items such as tissue typing and special antibody work fit very nicely into this combination of functions.

INPUT TERMINALS

Because of communication bottlenecks in the Blood Bank, a design was established to optimize a real-time physician dialog by utilizing an inventory function that would be available on all terminals. On this inventory system we maintain four parameters for every order: (*1*) the number of units ordered, (*2*) the number of units available, (*3*) the number of units used, and (*4*) the number of type and crossmatch tubes on file in the blood bank. These four elements had been the prime causes of distressed phone calls in years gone by. By providing real-time

input, our design hoped to minimize the number of calls and make the most effective use of our peripheral terminals. A special inventory terminal on a fixed-format keyboard was designed to allow easy input of this information as the status of the patient's order changes (Fig. 90). Complete interactive software to make this terminal functional is still unfinished; however, the same system does work less conveniently through an alphanumeric terminal currently present in the Blood Bank.

UNFINISHED TEST REPORT

The Blood Bank receives an unfinished test report which keeps laboratory records current and accurate on various patients in the hospital, and permits a chance to manipulate the inventory function until such time as the patient is discharged.

CHART REPORTS

Chart reports are designed to optimize the inventory system and also allow input of the free-format English information. The inventory uses

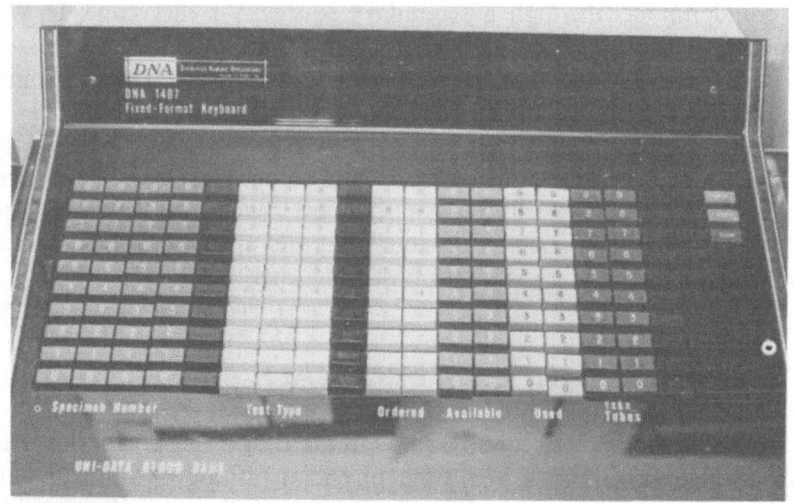

FIG. 90   The blood bank keyboard has been designed to allow entry of inventory items that are important for the physician. Categories such as the number of units ordered, the number that are available, the number that have been used, and the number of type and cross match tubes in the blood bank area are important parameters for physician update. These are achievable through the use of the keyboard and its associated software.

```
  SHANDS TEACHING*HOSPITAL/CLINICS                    LABORATORY CHART REPORT


  WARD:  SURG/SPL         DAILY           CHART REPORT                      PAGE 1
  NAME:  GXXXXX, MARGARET E                          MEDICAL RECORD #888888
  ROOM:  H549   31Y   F   00        DR:  AXXXX, S C

  PROBLEM:  NONE


  TEST           LIMITS            07/27
                                   13:45

  BLOOD BANK
  352ABO  GRP  RH  TP             07/27  13:45  A POSITIVE
      ANTIBODY SCRN               07/27  13:45  POSITIVE
      ANTIBODY ID.                07/27  13:45  ANTI KELL
      ANTIBODY TIT.               07/27  13:45  I:8
  3650ORDERED/AVAIL               07/27  13:45  10/5
      USED/Q.AD.UNT               07/27  13:45  5/0

  END OF REPORT
```

FIG. 91   The report from blood bank can be used to identify the type of test ordered.

a decimal system to separate parameters. As an example, 10/5 means ten units ordered and five units available (Fig. 91).

STAFFING

The Blood Bank experienced no staffing changes before and after the installation of the laboratory system since it was already on a 24-hour staffing pattern.

MARK-SENSE CARDS

The Blood Bank does not utilize a mark-sense card since each of its orders is free text and unique. No bills are generated with bank orders. The message file has been set up strictly to execute the order as for any other test, yet place no charge in the patient's billing area. We found this necessary because of the great complexity of blood-bank billing. It is virtually impossible to capture the exact charges at the time an order is placed since many crossmatches may have to be done to secure a unit of blood for a patient. All the additional charges for antibody identification, and so on, must be handled on a manual basis after the patient's work has been completed. We have designed special mark-sense cards for billing which will allow a patient's bill to be placed on one card (Figs. 92–94). These cards are completed at the end of the day by the appropriate clerk in charge of the billing area, and completely eliminate the hardcopy and keypunch routines previously used.

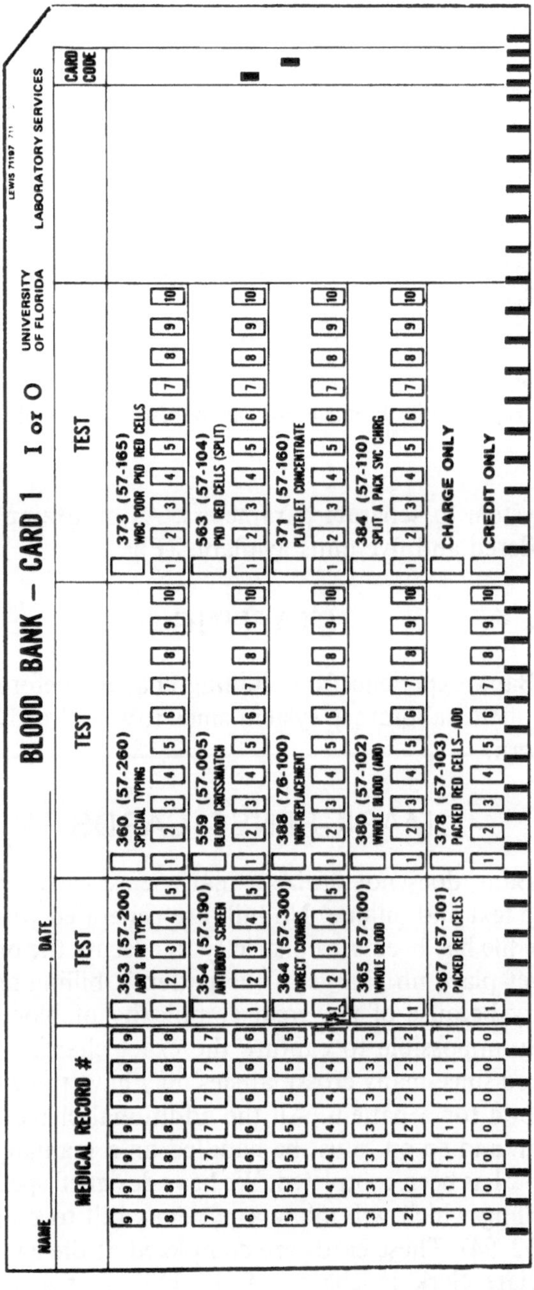

FIG. 92

FIGS. 92, 93, and 94. A special mark-sense card is used by the blood bank so that their billing can be accomplished. Most of the blood bank information can only be gathered after the completion of the order processing.

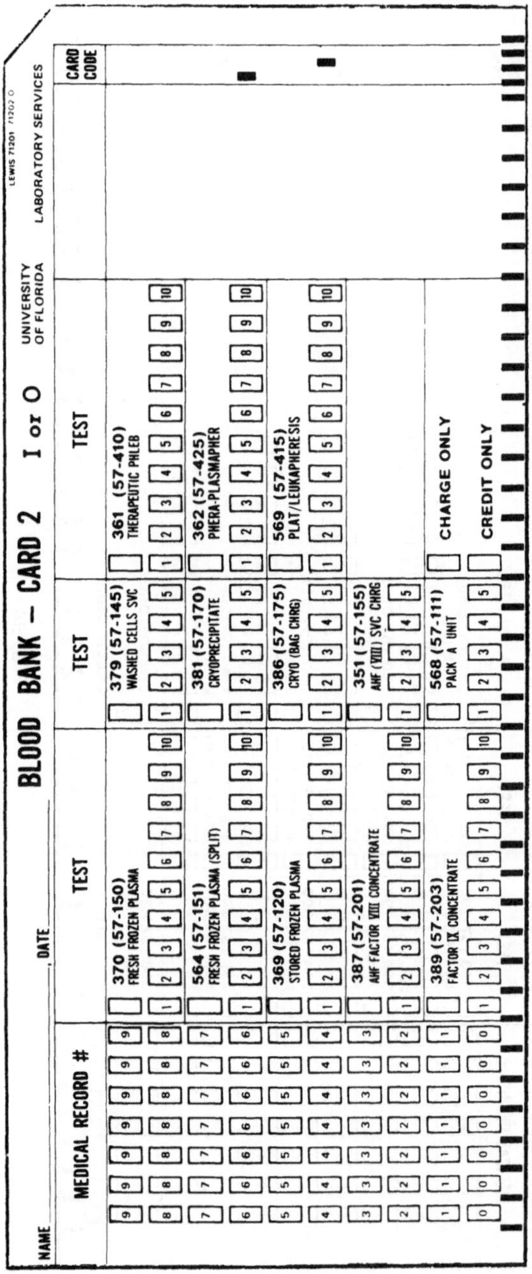

LEWIS 71201 71202 O
UNIVERSITY OF FLORIDA
LABORATORY SERVICES
NAME
DATE
BLOOD BANK – CARD 2
I or O
CARD CODE
MEDICAL RECORD #
TEST
TEST
TEST
370 (57-150) FRESH FROZEN PLASMA
564 (57-151) FRESH FROZEN PLASMA (SPLIT)
369 (57-120) STORED FROZEN PLASMA
387 (57-201) AHF FACTOR VIII CONCENTRATE
389 (57-203) FACTOR IX CONCENTRATE
379 (57-145) WASHED CELLS SVC
381 (57-170) CRYOPRECIPITATE
386 (57-175) CRYO (BAG CHRG)
351 (57-155) AHF (VIII) SVC CHRG
568 (57-111) PACK A UNIT
361 (57-410) THERAPEUTIC PHLEB
362 (57-425) PHERA-PLASMAPHER
569 (57-415) PLAT/LEUKAPHERESIS
CHARGE ONLY
CREDIT ONLY

FIG. 93

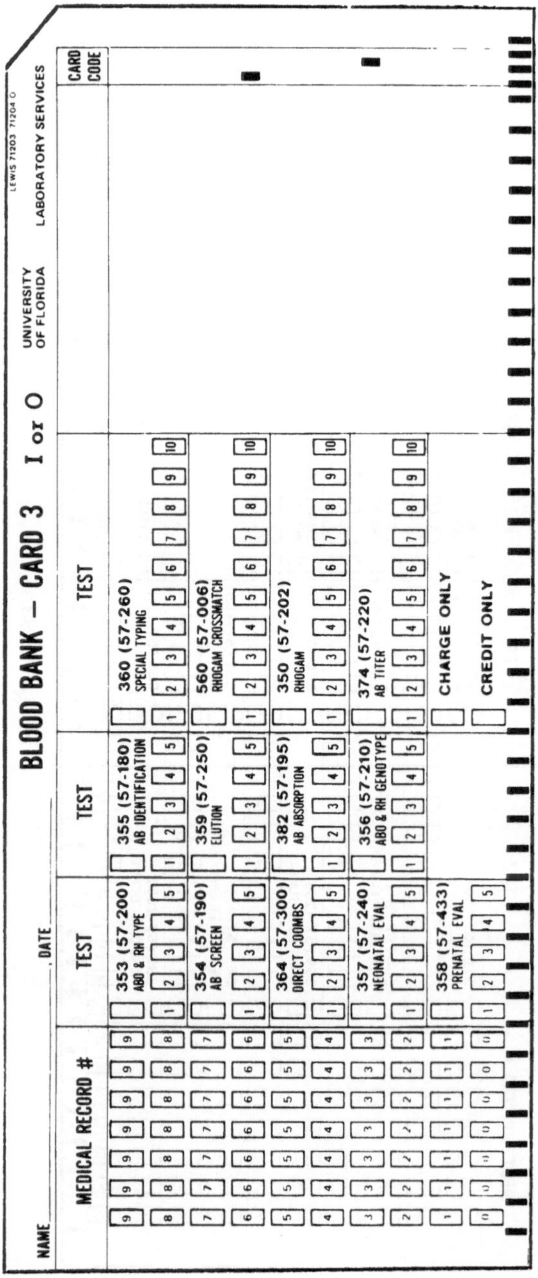
LEWIS 71203 71204 O
UNIVERSITY OF FLORIDA
LABORATORY SERVICES
BLOOD BANK — CARD 3 I or O
NAME
DATE
MEDICAL RECORD #
TEST
353 (57-200) ABO & RH TYPE
354 (57-190) AB SCREEN
364 (57-300) DIRECT COOMBS
357 (57-240) NEONATAL EVAL
358 (57-433) PRENATAL EVAL
TEST
355 (57-180) AB IDENTIFICATION
359 (57-250) ELUTION
382 (57-195) AB ABSORPTION
356 (57-210) ABO & RH GENOTYPE
TEST
360 (57-260) SPECIAL TYPING
560 (57-006) RHOGAM CROSSMATCH
350 (57-202) RHOGAM
374 (57-220) AB TITER
CHARGE ONLY
CREDIT ONLY
CARD CODE

FIG. 94

CRITIQUE

All the software needed totally to support the blood banking system has not been completed as yet. We can operate the system through the use of the alphanumeric keyboard and comment function, but currently are unable to use our fixed-format keyboard. Specific designs have been completed for mark-sense cards, which now provide complete retro-spective billing.

18

Anatomic Pathology

INTRODUCTION

Anatomic Pathology presents us with a historical instance in which the traditional lengthy, typed report, bearing the physician's signature, is standard and customary. Given this background, it is understandably difficult to identify and extricate the manual systems and to convince users to adopt an alternate mode of operation more compatible with an information system approach. It becomes quite apparent that lengthy typed pages are neither practical nor conceptually useful on an information system with limited storage. What we have attempted to do with Anatomic Pathology is to optimize basic information and minimize the risk of inappropriate interpretation. Two categories of diagnostics are supplied with each report. A PAD (provisional anatomic diagnosis) will give an indication to the physician of what is potentially possible for this patient. This is followed by an FAD (final anatomic diagnosis), which delineates the type and specific nature of the condition identified by the specimen and subsequent slides and staining.

REQUEST FORM

Requests for Anatomic Pathology, Cytology, and Surgical Pathology are included on the order sheets along with a small area for the addition of appropriate information about the patient (Fig. 20). We have tried to use the system in a communication mode to capture the initial basic-physical examination and history data, but found this to be too cumbersome and difficult for the floor clerks to enter. Moreover, it is imperative that the information be available for use by the cytologists and anatomic pathologists in properly interpreting slide material. To circumvent this problem, we have developed a small form that is completed when the slide or tissue is prepared. This is then wrapped around the bottle or the slide, and the order is placed on the system in the customary manner. The unit is transmitted to the laboratory where it is checked in and placed in a basket for Anatomic Pathology. These specimens are collected, logged, and subsequent slides and stains are performed until a diagnostic statement can be concluded.

INPUT TERMINALS

Anatomic pathology uses a standard telecommunication terminal which can perform the same functions as a free-format laboratory terminal. The ability to review the patient's chart (nursing station function) plus enter appropriate information (laboratory function) into the patient's test file renders this terminal polyfunctional. Such a capability provides unique service to Anatomic Pathology and is possible because of the terminal matrix map in the central files.

Special cards that report and capture charges on this billing system (Fig. 95) are used for Cytology.

UNFINISHED TEST REPORT

Anatomic Pathology, like the other laboratory areas, receives an unfinished test report and uses this to determine specimen status at any time. It can be used conveniently to determine the through-put time for various types of specimens and to evaluate changes in procedure which might improve efficiency and reporting.

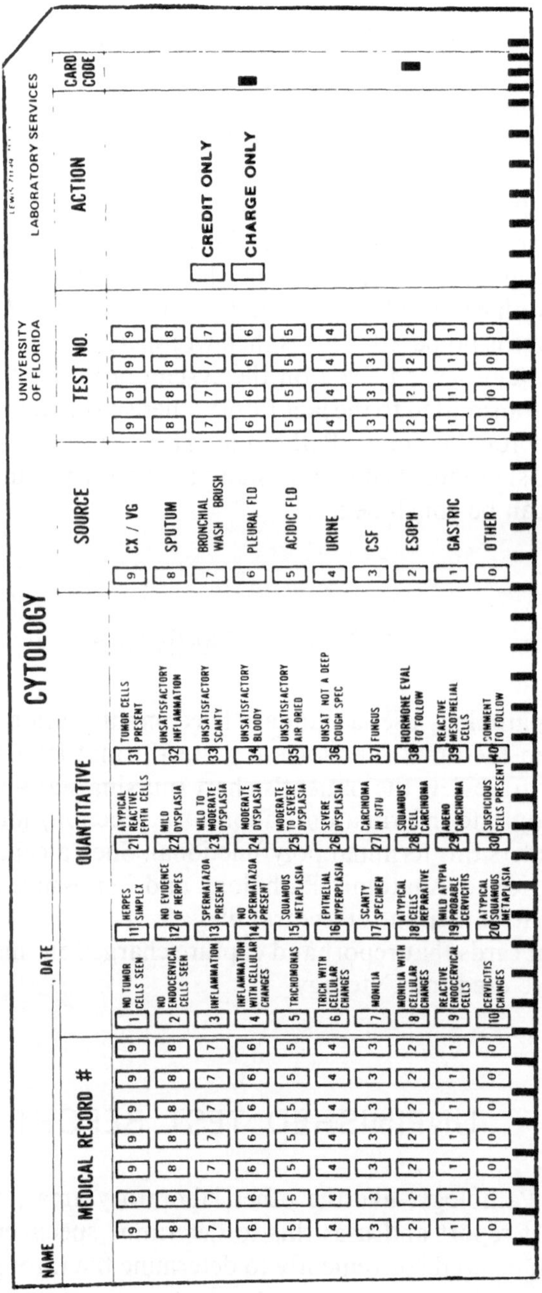

FIG. 95   A special mark-sense card is used for cytology and allows the direct entry of this information for patient reporting and billing.

CHART REPORT

The anatomic chart report is comment-oriented, since there is no quantitative data to be supplied (Fig. 96). Thirty-two characters of comment are allowed per line and each line must be separately input on the peripheral terminal. This is quite an inconvenient system, and has been modified to allow 64 characters per line and one identification step per transaction. It is anticipated that the final diagnostic pattern will be coded with SNOMED numbers that promise great utility in the long-term archive-retrieval program.

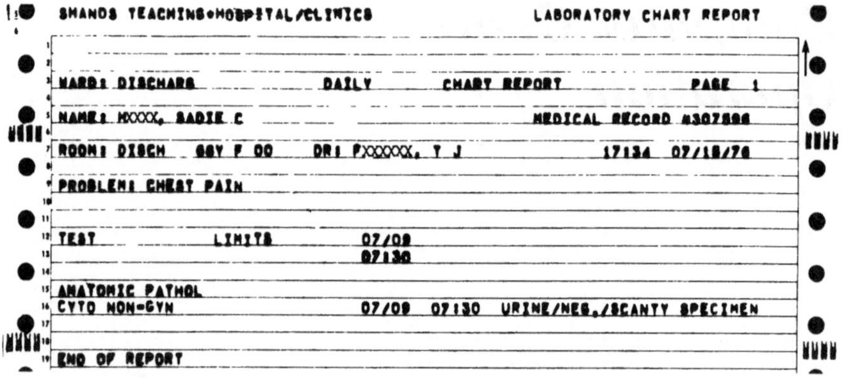
SHANDS TEACHING-HOSPITAL/CLINICS LABORATORY CHART REPORT

WARD: DISCHARG DAILY CHART REPORT PAGE 1

NAME: MXXXX, SADIE C MEDICAL RECORD #307898

ROOM: DISCH 68Y F 00 DR: PXXXXXX, T J 17134 07/18/76

PROBLEM: CHEST PAIN

TEST LIMITS 07/09
07130

ANATOMIC PATHOL
CYTO NON-GYN 07/09 07130 URINE/NEG./SCANTY SPECIMEN

END OF REPORT

FIG. 96 Anatomic Pathology has a report option which allows them to enter reports in paragraph format for subsequent chart distribution.

CRITIQUE

Anatomic Pathology has not totally abandoned its manual data handling systems. It continues to use the form and lengthy report sheet, but does periodically employ the communication system for Pap smears and some tissue specimens. A major problem in using the new system is the inconvenience of the short reports. Only time and specific changes in the operational mechanics of the department will make it fully convenient. Work is underway to automate billing and cytology using a mark-sense card to create simple reports and charges. [At press time, this package has now been completed.]

19

Computer Center Operation

INTRODUCTION

With the installation of an information system, the computer center now becomes the hub of the hospital environment and all the problems and essential data are handled through this central core. The laboratory communication system is no exception. This role of coordination and communication is the dominant theme of the computer center and must not be minimized or overlooked.

PERSONNEL

In seeking people to handle a system on a 24-hour, seven-day a week basis, one usually approaches the technologists in the lab in the hope that some of these individuals might be interested in a modified career. Our laboratory showed very little response since the pay scales for the computer operators and managers were lower than those of technolo-

gists. Therefore, there was little reason for them to divert their efforts to another area, one that generated either indifference or possibly hostility. Many of them felt they were poorly equipped and were hesitant about its future.

To be properly staffed, a key person is needed in the day-to-day hardware/software operation. Moreover, this individual should probably have a background in industry or production so that there is some understanding of the operational problems inherent in the work. We were fortunate to obtain such a person and began immediately to develop the operational staff to make this unit function. In our particular case, we had no choice in obtaining the needed computer operators— our clerks and secretaries had to be converted. No new staff lines were available from the hospital. This turned out to be a mixed blessing. Many of the personnel wanted a pay increase, yet the thought of working weekends and nights on a rotating basis was something that was displeasing to most of them. As an additional factor, most of the clerks and secretaries had never been placed in a highly responsible position before, and were now faced with making decisions on a minute-by-minute basis regarding the entire laboratory operation. This created an undue amount of stress on some individuals, and in time many left to be replaced by others who have found the work challenging and dynamic. Our current computer center staff has been drawn very heavily from our ward clerks and unit managers. These individuals have been found to possess the requisite experience, background, and personal acquaintanceship with many of the staff in the hospital, and for these reasons, interact easily in this particular environment. The system is a challenge to them as they work with the various options available, providing a broader and longer-range future than what they may have had on the floor.

In addition to the computer center operation, it is necessary to have another individual handling floor coordination, specifically, patient problems. We were fortunate to obtain an experienced individual who came to us from the hospital environment as director of ward clerks and was the ideal individual to help us integrate our program with the existing mechanical and procedural situations on each floor. Such an individual is essential for successful implementation.

In like manner, it is imperative that a physician become involved with the system at the very beginning to provide the necessary professional time and leadership, and assure that each one of these milestones is successfully accomplished. This individual cannot be left isolated, but needs the total support of the department and each of the individual lab sections to be successful. At times, this can become a strained relationship. The department chairman, in certain situations, must be very

active in coordinating the program, must become personally educated in the programs, and must negotiate disputes between vendor, hospital, and department in areas of personal opinion.

SCHEDULES

The scheduling of the computer operation is strictly a matter of optimizing system, people, and time. Computer operators run our system 24 hours a day, and we believe it is inappropriate to turn the system over to laboratory technologists since the specific details of daily operation are intricate. Our schedule calls for a permanent night team to handle the system from midnight to 8 AM. Our evening team can rotate, depending on demand and schedule, with the day crew. The chief computer operator works during the days and is available to fill in and teach on various shifts on a prescheduled basis.

TRAINING

Most of the people selected for computer operations are inexperienced, and it takes us approximately two weeks of one-on-one tutoring to bring them to a level of self-sufficiency. The supervision employs a training manual and, of course, puts trainees on during the day so that they can see the system in operation while learning functions through hands-on-control with close supervision.

It is important during the training process to evaluate new employees' attitudes and opinions about doctors and patient care problems. Many of the employees entering this area come from peripheral non-medical backgrounds. We very strongly stress in our training program that patient and physician come first, and that the system and laboratory are second. This means that if a procedural problem develops and a physician declares that a patient is in jeopardy, the system is placed second and the patient's specimen and results are handled on an individual basis in an expeditious manner. The lock step, categorical yes–no type of training program is not encouraged. The physicians must have a feeling that they can override the system if the circumstances dictate, and this happens approximately once a week in relation to some very critical patients on the floor.

Frequently, one of the interns or residents has been up all night and is in bad humor when arriving at the laboratory. It is inappropriate at that time for our operators to create a serious roadblock to the proper and appropriate specimen identification and handling. We do insist,

however, that after the crisis has subsided and the individual has been cared for, the system be properly updated and that all data be verified before a final chart is generated on the patient. This takes care of the necessary housekeeping to make the program reliable.

FUNCTIONS

Table 5 shows the daily schedule of the computer center and lists the times and the specific jobs to be performed during a 24-hour period. It should be noted that the system is copied four times each day to ensure that, should some disaster occur, we have lost only at most six hours of information input. A copy is taken directly before a billing tape is made. This eliminates any possible problems that might occur if the billing is destroyed or damaged during tape transcription. Our operational schedule is kept in the computer room and each operator on shift fills in the appropriate area on the form at the time the functions are performed. If problems should develop during the following shift or day, it is easy to see who has done what, and to go back and look at the audit trails to determine whether the function was properly performed, and whether the computer did what it was instructed to do.

SYSTEM CONTROL

Census

The census is one of the key features in the communication system which keeps the data base localized and accurate. Obviously, Admissions is handling its own census, but we do try to review basic reports each day to ensure that there are no inappropriate pieces of information in the patient's file, and that the patient is in the proper bed. In certain instances, when the system has malfunctioned because of software loops or halts, the census system has been affected. The computer center should check the census report daily to monitor the quality of information available.

Reports

For the laboratory, the daily charts and the final charts are very critical reviews of the system's performance. It is easy, with these powerful systems which handle large amounts of information, to be complacent about how they are operated and how the data is presented and

Table 5

Procedure Schedule for Computer Operations

Time	Procedure	Time started	Time finished	Operator
7:30–8:30 AM	Confirm spec. (draw team)			
8:30 AM	Worksheets (new) (1 part green, Chem., Hema., Immun., Micros., put in area basket)			
9:00 AM	Master worksheets (1 part green, Chem., Hema., Immun., Micros., Anat. Path., B.B., put in baskets)			
9:10 AM	Unfinished test (1 part green, Chem., Immun., Micros., Anat. Path., B.B., Microbio.)			
9:20–9:30 AM	SMAC tapes (stats) (place reports in SMAC room)			
10:20–10:30 AM	SMAC tapes (place reports in SMAC room)			
11:20–11:30 AM	SMAC tapes (place reports in SMAC room)			
12:00 PM	Ward report (2 part green, deliver 1 to floors, other goes in "Dup. Ward Report" basket)			
12:25 PM	Copy drum (mag. tape, place in green cabinet on 2nd shelf on right on bottom of stack)			
12:30 PM	Billing report (mag. tape, see intructions on next sheet, place in safe)			
1:20–1:30 PM	SMAC tapes (place reports in SMAC room)			
2:20–2:30 PM	SMAC tapes (place reports in SMAC room)			
3:00 PM	Abnormal test report (1 part green, place in "System Report" basket)			

Time	Task
3:20–3:30 PM	SMAC tapes (place reports in SMAC room)
3:45 PM	Census listing (put report on right side of counter at front window)
3:50 PM	Unfinished test report (Chemistry and Hematology only)
4:00 PM	Daily chart report (new) (2 part green deliver to floors, others to "Dup. Daily Chart" basket. Also do a repeat on area #50 for Dr. Kitchens.)
4:30 PM	Copy drum (mag. tape, place in green cabinet on 2nd shelf.)
4:40 PM	Billing report (Mag. tape, see instructions on next sheet, place in safe)
4:45–5:30 PM	SMAC tapes (place reports in SMAC room)
6:00 PM	ADTL report (1 part green, place in "Microfilm" basket)
7:00 PM	SMAC tapes (place reports in SMAC room)
8:00 PM	SMAC tapes (place reports in SMAC room)
10:00 PM	Unfinished test report (all areas, place reports in area baskets)
10:15 PM	7-Day chart report (new) (2 part blue, deliver 1 to floors, other to "Microfilm" basket. Outpatient, E.R., Discharge go in "Medical Records" basket.)
11:20 PM	Copy drum (mag. tape, put in green cabinet)
11:30 PM	Billing report (mag. tape, see instructions below, place in safe)
11:55–12:05 AM	DO NOT DO ANYTHING BETWEEN THESE TIMES AS THE MACHINE IS PURGING

(continued)

Table 5—*continued*

Time	Procedure	Time started	Time finished	Operator
12:10 AM	Print purged results (1 part green, put in "Microfilm" basket)			
12:20 AM	Census report			
12:30 AM	(2 part green, place 1 in "Systems Report" basket, other to "Admissions") Ward report			
1:00 AM	(2 part green, deliver 1 to floors, other to "Dup. Ward Report" basket) Archive entries/merge (use 2707 for entries, 1 part green, do a "Print" on Mondays and put in "Microfilm" basket)			
1:30 AM	Copy drum (mag. tape, put in green cabinet, 2nd shelf on right on bottom of stack)			
5:45 AM	Census report			
5:50 AM	(2 part green, place 1 in "Systems Report" basket, other to "Admissions") Unfinished test report (Hematology only, put in area baskets)			
6:00 AM	ADTL report (1 part green, put in "Microfilm" basket)			
6:15 AM	SCL tubes (new) (1 part green, ×2)			
6:25 AM	SCL labels (3-up labels, ×3)			
6:30 AM	Copy drum (mag. tape, put in green cabinet, 2nd shelf on right on bottom of stack)			

delivered. In our case, it is absolutely essential to have this information reviewed critically each day and looked at with a very careful eye toward hardware and software failures. These have a tendency to creep in, and and then suddenly cause a catastrophe. Unless the system is carefully monitored on a daily or hourly basis, there is no way of detecting such minor changes.

For instance, on New Year's Eve, 1975, we were given specific instructions by our vendor on how to execute the proper changes to transfer all the files over to the following year. We executed the instructions as given, and the following day noticed that the Microbiology reports were being printed in an improper fashion. A call was placed to the vendor and immediate assistance requested. After weeks of searching and evaluation, it was determined that the program that had been used to execute the change of year had not taken into account the fact that it was a leap year. This had a major effect on the test files and the way they were numbered. These are the strange and curious things that work their way into systems and have a way of creating a major disaster in short order. Once solved, the problem predictably went away and everything was forgotten.

Until New Year's Eve, 1976. How could anything go wrong? One day after New Year, the Microbiology charts went wild again! This time the programmers found a date-number problem which was then patched and repaired; we hope we have solved the problem after two years and two tries.

HALTS

When the computer itself is confused or is given wrong information, or tries to execute a command that is inappropriate, it often goes into a state of catatonic schizophrenia; in our system it also turns on a little red light that says Halt. At that point nothing else will happen. The computer operators must know how to handle the system when this occurs, and our original operators had plenty of practice.

LOOPS

Another game the computer will play is called the loop. This is a silent halt. In this case, no lights go on, but everything just slows down. What occurs is that the software gets itself into a circle and keeps going around using up all the access time that is required to service the other communication lines. Therefore, the speed of the system drops way down and

everybody sits and waits. When this occurs there is only one thing to do: halt the system, restart by bringing the programs back in off the drum, and reload. All of our original operators were trained in handling loops and had adequate experience in this area.

PHYSICIAN PROBLEMS

Physicians pose the greatest problem for operating the computer room. By the time they arrive in the computer center with a problem, they are angry and belligerent. This places great stress on the data processing personnel operating the computer room. We try to route all of these problems directly to one of the physicians in the pathology department to take the pressure off the computer center and operators by assuring that they do not have to deal with such situations on a one-to-one basis.

If one were to analyze physician complaints, in almost every case they result from a complex series of circumstances that start with improper assumptions and end with unwarranted generalizations. Such problems have greatly diminished as the systems have been on-line and the education program has been adequately implemented to reach the physicians. One of the greatest difficulties in dealing with this group is trying to educate them on how these procedures work. They refuse to attend lectures, they usually do not read what they are sent in the mail, and they always appear to be too busy to come to a conference or a meeting. We have found that there are certain ways of reaching doctors which we will discuss later.

FILE HANDLING

The maintenance and handling of the on-line files has been delegated to the chief computer operator, who is the only individual allowed to enter or modify this type of information in the system. The updating of the files is usually done with the help of the company hardware/software expert. In some cases, the files require manipulation through the CPU, and that can only be done through the on-site hardware specialist. By using this team approach, the changes we make in the files are company-sponsored, and will be protected if problems occur.

SPECIMEN HANDLING

Prior to the installation of our communication system, physicians brought the specimens to the individual labs. This was terribly con-

venient for the labs, but it turned out to be a disaster for the book-keeping and administration of records. Specimens were found everywhere. Most of the people bringing the specimens had no idea what they were or what they were supposed to do with them. The idea of a central check-in facility is essential, yet the physical plant necessary to support it is not customarily designed into hospitals.

Our computer room has now become the central check-in hub of the laboratory. Strict rules regarding specimen handling and through-put times are mandatory. Microbiology specimens cannot be left sitting about since the organisms will die. Hematology specimens cannot be held very long since the coagulation parameters will then be inappropriate. Chemistry specimens and Microscopy specimens must be handled in an expeditious manner in order to separate the cells and the sera. Immunology specimens, however, can usually be refrigerated to allow for

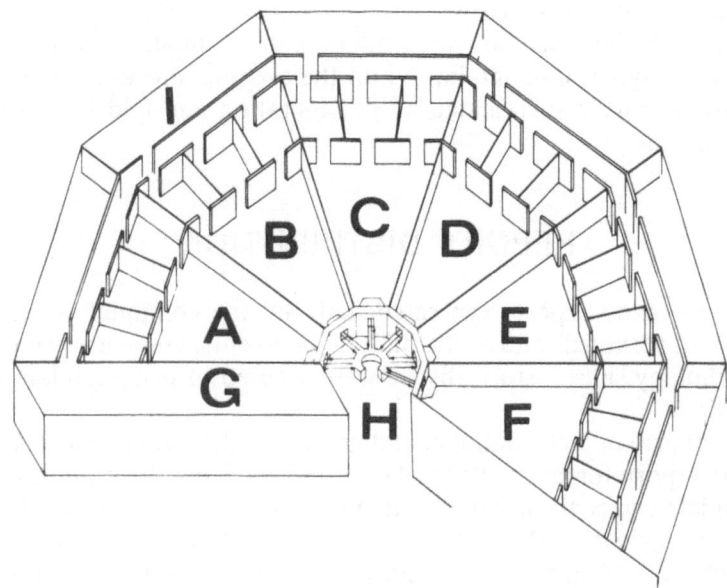

FIG. 97   The architectural design of a laboratory is critical to successful functioning. What is demonstrated is the need for specimen handling as well as direct communication between those handling the hospital communication network, and those that are critically involved in laboratory services. Laboratory areas A through F receive specimens from area H by conveyor belts. Support areas are allowed in section I for each of the laboratories to include reagent storage and offices for personnel. Area G is designated as the computer center and has direct visual contact with all laboratory facilities through glass windows and walls so that service can adequately be controlled at low staffing.

some delay in specimen pickup. The blood banking specimens are not handled by the central computer room, but are sent directly to the Blood Bank. Major architectural changes are required in the design of laboratories adequately to handle specimens through a central processing concept.

Our experience would dictate that the design of the laboratory would place the check-in area and computer center in close proximity to minimize the number of personnel required to operate both. It would also provide some very convenient means of transportation of urine jugs, tubes, and labels from the central area directly to the labs by a movable countertop (Fig. 97). A transport system equivalent to a grocery store checkout counter could be envisioned. A photocell detector in the lab would ring when specimens arrived, initiating immediate processing. This one architectural change would greatly simplify the internal operations of the lab and minimize the many footsteps that are required to handle specimens within a sprawling complex.

The architectural design should incorporate the use of a stat laboratory facility in close proximity to the computer area so that technology staff can be minimized on the evening and weekend shifts. We currently have such a stat lab configuration and find it extremely advantageous.

REPORT DISTRIBUTION

There are many reports generated daily by the computer system. It truly is "paperholic," and overproduces documents. This is a new posture for Pathology since historically we were accused of being too late with too little.

At approximately midnight and noon each day the system produces a ward report for every floor. This contains laboratory information accumulated since the last daily patient chart report was generated. This is usually tacked to the wall and utilized by those physicians on the floor who would like to review information up to that time. At about 5 PM we do the daily chart reporting on green paper and the computer operators make the delivery between 5:30 and 6 PM to each ward area. After ward delivery, these charts are kept in a central basket on the floor, and then taken by the ward clerks and placed on the patient's chart. About 11 PM, seven-day/final charts are produced on blue-lined paper, which are transmitted to the floors by the computer operators.

Using our computer technicians as couriers provides an opportunity for them to visit the floor areas and meet some of the clerks and

personnel. This develops a mix between our people and the floor, where they have a chance to talk to each other and discuss common problems. It also provides an opportunity for them to look at the peripheral terminals and evaluate those that may be marginal. It is my personal belief that people who are working in a highly structured and production-oriented system should spend some time in the actual patient care areas so they gain some feeling for the necessity and the importance of their job to the patient. This experience will provide them with a feeling of the importance and value of their work on an individual basis.

SERVICE

An in-house service technician is supplied by the company under contract and has proved to be an extremely valuable asset to the entire program. Initially, it was our intention to employ this individual in the evenings and weekends, when the system was not highly utilized, for preventive maintenance. During our first nine months of operation this was impractical, and it was decided that the best time to have such service available is when the laboratory was working its hardest. Most problems develop when through-put is high and the demand on the terminals is great. This is also the time when the laboratory is most vulnerable to peripheral failure and requires a high level of expertise to keep the system operating. Our initial service contract stipulated that our CE (Customer Engineer) was to be on-site 40 hours a week, and provide coverage in the evenings on an overtime basis and on the weekends through a similar mechanism. All parts required to maintain the system were supplied under contract by the vendor. Our new contract includes two CEs working ten hours a day, seven days a week. This change was necessary to allow for full coverage on weekends and to decrease our overtime expenses.

NEW PROGRAMS

For those who have not been initiated to the joys of computer systems and thus have not had to recover from a serious programming fault, let me caution you that new programs should never be loaded during a time of utilization. It is easy for an enthusiastic serviceman or engineer to arrive and load in a new program in the middle of the morning run. It certainly is convenient for him to get the job done and get back to the plant. Do not let it happen. And do not let more than one new program be loaded at a time.

Through bitter experience in this area, we have learned our lesson. It is very important when new programs are loaded to have all the responsible people available to evaluate each program, one at a time. For each new program that is being entered, set up a test protocol before it is ever put on the system. Decide, beforehand, how you are going to determine whether it is successful. If it requires overtime to do it, then that is the cost of running the system. We usually try to use the evening to load programs, so that we can shut the users off for a short period and run our protocols through to ensure it does exactly what is anticipated. In some cases we have had to redo a program three or four times until it successfully implements what was planned. This is an extremely hazardous process, and when dealing with a communications system, you cannot afford to make mistakes. We have had situations in which programs were loaded, and immediately caused four to five hours of hair-raising file manipulation to recover. This only increases the gastric acidity, gray hair, and the mumbling all too commonly associated with hospital information systems.

NOISE

Noise is a constant problem for the laboratory and the computer center. Most equipment available today is quite unacceptable in this regard and needs to be repackaged in a form with which we can live. The logging terminals in the laboratory have constantly given my ears problems, along with others who work around these daily, and the hospital has had to build special soundproof units to minimize the noise. Figure 40 shows such a box; its plexiglass top is lifted off the terminal for paper changes. This box creates a drop in the noise level below 55 dB and allows people to talk on the phone, whisper, and discuss patient problems without interference.

In a computer room, the line printer is a continual source of noise and special attention methods are again necessary. Plexiglass shields can be arranged in front of the paper head and around the unit to baffle the noise and divert it to the walls. A very heavy vinyl-coated curtain is used in our computer room to soak up as much noise as possible. It would be nice to carpet the floors, yet most computer equipment is very heavy and is housed on small rollers which may tend to tear the carpeting. The fans from the CPU create another type of noise, and these again can be baffled by plexiglass screens hung over the face of the unit to divert the sound. Specifications need to be developed in this area to limit the amount of noise produced by any of these devices.

20

Equipment and Configuration

DESCRIPTION

Table 6 shows the first stage of equipment employed in the communications system. Obviously, there is no room available for additional terminals or functions. This is one of the serious problems we faced as the system began to expand. The computer equipment, terminals, and software are all produced by Diversified Numeric Applications and the software is written in Medcoder assembly language.

RELIABILITY

The reliability of the system has been exceptional and the hardware has given us few problems compared to the total number of hours we have been operational. One serious hidden difficulty in dealing with a communications system is that minutes become hours, and hours become months in the eyes of the users. What this translates to is simple—when the computer center is down, every second is significant and the whole

Table 6

Initial Communication System Equipment List

Quantity	Item
1	Central processor with: Direct memory access Real-time interrupt subsystem Power failure interrupt Hardware multiply/divide
1	System operator console
1	Core memory module
1	Console typer
1	Drum memory system
1	High-speed paper-tape reader
1	Line printer subsystem consisting of: Printer module with self-standing enclosure Printer controller
1	Mark-sense card reader subsystem consisting of: Card reader module with self-standing enclosure Card reader controller
1	Analog/digital converter
1	Autoanalyzer interface
1	Disc cartridge subsystem consisting of: Disc cartridge drive Disc cartridge drive controller
1	Communications controller (24 channels) consisting of: Communication controllers Transmit multiplexers Receive multiplexers Communications input/output terminal panels
1	Request/inquiry subsystem consisting of: Fixed-format request/inquiry keyboard Desktop page printer STAT label printer
1	General chemistry subsystem consisting of: Fixed-format chemistry keyboard Desktop page printer
1	AutoAnalyzer control subsystem consisting of: Fixed-format AutoAnalyzer keyboard Desktop page printer Desktop page printer (audit trail)
1	Bacteriology reporting subsystem consisting of: Fixed-format bacteriology keyboard Fixed-format bacteriology smear keyboard Desktop page printer
1	Coulter Counter Model S interface consisting of: Fixed-format Coulter S control keyboard Desktop page printer Coulter S telecoupler

Table 6—*continued*

Quantity	Item
2	Gas plasma differential cell subsystems consisting of: Free-format keyboards Plasma display modules
1	Clinical immunology inquiry subsystem consisting of: Alpha/numeric/function keyboard Desktop page printer
1	Blood bank logging subsystem consisting of: Desktop page printer
11	Ward terminal subsystems consisting of: Alpha/numeric/function keyboards and printers

time frame of hospital operation collapses to an expectation of seconds. If the terminal fails to operate when any individual approaches, the system becomes suspect. There are certain times of the day that the entire system must go down so that we can copy the files. During this period we send messages to all the terminals informing them that we are going to be down for two to three minutes to copy the drum. After two years, we have finally accustomed our users to this short interruption.

SERVICE

The service of the hardware and software is a major responsibility in the everyday operation of the system. Broken terminals, blown fuses, and disconnected communication lines all add up to down time in the eyes of the hospital. This is the reason we have established an exchange cart system for all of our terminals. There is enough hardware on hand to wheel in a replacement unit within five minutes. The idea that this equipment is available is very reassuring to the floors and gives them a level of confidence which is important. Table 7 shows our experience in dealing with the hardware and the number of failures we have had for the past nine months.

Initially, many teletype unit failures were the result of improper lubrication at the factory. Subsequent use of heavy instead of light oil for gears and cams has solved this problem. In addition, we have asked for, but not yet received, the capability to shut off these terminals and their print motors when the lines are not used for communication purposes. Although a normal teletype will do this, our communication terminals cannot. In a practical sense, a series of pusher bits are sent

Table 7
Hardware Service Record

Type of device	Function	Units in system	Average failures per month	Average repair time per unit, h	Backup units	Common problems
1415	Hard copy print-out of laboratory information	20	7	1	2	Terminal printing erratically; double spacing; no power
1404	Printer used in conjunction with 1406/1407 keyboards	8	2	2	None	Printing erratically; noisy
1407	Fixed-format keyboard for fixed-format results	8	$1\frac{5}{8}$	1	None	Noisy; keys sticking
1411	Cathode ray tube, visual display of laboratory information	3	$2\frac{3}{5}$	$1\frac{1}{2}$	None	Display altered; no power
1496	Alphanumeric keyboard; located in Immunology, Microbiology; free-format results	2	$1\frac{1}{6}$	$2\frac{1}{4}$	None	Printing erratically
1420	Diff pad cell counter with morphology keyboard	2	1	$1\frac{3}{4}$	None	Not counting properly; no power
2707	Main console	1	$1\frac{2}{5}$	$1\frac{1}{5}$	None	Not displaying functions; operator error
Cartridge disc	Store data	1	1	2	None	Noisy
Line printer	Print reports one line at a time	1	$1\frac{1}{2}$	1	None	Printing poorly; dead
Label printer	Print labels for lab work	1	1	$1\frac{1}{2}$	None	Double spacing; not printing labels

to the terminal to turn it on and get the motor up to speed before any messages are sent for printing. This requires hardware and software modifications for both the peripheral terminal and the CPU, and as yet has not been accomplished. Such a change would extend the service time of the teletypes by approximately eight to ten times the current service cycle.

DOWN TIME

During the past 18 months, we have not had to shut the system down totally for any length of time. However, we have had some major failures with peripheral equipment. On one occasion, the main high-speed line printer failed. This unit was out for 24 hours, yet our peripheral terminals carried us through. Those remote terminals printed ward reports, patient data, census lists, and physician inquiries without the use of the central line printer.

SPARE PROGRAM

Our service contract allows for in-house hardware to service every piece of equipment, except the high-speed drums. These units are expensive and are centrally stored. If our site should lose one, it can be shipped in a matter of hours.

SOFTWARE MAINTENANCE

It has been our uniform policy since the beginning that the software necessary to support the system and improve it is an obligation of the vendor. During the development of our system, in-house programmers were not used. A special hospital programming group sounds terribly attractive, yet the logistics and dollars involved in such a venture are not realistic. In our case, the system runs 24 hours a day and there is no time for programming. One cannot just shut the system down for a couple of hours to develop a new package. The system is totally utilized. Therefore, there is nothing that the programmer can do until he has a finished product. As an additional problem, the type of programmer required for assembly language programming and the detailed and intricate work of establishing an online communication system and their subsystems software, is such that the hospital cannot afford to hire this

type of talent. It is difficult to find or keep happy such an experienced person in this type of setting, since there is very little upward mobility or latitude for growth. It is my personal belief that no hospital facility should become dependent on a group of programmers who can control and dictate the hospital's future operations. This can happen with an in-house group.

With this in mind, we elected to encourage our vendor to develop a software maintenance contract so that we could write specifications for changes in the software and receive a price, delivery date, and guarantee that the changes would not affect the system. Any problems that occurred would be the obligation of the company for one year. In addition, the agreement guarantees that we own the software; any later customer using our software would return our investment dollars. Theoretically, this provides the ultimate choice of hospitals, and especially laboratories, in dealing with these complicated machines. It also guarantees the long range support of the vendor and the viability of new software, so that the vendor maintains documentation and is in a direct position to service such software if problems should develop. All too often, homemade programs on turnkey systems somehow eventually cause problems and result in the company taking a very positive stand against the individual customer. It would not be our intention to place the hospital or the laboratory in such jeopardy. Through the use of this same mechanism, we can insure the long term integration of our particular software package with others that are developed within the growing field of systems. With the viability of the company, our contract software insures the long term success of the hospital and laboratory systems.

If the company fails, a software maintenance contract is worthless. At that time, in-house programming becomes mandatory, and the parent company staff must be approached. This is part of the risk of operating in such an environment, and should be appreciated at the outset. At press time, we can only reinforce this last paragraph. DNA no longer exists as a viable business. Their parent company AVNET stopped all support in early 1978 and left the field. We now have in-house programming and maintenance and continue system operations. The transition was painful and traumatic, and has resulted in serious scars which will not be quickly forgotten. The patients, however, were never affected and the service to the hospital has been uninterrupted.

MEDICAL INFORMATION SYSTEMS

RALPH R. GRAMS

CORRIGENDUM

p. 42   Fig. 19. The top of the figure is on the right inside margin. Rotate 90 to view properly.

p. 147   Fig. 68. Rotate the figure 180° to view properly.

p. 157   Fig. 76. Rotate the figure 180° to view properly.

p. 167   Fig. 86. The omitted figure is printed below.

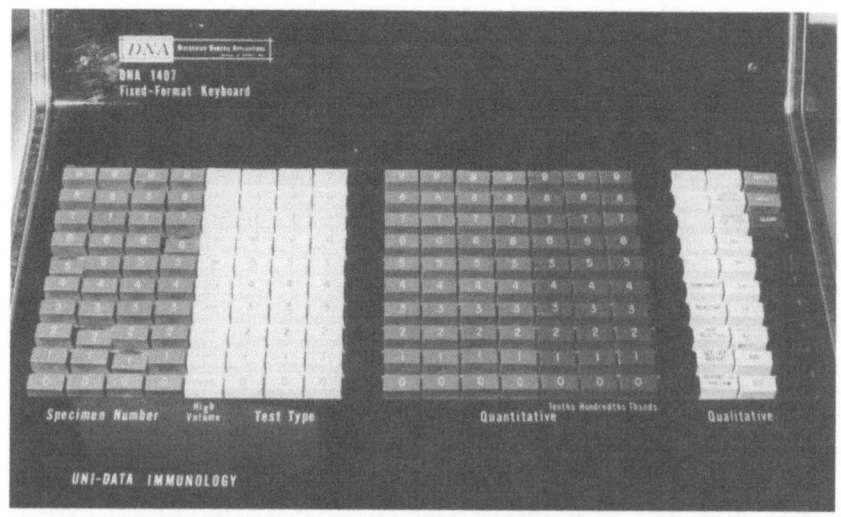

p. 277   Exhibit II C5, which appears on p. 280, should appear following Exhibit II C4 on this page.

21

Back-up System

INTRODUCTION

An alternate system which can be used in cases of hardware or software failure is absolutely essential in developing a well-integrated program. It is inappropriate for a hospital to rely upon computer equipment even if it is 100% redundant, since a time will come when this is not enough. It is much more reassuring to know that a system exists which can handle the hospital in case of failure. It is also appropriate in the development of a reserve system to provide a military (SAC)-like testing phase for the hospital such that each individual is aware of the necessary requirements for manual systems success. After many months of working with our system, it has been possible to develop several levels of back-up which we hope will never be used, but which are always ready for action.

HARDWARE ROTATION

It is very important in a communications system to be able to divert functions from one peripheral unit to another. We have found that

peripheral units such as printers, tape drives, and label makers have a much higher degree of failure than do the central CPU, controller, power supply, and drum units. It is very helpful to be able to divert from a high-speed line printer to a medium- or low-speed printer if the case should arise. Such alternatives will certainly not be as fast, but should do the job until the main hardware is fully repaired. Our system design planned for the ability to rotate a report usually produced on a line printer, to a label printer, a magnetic tape, or a disc cartridge. Using this process the system can copy any of the main documents and bring them back after the peripheral terminal is repaired. The system can also divert from magnetic tape to disc cartridge. If the tape drive should break down, the operations supervisor can execute a transfer to the disc cartridge and still keep the system on-line. As additional protection, any of the peripheral terminals can be switched with our back-up units on carts. Within the laboratory, most terminals can serve double duty in terms of data entry, so that if one particular terminal should be disabled, a parallel terminal in another laboratory can be used.

SCHEDULING OF SPARE PARTS

It is important to evaluate with each vendor the number of spare parts required to maintain full operation. One should have a complete inventory of elements, such as boards, chips, and resistors. In this regard, our system has a very unique problem in dealing with a spare drum that is in storage in Atlanta, Ga. After checking with Eastern Airlines, the drum was found to be too large to be flown to Gainesville. A smaller box must be used to accommodate the cargo doors on our arriving airplanes. Such problems are not uncommon and one would be wise to plan ahead to make absolutely certain that parts can be delivered on time and in one piece. Similarly, it is important to have the service staff well aware of the flight schedules in and out of the site since each installation is dependent on the airlines for many of the more expensive pieces of repair equipment.

SERVICE CONTRACT

Our service representative maintains a periodic maintenance program for all the peripheral terminals so that they are properly oiled and cleaned, and that parts are preventively replaced before they fail. Such a program has been highly successful and has decreased our overtime service expense.

MANUAL SYSTEMS

Our original concept of the back-up system has changed over the last six to eight months. We had intended to use our mark-sense cards for manual input once the system was running so that we could reload the patient data files and execute all the proper steps necessary to recreate the charts if ever necessary. Analysis was done on the actual time required to handle the cards, execute admissions, discharges, and transfers on a daily basis, and do the necessary housekeeping of the system. This study showed it required four to six hours on the system to catch-up for each day down. This could be dropped drastically if other means were available for manual input. Without another computer system or more highly-automated input factor, the mark-sense card was probably the cheapest loading form, yet too slow in comparison to the dynamics of the whole system. What this has done is create the necessity of two back-up systems; one which exists for approximately 24 hours or less, and the other which becomes active after 24 hours (Appendix V).

Less Than 24 Hours

Of course, we never know what the time delay is going to be during down time; therefore, we plan for the worst case. The following system begins immediately when the hardware fails and the system is inoperative.

First, all orders placed on the system use exactly the same forms for input. The doctors evidence no change in their daily activity. They circle and check those tests they require and place the sheets on the charts as usual. The clerks take those sheets and decide whether the order is stat or routine. If the order is stat, the notation on the sheet is observed for the tube required and the appropriate tube is drawn, labeled with the patient's name through the addressograph plate, and taken directly to the laboratory. For those items on the blood drawing list, the form is placed in a special basket on the floor. In the laboratory, the check-in window screens specimens and order sheets to make sure they contain the physician's name, the ward on which the patient is located, and the proper data. A portable Xerox machine transported to the check-in area now creates a billing copy from the order sheet. The tube and the primary order are then passed to each separate laboratory. A separate order sheet is used for each major laboratory. The labs receive the tubes plus the order sheet, which has full identification data, and transcribe this onto work sheets. The results are recorded directly on the order sheet in the box titled results. Those orders that are stat are called

directly back to the floor. While answers are being transcribed, a mark-sense card is coded with the appropriate information and placed in a deck for each lab area. Certain areas have difficulties with this system, and automatically switch over to the manual cumulative reporting card which is conveniently arranged for their data. Microbiology experiences this problem, as does Hematology with the differential count. In the case of Hematology, we staple or tape the Coulter card with the appropriate differential information directly to the order form for subsequent transmittal.

At the end of the day, the completed order/result forms are stamped "FINAL REPORT—DO NOT DESTROY." The original can now be sent to the floor, and the laboratory then uses its work sheets for reference. When all areas are finished, the reports are delivered for charting. The physicians can then review their data in a less than optimal manner, yet in a form which is consistent with the requirements of the manual system. In the admissions area, a Xerox copy of admissions, discharges, and transfers is kept during the period of failure.

This approach will sustain itself for about 24 hours. After that point, the only change made in the back-up system is to disregard the rebuilding of the patient files.

Greater Than 24-Hour System

If the package goes down and stays down for more than one day, we believe it is impractical to try to play catch-up since every hour only puts one further behind. In this case, we would elect to wipe the system clean and readmit the entire hospital population and start the ordering process anew. Prior to doing these two functions, we would reload the last complete system and print out all chart data on file. This would clear the data files and release the system to start anew. The old census could be retained for correction and update and the files cleared for new requests and their associated results.

Limitations

Our system relies heavily on the fact that these two back-up programs can keep us going and maintain some semblance of order. There are many problems related to this approach which cannot be fully discussed since there are intricate details involved with each step. One difficult problem is the recovery of information which is in the system at the time of failure. If the disc did not fail, it should still be viable and allow us to empty the files before reloading the system. Alternatively, we can

go back to the last drum copy that provides a complete system and take what necessary billing and chart copy we need to complete the last known information on the system. There is no question that our complex systems are extremely tricky, and the larger the system and the more complex its integration, the more painful becomes the period of failure, and the more difficult it is to bring the system back. A great deal of thought should be given to a back-up system before the purchase or implementation of any package; a poor back-up can prove a cruel Achilles' heel, and sooner or later one will be needed.

22

System Reports

WARD REPORTS

A ward report lists those studies that have been completed or are pending since the last daily chart report was issued. Figure 41 illustrates this particular document, which is distributed to the floors at noon and at midnight by the computer operations group. The format is quite different from that on the chart report and is used to minimize paper and maximize content.

DAILY CHARTS

Daily charts are produced on green striped paper to be color coded and different from that of the final charts. We use the cumulative reporting approach in some areas, and paragraph format in others. The chart program is one of the most difficult and complex parts of the whole system, and has required many months to optimize for our particular facility. We have attempted to keep the system simple and readable so that the physician does not require code numbers or extensive short-

208

hand to interpret the final document. Our system provides one page for each lab section. This is done to minimize misinterpretation. When the daily charts are brought to the floor, all old green sheets are removed and a new set is inserted. Each patient should have only one set of green barred paper of daily charts and, therefore, a maximum of six to seven separate pages per patient (see Figs. 61–63, 69–72, 79–81, 87, 88, 91, and 96).

SEVEN-DAY OR FINAL CHARTS

At 11 PM each day the system generates the seven-day/final charts, which purges the files and allows the patients to have additional data entry and requests. A patient can have up to 48 requests pending and a maximum of 165 results before the file capacity is exceeded. The 48-test maximum is an important part of the whole system since 12 or 24 is insufficient for many of the patients on medicine or in the surgical ICU areas. Request overflow usually occurs because of the high number of pending microbiology orders. Any of these may take five to ten days to clear the system.

ADTL

The Admission/Discharge/Transfer/Leave report is printed twice a day and gives a current listing of all the changes in regards to these four functions. This can be used by hospital admissions and accounting to make the necessary updates in their systems (Fig. 98).

ABNORMAL TEST REPORT

The abnormal test reports are only called on demand. The utility of this report has not been appreciated since almost all of our patients have some abnormal data and are on the report.

SMAC-SEQUENTIAL MULTIPLE ANALYZER WITH COMPUTER

Our SMAC paper-tape interface creates its own report on the high-speed line printer as the paper tape is processed. This particular function is

```
              ADTL  REPORT     ADMIT                    07/21/76

  307010  AXXXXX, SIDNEY E             1908505 H561C  00 M 19Y  SYBAVITIS L-KN
  510                                  07/19/76  10:40

  249962  SXXXM DWIGHT L               1908588 H561B  00 M 26Y  INFECTER OSTEO
  510                                  07/19/76  10:41

  268179  XXXX, LEWIS                  SS-0000 OPCLU  00 M 75Y  NOT GIVEN
  794                                  07/19/76  10:43

  106354  HXXXXXX, DEBBIE R            1908561 A634A  00 F 12Y  NONE GIVEN
  999                                  07/19/76  10:45

  308855  KXXXXXXXX, JOAN              00-0000 OPCLO  00 F 23Y  DIABETES
  223                                  07/19/76  10:53

  308858  KXXXXXXX, MARGUERITE         MM-0000 EMRMX  00 F 64Y  LUMPIN THROAT
  657                                  07/19/76  10:54

  308803  WXXXXX, RICHARD N.           00-0000 EMRMX  00 M 43Y  KIDNEY
  514                                  07/19/76  10:55

  308848  BXXXXXX, KATHY J             1908898 A312B  00 F 05Y  W/BT-CLS HUMERUS
  510                                  07/19/76  10:56
```

FIG. 98 The admission–discharge–transfer–leave report can be printed at any time, and lists those patients who have changed status since the previous report.

called from the master console and each individual element of the SMAC profile is matched against the patient's request file to determine whether that particular test has been selected. If it has, the test is read into the file, verified, and passed immediately to the patient's report file.

DISC COPY

The disc copy creates a replica of all the files and programs on a magnetic tape which can be dismounted and kept in a locked cabinet. A fireproof vault is used for this purpose in the event that there should be a fire in the computer room or lab area which would quickly destroy any tape. The system has the ability to divert the copy to the disc cartridge unit and utilize a removable disc-cartridge platter for storage.

DOCTOR REPORTS

The central processing unit was programmed to allow physicians a ward report by doctor number of all their patients in the hospital, clinics, and emergency room areas. This was designed to be used for rounds by major services in the hospital and was a direct result of the system study which found hundreds of medical students, residents, and interns in the laboratory digging through all of our data files trying to come up with results for rounds. Now it is strictly a matter of calling in the doctor

```
SURGICAL              WARD REPORT              07/23/76        14:42      PAGE 1
DOCTOR:  DXXXX, D


H635A    OXXXXXX, ASTON,                  MEDICAL RECORD # 147138

HEMOGRAM                        07/23/76      07:45
    HGB    GM            9.7* GM               07/23/76   07:45
    HCT    %            29.7* PERCENT          07/23/76   07:45
    RBC    10X6/CMM  3.50* 10X6/CMM            07/23/76   07:45
    WBC    10X3/CMM    9.7 10X3/CMM            07/23/76   07:45
    MCV    CUB MIC      85 CUB MIC             07/23/76   07:45
    MCH MC MC GM       27.7 MC MC GM           07/23/76   07:45
    MCHC   %           32.7 PERCENT            07/23/76   07:45
NA     MEQ/L            137 MEQ/L              07/23/76   07:45
K  MEQ/L                4.4 MEQ/L              07/23/76   07:45
CL MEQ/L                100 MEQ/L             07/23/76   07:45
CO2    MEQ/L             26 MEQ/L              07/23/76   07:45
BUN  MG/DL               14 MG/DL             07/23/76   07:45
CREATININE  MG/DL       1.3 MG/DL             07/23/76   07:45
BLOOD CULTURE      REQUEST RECEIVED           07/17/76   17:30
BLOOD CULTURE      REQUEST RECEIVED           07/17/76   10:15
```

FIG. 99   The physicians each have their own doctor number and can call their own ward reports. This document lists all the patient information since the last chart report was generated. This is usually called in the computer room, but can be made available on the nursing station.

number, giving us approximately 15 minutes to run the individual report, and then picking this up at the appropriate time (Fig. 99).

CORRECTING THE PATIENT'S DATA FILES

The only persons allowed to access the patient data files are the computer operators and the service representative from the company. This function is exercised only if mistakes have been made in data entry or problems have occurred in the software which require file manipulation. These are carefully documented to ensure that any information changed or modified is in fact the correct material and is not a clerical problem. It is very important to protect this function since it is a security issue and could be of legal significance (Fig. 100).

WORK SHEETS

Work sheets are called in the morning immediately following blood drawing and are separately executed for each lab. This allows the divisions to schedule work sheets in close proximity to the daily work schedule (see Figs. 28, 29, 56–58, 66, 67, 84, and 85).

OB/GYN   JXXXXX, GERALDINE *   15189R   RESULT LISTING

#	Code	Test	Value	Units	Date	Time
0001	444	QUAL HCG			09/12/76	12115
0002	753	SP/GR-U	1,035		09/12/76	12115
0003	754	HCG-QUAL	NEG		09/12/76	12115
0004	75	NA MEQ/L	136	MEQ/L	09/12/76	12115
0005	76	K MEQ/L	4.1	MEQ/L	09/12/76	12115
0006	77	CL MEQ/L	92*	MEQ/L	09/12/76	12115
0007	78	CO2 MEQ/L	24	MEQ/L	09/12/76	12115
0008	79	BUN MG/DL	8*	MG/DL	09/12/76	12115
0009	80	CREATININE MG/DL	0.9	MG/DL	09/12/76	12115
0010	84	GLUCOSE MG/DL	129*	MG/DL	09/12/76	12115
0011	85	T PROT GM/DL	7.1	GM/DL	09/12/76	12115
0012	86	ALBUMIN GM/DL	4.0	GM/DL	09/12/76	12115
0013	89	T BIL MG/DL	2.2*	MG/DL	09/12/76	12115
0014	90	D BIL MG/DL	0.3	MG/DL	09/12/76	12115
0015	91	ALK PHOS IU/L	48	IU/L	09/12/76	12115
0016	92	TOT LDH IU/L	173	MIU/ML	09/12/76	12115
0017	93	SGOT IU/L	11	IU/L	09/12/76	12115
0018	94	SGPT IU/L	6	IU/L	09/12/76	12115
0019	1	HEMOGRAM			09/12/76	12115
0020	5	WBC 10X3/CMM	5.0	10X3/CMM	09/12/76	12115
0021	4	RBC 10X6/CMM	4.98	10X6/CMM	09/12/76	12115
0022	9	HGB GM	14.0	GM	09/12/76	12115
0023	3	HCT %	41.9	PERCENT	09/12/76	12115
0024	997	MCV CUB MIC	84	CUB MIC	09/12/76	12115
0025	996	MCH MC MC GM	28.1	MC MC GM	09/12/76	12115
0026	995	MCHC %	33.4	PERCENT	09/12/76	12115
0027	11	ESR			09/12/76	12115
0028	974	ESRU MM/HR	44	MM/HR	09/12/76	12115
0029	973	ESRC MM/HR	FL NTF		09/12/76	12115
0030	994	DIFF-POLY	50	PERCENT	09/12/76	12115
0031	993	BANDS %	37	PERCENT	09/12/76	12115
0032	992	LYMPHS %	9	PERCENT	09/12/76	12115
0033	991	MONOS %	4	PERCENT	09/12/76	12115
0034	979	MORPHOLOGY	VAC IN CYTO		09/12/76	12115
0035	979	MORPHOLOGY	RBC + PLAT NORM		09/12/76	12115
0036	1	HEMOGRAM			09/13/76	08115
0037	5	RBC 10X3/CMM	12.1*	10X3/CMM	09/13/76	08115
0038	4	RBC 10X6/CMM	4.61	10X6/CMM	09/13/76	08115
0039	2	HGB GM	12.9	GM	09/13/76	08115
0040	3	HCT %	39.0	PERCENT	09/13/76	08115
0041	997	MCV CUB MIC	85	CUB MIC	09/13/76	08115
0042	996	MCH MC MC GM	28.0	MC MC GM	09/13/76	08115
0043	995	MCHC %	33.1	PERCENT	09/13/76	08115
0044	994	DIFF-POLY	70	PERCENT	09/13/76	08115
0045	993	BANDS %	21	PERCENT	09/13/76	08115
0046	992	LYMPHS %	9	PERCENT	09/13/76	08115
0047	979	MORPHOLOGY	RBC + PLAT NORM		09/13/76	08115
0048	979	MORPHOLOGY	PLATLTS CLUMPED		09/13/76	08115
0049	89	T BIL MG/DL	1.9*	MG/DL	09/13/76	08115
0050	90	D BIL MG/DL	0.4*	MG/DL	09/13/76	08115
0051	91	ALK PHOS IU/L	50	IU/L	09/13/76	08115
0052	92	TOT LDH IU/L	149	MIU/ML	09/13/76	08115
0053	93	SGOT IU/L	17	IU/L	09/13/76	08115
0054	94	SGPT IU/L	4*	IU/L	09/13/76	08115
0055	11	ESR			09/13/76	08115
0056	974	ESRU MM/HR	99	MM/HR	09/13/76	08115
0057	973	ESRC MM/HR	FL TF		09/13/76	08115
0058	292	VDRL	+ RCT		09/13/76	08115

FIG. 100 For auditing the patient's record on computer storage, a special result listing provides all the significant data in block format so that any corrections or errors can be handled through the system software.

CENSUS

Census reports are called daily and distributed to Admissions, Pharmacy, and Dietary. A copy of the census list is also sent to the information desk at the hospital, and provides a convenient means of tracking patients and answering phone calls (see Fig. 32).

ARCHIVE INPUT

In order to maintain an accurate archive file of patient microfilm data, it was necessary for the night and evening computer operators to load into the files the appropriate patient information along with the magnetic cartridge and page number for subsequent retrieval. This operation averaged approximately four hours a day for the inpatient service (Fig. 101).

When we tried to extend this manual input to outpatients and Emergency Room patients, there was too much work involved. This problem forced the creation of an automated system for data handling [31].

```
02:11 ENTER KEYBOARD     06/13/76

02:11 F   385731   MXXXXXX, IRENE * 14   06/13/76

ENTRY ACCEPTED

02:12 ENTER KEYBOARD     06/13/76

02:12 F   385731   0012   0115   04/07/76   I   PYLONIDAL CYST   06/13/76


ENTRY ACCEPTED

02:12 ENTER KEYBOARD   06/13/76

02:12 F 482915   GXXXX, MELISSA J   F   06   06/13/76

ENTRY ACCEPTED

02:12 ENTER KEYBOARD     06/13/76

02:12 F 482915   0012   06404/23/76   I   MYOCARDIAL   INFARCT   06/13/76
```

FIG. 101 The maintenance of the archive can be done manually through keyboard entry in which case, the name, medical record number, age, and sex are captured initially. This is then followed by the cartridge, page number, date, time, problem, and inpatient or outpatient designation.

23

Billing

INTRODUCTION

There are many different techniques of interfacing billing. The most exotic is direct hardware connection in which we send the data instantly to another computer system so that they can accomplish our billing. In looking over the cost of direct connection and the great complexity of interfacing two data centers, it became apparent that the only convenient mode of exchange was the use of magnetic tapes.

TAPE HANDLING

Twice a day we generate a magnetic tape which contains all the billing information required for both hospital and professional fee billing (Fig. 102). The tape is called twice a day so that the volume of charges does not overflow the system. Files are set up to hold approximately 1800 charges before the buffer is exceeded and the data are lost. On slow days, only one tape is required.

214

```
 BILLING REPORT      12:46        11/24/76
 I1539749  038573640   304967  SXXX, MAY                DIABETES MELL
 I1539687  038578294   395683  WXXXXXXXX, SHIRLEY A      FAMIAL PARALYSIS
 I1539689  038578294   395683  WXXXXXXXX, SHIRLEY A      FAMIAL PARALYSIS
 I1549386  035874930   495827  GXXXX, HERBERT *          POSS/FX FEMUR
 I1539683  035783920   395861  LXXXXX, GARY R            XPULMONARY DIS
 I1539683  035783920   395861  LXXXXX, GARY R            XPULMONARY DIS
 I1539482  035874622   496827  FXXXXXX, JOSEPH *         STROKE
 I1549386  035874930   495827  GXXXX, HERBERT *          POSS/FX FEMUR
 I1539749  039573640   304967  SXXX, MAY                DIABETES MELL
 I1538596  038592746   388726  SXXXXX, PATRICIA A        RETINAL EMBOLUS
 I1548396  038579402   496821  FXXXXXX, CASSANDRA Y      RENAL RAILURE
 I1549285  038574920   395861  PXXXXX, WANDA G           PELVIC ABSCESS
 I1549285  038574920   395861  PXXXXX, WANDA G           PELVIC ABSCESS
 I1549285  038574920   395861  PXXXXX, WANDA G           PELVIC ABSCESS
 I1549285  038574920   395861  PXXXXX, WANDA G           PELVIC ABSCESS
 I1538499  038579208   069284  VXXXXXXX, JAMES           CORORY ART-DIS
 I1539582  038569384   404287  OXXXX, EARL J             CHF
 I1543295  038539204   204851  WXXXXXXXX, RUTH A         MYELOFIBROSIS
 I1523859  038574320   391148  SXXXXX, ROOSEVELT *       CHEST PAIN
 I1523859  038574320   391148  SXXXXX, ROOSEVELT *       CHEST PAIN
```

FIG. 102   Billing is done daily onto magnetic tape with the hardcopy verification available after the tape is made. The problem is captured on the bill by order and subsequently reviewable by a third party if requested. Special information is carried in the billing header to indicate whether the test is a stat procedure or whether the item is a credit.

The tape handling procedure is simple, yet critical, since this particular step is one of extremely high visibility. All one need do is lose a billing tape just once to see the wrath of the hospital accountants. There is nothing glamorous about going through a whole set of order sheets with a key punch operator trying to figure out what and who to charge.

To minimize this possibility, we have designed a tape handling routine that gives us maximum assurance of the final product. When the program is called to create billing, the appropriate billing information is transferred from the files to the magnetic tape. Then the entire reel is rewound and what is on the magnetic tape is read back to the line printer. Therefore, if there is nothing on the magnetic tape, nothing will print. Likewise, if the appropriate billing is on the tape, the line printer will verify this fact. We then keep a copy of the billing print-out and send the duplicate with the tape to the hospital and the professional fee services.

When the system was just starting, about four or five tapes went down to the hospital billing group and were called blanks. Our systems group provided hard copy audit trail and insisted that the tapes were valid. Subsequently, the hospital tape drives were inspected and found to be malfunctioning. One small special sequence of write, read, and print instructions in the billing cycle renders the whole process simple and reliable.

INTERFACE

Our tape drive is 1600-BPI phase-encoded 25-ips IBM compatible and the tape is sent directly to an Amdahl 470-V6 system using a SHAS hospital accounting package. This bookkeeping package subsequently spins off another tape which is sent to a remote site for Pathology professional fee billing. This whole tape-interface system is so convenient that we would never consider going to hardware on-line interfacing. The fact that the tapes can be handled, batched, stored, read, and reread with minimal effort produces a highly reliable operation. In a practical sense, our system has no other data center to halt our active schedule, yet the minicomputer can talk to all of them by tape through batch-mode processing.

Archive Retrieval

INTRODUCTION

With the use of communication systems, heavy loads are placed on the medical record room to keep pace with the volume of paper generated. It is easy to produce large stacks of documents and pass these on to others to handle. Because of the manual system overload, a new approach has evolved that could ultimately replace manual charting and storage of historical medical documents.

INPUTS

The archive retrieval system designed for the laboratory incorporates a basic principle that can be extended to the entire hospital medical record system, yet is only being used at this time for laboratory work. Once a patient is discharged, the now inactive files are entered into our archive system through manual keyboard entry in the central computer room. The following data is stored: name, age, sex, problem, date of service, outpatient or inpatient code, and microfilm page and cartridge number on which one would find the appropriate laboratory information.

OUTPUT

When an archive entry is made, it is merged by computer with similar information, which is kept on a long-term archive file on disc cartridge. This is sorted in such a manner that multiple entries for the same patient are placed together. During the retrieval process on a peripheral terminal the doctor will find that for a selected medical-record number (see Fig. 50) the data is arranged so the most recent entry is first on the list. Using only the problem field, it is possible to do a quick problem-oriented review of the patient's history. From this copy those pages one would wish to review are then selected. Using a peripheral reader-printer and the proper cartridge, entry of the page number will result in the patient's data being displayed on a screen (Figs. 103 and 104). Our reader printer allows hard copy within 20 seconds if requested.

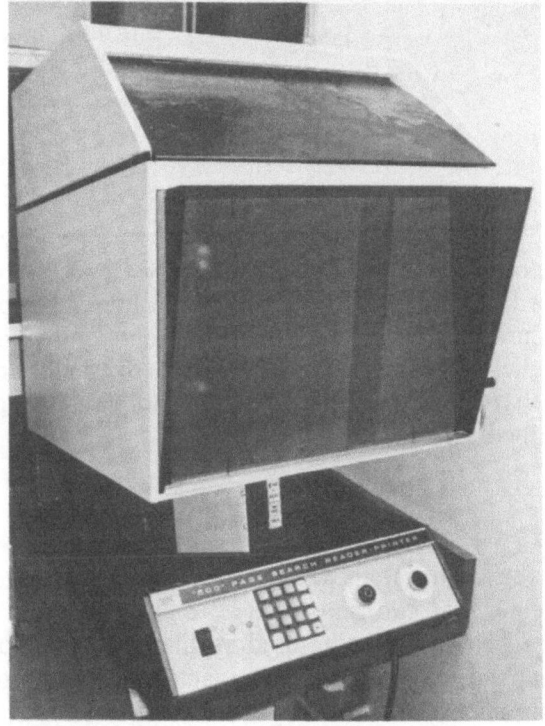

FIG. 103 For review of archival records, a microfilm reader printer is available in a security facility that maintains 24-hour/day access for physicians or qualified individuals.

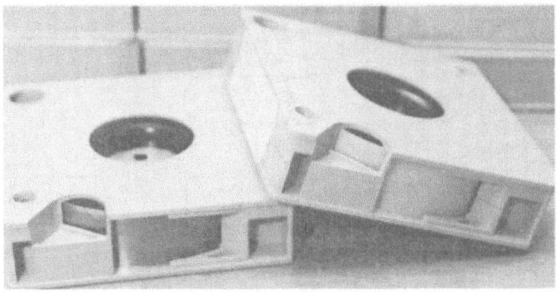

FIG. 104   The microfilm cartridges are small convenient media of storage and can maintain up to one month's total transactions per cartridge.

MICROFILM PROCESSING

To make this program function, we originally used the carbon copy of the seven-day/final chart reports and sorted these into hanging files in a file cabinet by medical record number. When the patient was discharged and a final chart appeared, the patient's file was pulled and run through our microfilm camera located in the laboratory. The camera designates a page number by blip coding the bottom of the film. A log sheet was made for each particular patient, which was then transmitted to the computer operators for entry in the archive system. Along with the filming of the seven-day/final charts, we also filmed a copy of each day's ADTL report, each day's purge results, all laboratory work for outpatients by day of the week, and all laboratory work for emergency room patients. Originally, we did not catalog outpatients for long-term archive retrieval because of the sheer volume of manual input.

MICROFILM/COMPUTER INTERFACE

Today's modern technology offers a whole host of alternatives in automating this entire manual archiving system. We have currently achieved a tape copy of our seven-day/final chart which is then transmitted to an IBM 370 system and a separate file is then made of all these particular documents for long-term archive retrieval. From that secondary tape comes another tape which sent to a special COM (Computer Output Microform) machine which can generate microfilm from computer tape. In the process of generating that secondary COM tape, we also produce an IBM 370 archive index of unlimited size. By

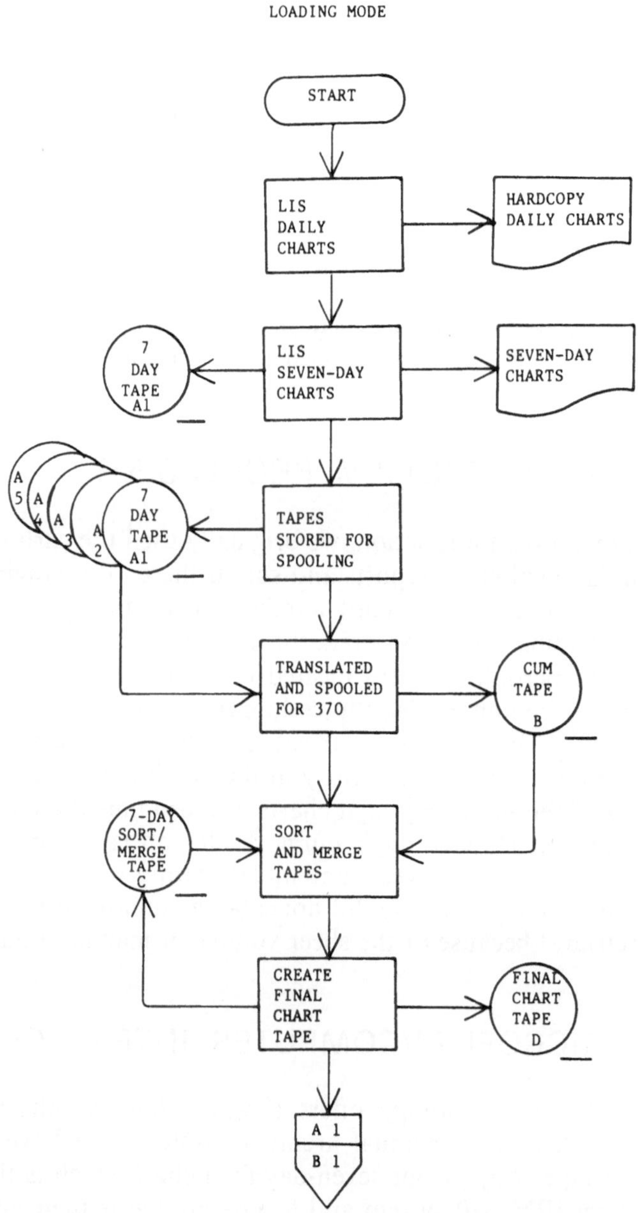

LOADING MODE

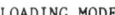

```
                        ┌──────────────┐
                        │    START     │
                        └──────┬───────┘
                               │
                               ▼
   ┌────────────┐       ┌──────────────┐       ┌──────────────┐
   │            │       │ LIS          │──────▶│ HARDCOPY     │
   │            │       │ DAILY        │       │ DAILY CHARTS │
   │            │       │ CHARTS       │       └──────────────┘
   │            │       └──────┬───────┘
   │            │              │
   │            │              ▼
  ┌──────┐      ┌──────────────┐       ┌──────────────┐
  │  7   │◀─────│ LIS          │──────▶│ SEVEN-DAY    │
  │ DAY  │      │ SEVEN-DAY    │       │ CHARTS       │
  │ TAPE │      │ CHARTS       │       └──────────────┘
  │  A1  │      └──────┬───────┘
  └──────┘             │
                       ▼
 ┌──────┐       ┌──────────────┐
 │  7   │◀──────│ TAPES        │
 │ DAY  │       │ STORED FOR   │
 │ TAPE │       │ SPOOLING     │
 │  A1  │       └──────┬───────┘
 └──────┘              │
    │                  ▼
    │         ┌──────────────┐       ┌──────┐
    └───────▶ │ TRANSLATED   │──────▶│ CUM  │
              │ AND SPOOLED  │       │ TAPE │
              │ FOR 370      │       │  B   │
              └──────┬───────┘       └──┬───┘
                     │                  │
 ┌──────┐            ▼                  │
 │7-DAY │     ┌──────────────┐          │
 │SORT/ │◀──▶ │ SORT         │◀─────────┘
 │MERGE │     │ AND MERGE    │
 │TAPE  │     │ TAPES        │
 │  C   │     └──────┬───────┘
 └──────┘            │
    ▲                ▼
    │         ┌──────────────┐       ┌──────┐
    └─────────│ CREATE       │──────▶│FINAL │
              │ FINAL        │       │CHART │
              │ CHART        │       │TAPE  │
              │ TAPE         │       │  D   │
              └──────┬───────┘       └──────┘
                     │
                     ▼
                ┌─────────┐
                │  A 1    │
                │  B 1    │
                └────┬────┘
                     ▽
```

FIG. 105 The handling of the archive system begins with the creation of the daily charts. As the result file fills up or the patient remains beyond seven days, the Laboratory Information System then creates a blue copy or seven-day chart and sends this to magnetic tape which is subsequently printed on paper. The paper charts are distributed to the floors and the magnetic tape is stored and spooled on an Amdahl 470. The cumulative tape B goes through daily sorts and merges to create a series of highly organized records that are available on final chart tape D.

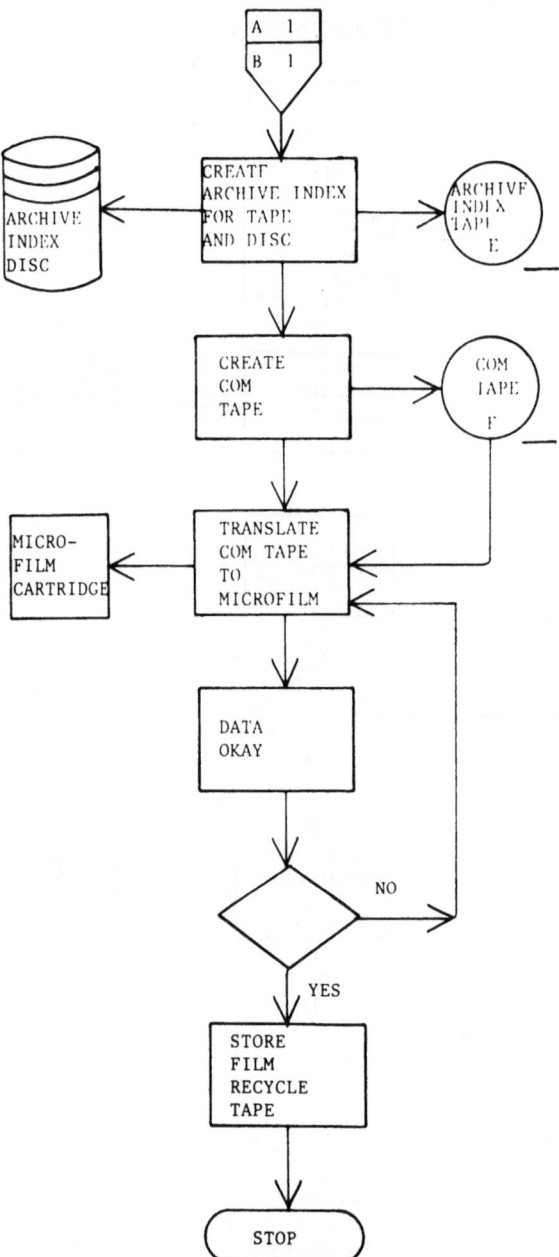

FIG. 106 From the final tape, an archive tape is created and kept on disc pack which allows access through both the medical record number and name. From this archival information and this data tape, a computer on-line microform (COM) tape is created and sent to a COM facility to create the microfilm cartridges. The data is verified and the film is entered into our archival storage room for permanent access.

INQUIRY MODE

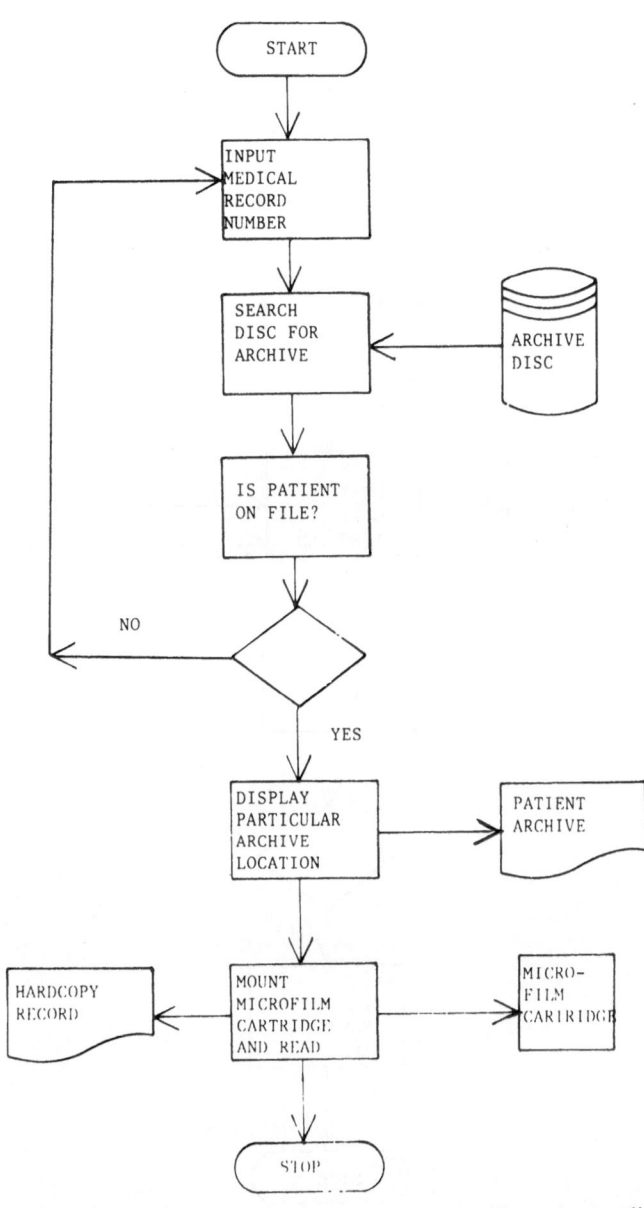

FIG. 107 The inquiry mode of the archive system utilizes the medical record number which then searches the archive disc for the appropriate patient file. This then displays the appropriate archival location and the microfilm cartridge is utilized to achieve either a visual or hardcopy display of information.

linking our minicomputer to a 370, one can access the archive when needed as well as the IBM resident patient data (Figs. 105–107). Through this process, we have accomplished the following objectives:

1. A completely-automated hands-off system for capturing all laboratory data on microfilm.

2. A completely-automated indexing system that will sustain the laboratory record system indefinitely.

3. A long-term archive system maintained on IBM-370 tapes which can be manipulated for quality control purposes, special medical data studies, laboratory utilization reviews, and epidemiologic reports.

In addition to the obvious uses for this mass storage and manipulation capability, we find we have additional flexibility in being able to relieve the real-time system of this kind of bulk information, yet still not totally lose control of it. Any number of scientific studies can be conducted on this data base, which will of course hold all the critical parameters during a patient's stay in the hospital, clinic, or emergency room. Such information will prove invaluable in looking at epidemiological problems, research of clinical areas, quality control programs within the laboratory, and general statistical routines handling the evaluation and utilization of laboratory information.

25

Departmental Requirements

INTRODUCTION

In looking at the medical data-processing field—the equipment, the requirements, and the expectations—it seems certain that every laboratory of any major size eventually will have to go through an integration program with a communication system. We believe we have accomplished this phase of our growth and development, and have only been able to survive and persevere because of the individual input of every member of the department, and their concern and desire to see this program accomplished.

ORGANIZATION

The department chairperson becomes the key figure in the installation of a laboratory system since it will require all the authority, power, and dominance of the position to guide and control the individual participants in the program. The chairperson must have unwavering faith in those selected for the job, and must be willing to put the requisite time

and effort into supporting these people and providing the necessary manpower to get the job accomplished. It takes a minimum of one physician and one full-time experienced systems analyst to put together the necessary files and organizational structure for the department to make it a success. At the time the system is installed, the full time services of a coordinator will be necessary to handle the integration of the laboratory and the various nursing units. This team of three should be tied in with the service representative and the chief computer operator to make a viable unit of five to support and sustain the operation. Any fewer than this creates a serious crisis of control and management which could place the project in jeopardy.

CONTROL AND MONITORING

The initial design and installation group should not shrink in size after the job is done. If the system is to be viable, it must be constantly monitored and evaluated for changes that occur in the hospital environment. As the system matures, changes will be requested, and these must be discussed in terms of the systems concept of the entire program to determine whether these are viable, hazardous, or of marginal benefit. Only an experienced systems staff can make realistic recommendations for software and hardware development.

START-UP AND TRAINING

To maximize our effect, the systems group attempted to indoctrinate, sell, train, brainwash, and otherwise stimulate every faculty member of the department of pathology to understand and cooperate with the implementation of the entire systems program and approach. One week before start-up, all faculty members were gathered in the evening for hands-on training on the system. They were taught how to order lab work, how to check it in, how work sheets were called, and how to input patient results. This turned out to be a fascinating experience for most, since many had been peripherally involved in the system and contributed in some way to the test files, but yet had never had their hands on the hardware to see what it was really like. Enthusiasm was high.

The second part of the program was the implementation of a call schedule for the entire department. Every member of the faculty was scheduled in the hospital for a block of time making rounds on the floors to review the operation of the system. Even the Pathology

Department head participated. The internists and surgeons were shocked to find pathologists making rounds at two and three in the morning on Saturday and Sunday. To make this a scientific venture, we provided each one of the rounding teams with check lists so that they could evaluate every terminal in the hospital, every nursing station, and record any complaints that arose. The problems that developed were brought back to the systems group for immediate discussion and, in some fashion, resolution. The program was a success in creating a highly positive environment in the hospital.

HOUSE STAFF ORIENTATION

Approximately two months before the system was initiated, the house staff was mailed a detailed handout regarding the entire operation. What a failure! Hundreds of these must have ended in garbage cans, since by the time the system was ready to be launched, no one in the residency group was even aware that it existed. We suffered greatly during the first month of operation because of this lack of education.

KNOW YOUR COMPANY

The undertaking and the installation of a computer system requires the marriage of a company and a hospital on an extremely intimate basis. For the project leader it is even more critical, since the company is not a nameless entity, but is a select group of people who have to be dealt with daily. In some cases, on a very crisis-oriented basis. As program director, one must know the financial backing of the company to be certain that the project will be completed and the corporate group will not file bankruptcy halfway down the line. Of course, there are no guarantees in this area. Those who have a strong parent company and corporate backing are certainly in a much better position to survive, yet this is still no absolute protection. Large conglomerates often divest themselves of corporations and send their customers packing. Caveat Emptor still is a good watchword.

Understand the service obligations of the company and learn how they work. Our particular approach requires that equipment be kept on-site for repairs, and in this particular situation, the serviceman becomes a key person. Be very careful in your selection if you have the choice, since this person becomes an essential member of the laboratory team working daily with the technologists and physicians when the hardware

and software malfunction. Since it is such an intimate relationship, it is my belief that the service contract should contain an additional clause allowing the laboratory to help select an individual for its site.

Further, the project manager should maintain a very close surveillance of the corporate structure and know who is being promoted and what projects are being accepted by the main vendor. Keep track of the names, phone numbers, and addresses of all the corporate principals as well as the sales force, and try to understand the normal chain of command. I would not be satisfied unless I had the name, address, and telephone number of the corporation president.

Why gather this kind of data? When the chips are down, the system does not work, the patients are suffering, and the doctors are gathering for a lynching, the project leader has no choice but to pick up the phone and call anybody who will listen. If you have selected a responsive company, this may never come to pass. In all likelihood, this list will be invaluable as one works through the various levels of difficulty in ironing out some of the problems involved with any of these complex systems.

CORPORATE PROBLEMS

Corporations should not be viewed as good or evil. They exist with one thought in mind—to make money. You cannot fault them for this objective since you and I buy stock in them and insist that they have high gross earnings and be profit oriented. In many cases, the hospital and its pathologists do not understand this and make the wrong supposition in trying to interpret a company's motives and actions. Most companies in hospital systems are not making big money, but losing money because of the extreme demands and high expectations. Most corporations have not learned how to handle 24-hour a day coverage of hardware and systems, and have not learned to build hardware cheaply and redundantly enough that it will sustain itself during periods of failure.

Like our own health system, most larger corporations are highly bureaucratic and are not geared to pick up and solve problems expeditiously. It is common to find them procrastinating on issues, passing the buck, and producing nothing. One difficult area to deal with is the hardware–software issue, which turns up time and time again. In a typical scenario, the machine does not appear to be printing documents correctly, or it does something undesirable to the files. You call the vendor and state that you have a problem. They send a programmer out to look at it. (If you are fortunate.) The programmer reviews the

information, tests the system a while, and says it is perfectly all right. Therefore, it is obviously a hardware problem. The hardware expert is summoned, puts on some test programs, checks a few voltages, pulls out a number of bays, hooks up a scope, and suddenly declares that the hardware is functional, and that it must be a software problem! Around and around the merry-go-round goes. Caught in the middle is the pathologist, trying to fend off angry physicians and their compromised patients. This situation becomes even more difficult when companies are dealing with primary software, and have no hardware production capability. Here you must deal with two corporations who do not necessarily agree to cooperate. I wish I had an easy solution because this problem certainly exists today, and I expect it will continue to bedevil us in the future.

Another interesting tactic that computer corporations use is the "turn it off syndrome." If anything goes wrong, their first recommendation is to shut the system down and then start it up again. For us this means a tremendous amount of work, loading all the files, reloading all the patient admissions data, and trying to recover from the whole mess. The programmers like to suggest this if they think anything has gotten into the file structure and might be working its way through destroying other parts of files. This is rather like an infection without antibiotic coverage. One area can begin and infect another until the entire set of files is destroyed. We have had this recommendation made on our system twice, and have stayed up all night evaluating all the files only to find that they were perfectly all right and that the culprit was a non-destructive software problem. This does not mean that such a problem will not happen in the future, but in our experience, shutdown should be considered only in terms of the actual facts of the problem.

Physicians and hospitals have a great deal of difficulty in understanding why corporations do not care about patients. The altruistic goals of the hospital do not match those of a corporation. In many of our contracts, the corporation is limited to the amount of expenditures or dollars on the contract, and there is no clause that claims that patient care negates the dollars involved. This therefore limits the responsiveness of the corporation and places the hospital in a position of jeopardy.

Hospital service for both hardware and software is drastically different from industrial computer operations. Customer service groups for the hospital computer industry are going to have to be maintained 24 hours a day, seven days a week with alert, intelligent people who understand the various systems and are in a position to make some knowledgeable contributions. Parts depots must be set up for convenient transmission of basic materials to centers to support their operation.

These things are beginning to happen, but have not yet arrived in full bloom in the medical systems area. Similarly, we certainly foster and promote the concept of software maintenance houses tied to the various corporate groups dealing with the medical-information data base. These are going to become invaluable in the future in terms of conserving patient dollars, optimizing productivity, and producing the kind of working environment in which hospitals can function conveniently.

The hospital is not the natural seed bed for programming and hardware support. Its primary role is patient care. The only way the technology can easily interface with this kind of setting is to come to us with a full service program which is able to handle the problems, yet provide a realistic price for service. Likewise, hospitals must accept the fact that the costs associated with this kind of operation are not low, and will require a major budget allocation each year [32]. The alternatives are even more costly, time-consuming, and counterproductive when reviewed with respect to the totality of patient care programs.

THE MARRIAGE CONTRACT

The development of a contract for a system is a talking document which establishes a price, date, and time. Once the system is in and running, all the good words and deeds are thrown by the wayside, and only the working relationship between the individual hospital and the corporate support team will survive. A lawsuit by the hospital hung on the end of a malfunctioning computer system is totally destructive to both the vendor and the hospital. It is up to each party to resolve the issues and put the pieces back together again and proceed. This is why the selection of the vendor is extremely important, since this type of dialog and cooperative venture requires a viable corporation with long-term survival.

26

Hospital Implementation

INTRODUCTION

The narrative part of our development is being presented to give a factual account of how our system has evolved to its current state, and the types of problems and challenges that the staff and faculty faced at each juncture. This kind of information is necessarily anecdotal in nature, but I hope will be of value to those now beginning to venture into this area, and provide some yardstick by which to handle both the internal and external problems that must be anticipated in working with these large systems.

Staff

In 1973 through January 1974, the Department of Pathology systems group consisted of one physician and one experienced hospital data-processing expert. Between 1973 and 1974 a concerted effort was made to establish a contract with very tight specifications and to begin the necessary work in the hospital to start orienting the physical plant and personnel sections. It took one painful, agonizing year to obtain a

mutually agreeable contract between the State of Florida and our vendor. Each time we thought we had things worked out, one party would step off to the side and refuse to participate. Appendix I shows a copy of this contract which required uncounted hours to finalize, and which has subsequently proven to be a fairly successful prescription for the integration of a corporation and a state medical institution.

In January 1974, the contract was finally signed and the company began programming. We immediately started preparing our site so that all of the necessary materials would be available. During this period we had a chance to visit the manufacturer, view the software, match it up against our specifications, and insist on the necessary changes. Careful monitoring at this stage was critical.

A very common problem experienced with software development is the simple fact that a programmer will write whatever is personally convenient, and fail to recognize the special needs of the customer or user at the other end. A practical user-oriented piece of software is usually more expensive and time-consuming to generate than a quick and dirty program. By making frequent site visits we kept ourselves in a good position to monitor our programs and detect problems before they became insurmountable.

CASE HISTORY

During 1974, all the necessary plans and specifications were written for the computer room and the UPS battery area. This begins another incredible story about our physical plant and its ability to move on projects. Numerous letters and complaints were exchanged over this issue, and in December 1974, after 12 months of inactivity, we still had nothing to house the equipment expected in one month. By some miracle, yet to be explained, the transformation of our site occurred within two weeks; the walls went down, the ceiling went up, the draperies went in and the paint went on. On the last day, when the floor was being laid, the hardware arrived. Such split second timing was never anticipated, yet the crisis approach to planning did bail us out in the end.

The phone company had been very reliable and had promptly installed the communication lines well before the delivery of the equipment. This took approximately four months to schedule, since special cable had to be pulled throughout the hospital for a major communication systems network.

To provide a little better perspective, our systems group did have a chance to evaluate most of the programs at the factory, but many of

those did not work and we were quite concerned that the system was being shipped ahead of its final debugging. Unfortunately, the contract called for a specific time and date for delivery, and our vendor shipped according to contract.

Since an excess of 50% of the programs on the system were brand new, we very cautiously planned a long stage of development and testing to be absolutely certain that the package was going to work and that the design and plans were sound. At about this same time, we were fortunate enough to obtain the services of the patient unit coordinator for the hospital, who joined our department as a floor coordinator for the entire system. The coordinator's initial task was to prototype and test our system within the Medicine Department and the Emergency Room. This data would provide the preliminary criteria for evaluation. During this same time, each lab area was making final its test files, since the facility had just finished a major revamping of equipment and methods.

While the files were being completed, each laboratory tested its terminals. As a bit of a surprise, the hospital approved the purchase of a SMAC for delivery in the spring. This was greeted by mixed feelings, since all of us knew we needed the instrument to handle the workload, yet we had no idea how this device would interface with our communications system. This decision also necessitated the changing of all the files to match this particular device. As the files were changed again and the order sheets were modified, some of the nursing staff began training on our prototype unit. It became extremely difficult to do adequate model testing because of the staffing problems in the laboratory. We were still running a Xerox cumulative report and required secretaries in all areas. There were not enough people to staff the computer system 24 hours a day and still maintain the manual systems. During the testing phase, each lab area complained bitterly because of the lack of support.

Our initial evaluation of the system in the nursing station/emergency room area was disappointing. Many of the functions that we had anticipated would work smoothly caused problems and dissension among the laboratory personnel (see Table 1). After a week of heated debate, it was agreed that the software had to be changed if the system was to survive. As a starting point, the vendor had underestimated our requirements for files, and the system needed a second drum. The files had to be expanded to include 48 pending tests per patient since the initial prototype of 12 tests was totally unsatisfactory. We initiated the necessary correspondence in hopes of rapid resolution. As a point of fact, no additional monies were available, and the vendor elected to supply the necessary hardware to complete the contract. At this same time, our data processing department had finally decided on what kind of tape drive would be

compatible with its IBM system, and insisted that we get a 1600 BPI unit to service its billing package. Concurrently, the hospital was growing and additional wards and outpatient clinics were being added weekly. This meant that the file sizes were too small and the basic configuration was inadequate.

Looking at this from the vantage point of an active participant, I was quite sure that our communication system was burning and there was nothing we could do about it. Every new piece of information seemed to be another disaster headed our way. About midway through the Summer of 1975, our vendor agreed to continue programming and make the necessary changes to bring the system back to total capability. We did not receive the additional hardware, tape drive, or software until the end of August. At that point immediate testing of the system began.

Concurrently, the SMAC unit arrived and we were struggling to keep it operational. This unit was purchased to carry the major share of Chemistry's load, and had to be interfaced because of its large data output. We explored options and chose to use paper tape and an existing program that the vendor made available. On our initial evaluation, the standard program for our SMAC unit would not work. It had something to do with the files and the way it had been programmed at Technicon, which meant we had to rebuild the SMAC program. Finally, after getting that organized along with the necessary updates for the proper file sizes, we went through the prototype stage again and ran the nursing station and Emergency Room. This time we were considerably more successful and found that our greatest difficulty was in handling the SMAC tapes. We experienced a number of halts and loops on the system, which of course had been present since the initial installation, but had not been fully evidenced since the system had not been actively used on a daily basis.

These halts and loops were impossible. Every time the laboratory got rolling, the floors settled down, and the ordering process seemed smooth and operational—the system would suddenly die. In some cases, it would go into a state of total spasm and start an automatic core dump in which all of the core and registers were printed out on the line printer. This is similar to a state of seizure in which the electrical wires within the CPU empty out the entire bowels of the memory bank. Repeated calls and mail shipments of print-outs back and forth between our hospital and the vendor produced very little sympathy. We were learning to work with the system, but every time we got something going and believed we were making progress, a whole series of halts and loops would occur and set us back again.

At the same time, there were divergent forces within the hospital

demanding that this toy the department had purchased be turned on and utilized. The laboratory, in addition, was faced with a constantly growing workload and the technologists were anxious to get their manual systems unloaded. The secretaries and clerks wanted their raises as computer operators, and the only thing that seemed to be practical was to turn the system on.

During this time, we had been working with the hospital data-processing group to establish the viability of our magnetic tape billing system. We believed we had this fairly well documented and had a feasible program.

Around the beginning of November, it was decided that only one choice remained, turn the system on and go. This was not an easy decision since many heads were on the chopping block, mine in particular. We sent memos out to everybody in the hospital notifying them that Saturday, November 15 would be the starting day. We went through the training program for the department. Call schedules were published and protocols distributed for review.

One month before the system was to come on-line, we unilaterally initiated Emergency Room and Admissions so that they would have an adequate lead in terms of establishing their program. They were the first ones to start and were kept on the system on a permanent basis after November 15.

The day before full operation of the system was to begin, everyone was nervous, panicky, tense, and irritable. At about 1 PM, I received a frantic call from the acting hospital director informing me that I must be down in his office immediately for a serious conference. Arriving, I received an uncomplimentary verbal epithet for not adequately notifying hospital administration. I was told categorically that the system start-up must be postponed until the chief accountant of the hospital had approved our billing process. I related the fact that we had gone through an extensive program of evaluation for our billing tape and that I was satisfied that it would work. This did not seem to console them and I listened to a half hour of dialog that led me to believe that his whole program was something less than enthusiastically accepted. I left the office disgusted but determined to go ahead and told them there was nothing that was going to stop the system at this point.

November 15 arrived, the system started, the billing tapes rolled, and we were in business. Tranquility reigned on Saturday and Sunday as the reports were first generated, the ward reports were first delivered, the faculty made rounds, and everything was on schedule. The system started off with one or two halts and a couple of loops on Saturday. On Sunday the halts got worse.

It is important to mention again the conceptual change that had occurred in setting the laboratory up with a central check-in desk. We had estimated the volume involved in this centralized operation, but had not anticipated the through-put or the timing of these within the day. Monday morning came and the full load of the hospital hit the laboratory. We were up to our elbows in stools, urine, serums, plasmas, and everything else. The entire hospital laboratory load hit us like a sledgehammer. Three carts were stacked with orders, tubes, and jugs sitting in the middle of the computer room. I vividly remember the fragrant smell and the eccrine stimulation as we tried to check through the incredible pile of specimens. Every time we turned around, another courier would arrive with a cart full of goodies for the laboratory. Our initial plan was to do all the central ordering and specimen check-in for all the hospital areas until we could get the nursing station personnel trained on the system. What a mistake! We worked day and night trying to keep up with the ordering and confirmation process for the entire hospital.

The third day was a categorical flop and we had angry doctors and angry technologists everywhere. We immediately dispatched our patient coordinator to the floors to begin a crash program of training to get the floor terminals operational for ordering. Our residents were mobilized for immediate training of ward clerks. The load started to lighten and the central operation started to pick up a bit. Simultaneously, we were still experiencing an incredible number of halts, on the average of 10–15 a day and each one of the halts was followed by a 5–10 minute core dump which shut the system down completely in the hospital. This spastic activity discouraged everyone and created an environment less than optimal. As the floor terminals were starting to operate and handle their own information, we noticed another serious problem in planning —the Outpatient Clinic. We had not anticipated the volume coming from this area, and the times at which their work could be delivered. We would periodically find our own laboratory people unloading hundreds of specimens which had suddenly arrived from the clinic. These would all have to be checked in and split up among the various labs.

At that point, the outpatient area was established as a separate ordering and specimen check-in site. This allowed the outpatient lab to do its own splitting and delivery to the various areas. This took the workload off the central computer facility and gave us some breathing room.

We also experienced tremendous difficulties with our chart programs, which for some reason refused to run without halts. After three weeks of agonizing effort, we were ready to return to the manual paper system and forget we ever heard of a computer. There was no question

in our minds that this particular beast, unless it was properly tamed, was going to destroy us all. We had been working 18–20 hours a day, seven days a week slaving over this machine and receiving virtually no help from our vendor.

It seems that the company had undertaken its own series of space age problems by attempting to handle the development of a whole new software and hardware package for laboratories along with a complete hospital information system. By making these commitments, they had diverted all their resources for programming and hardware into these two areas and left us with nothing. Repeated phone calls to the plant brought absolutely no results to resolve some of our problems. After one month of screaming and hollering, the chief programmer did finally arrive from the company and within a matter of three to four hours, we had eliminated about 70% of the halts and loops. Bliss reigned supreme. The SMAC tapes, which had been impossible, now became just difficult. The chart program started to run, and the computer operators rescinded their resignations and decided to stick with it for another 30 days. At this point we regrouped our forces and decided to go through every system we had to see whether we could find procedural ways of solving some of the hardware and software problems.

The outpatient area was having trouble with specimen handling, and we solved this by containerization. When specimens were brought from the outpatient lab to the central area, they were kept together, along with the appropriate labels, from the time they left the outpatient facility until the time they arrived at the central lab. This made it much easier for the outpatient people to check their samples in at the various areas. In Admissions, we found that there were inadequate people resources to support the accurate upkeep of the census system, and we had to request additional personnel to supply eight hours of computer operator time a day to handle our system. In the Emergency Room, the teleprinter terminal was too slow to handle the volume, and we ordered a CRT to satisfy them. On the floors, we had completed the training of all the individual ward units, and now were trying to iron out some of the difficulties with the remote areas, such as dialysis, cancer research, and some of the remote patient-care facilities. At this same time, we were finding a tremendous number of individual services which did not fit within the system. We held a very firm position on this and stated that if we could not handle them through the system we would refuse to do the work. This made it quite easy and convenient to decide which of the outpatient services we should continue to provide and which should be diverted to private labs or other sources. Many peripheral problems had been hiding in the bushes, very difficult to find. By the installation of a

system for sample reception and data retrieval, these became obvious outliers, and made it possible to delineate the problem and come up with an appropriate solution.

Within the lab, our label printer was too slow and had to be replaced with a faster model to keep pace with the volume. It was also obvious that we needed a CRT in the check-in room to increase the speed of ordering for some of the outlying clinics and wards that did not have a terminal. Within the laboratory, we had adequately guessed what was required and made no major changes.

During the month of December, the system received additional programming help, which eliminated a few basic problems and one or two halts stopped. In January through April 1976, minor changes were made by the company on the software, but some halts and loops continued. They were not disastrous, but extremely annoying. Many good letters were sent telling us about how these should be stopped in the near future. The only letter that counts is the one that says when it will be done.

The system in its current configuration has resolved many of the problems we initially experienced and has gone through a great stage of siege with a final successful burst in the end. The team work and dedication of the department, the technologists, and the staff of the hospital sustained the system when it was most fragile and vulnerable. To them I owe a debt of gratitude for a job well done. We have matured and I hope our vendor has learned through this experience. We know what we need to do in the future, and we recognize the mistakes and problems that cannot be repeated again. Companies that advertise to work in this area must understand the tremendous pressure that is placed on the department and the hospital when they finally flip the switch and become devoted to its data processing systems. In the end, money became an insignificant factor, and the simple fact that the company had no resources to dedicate was the primary problem. The training time for programmers and experts in hardware on our system was outside the range of response, and the management had not adequately anticipated our needs. We trust that this will never happen in the future, but expect and plan for the worst.

ADDITIONAL PROBLEMS

System MD Challenges

During the first two weeks of operation, when the hardware and software were grossly inefficient, we were seriously challenged by the Medicine

Department and its residents. It may have not been a conscious challenge, but it certainly was verbal. Any problem regarding the system was immediately down in my office in living color to be tacked on the door—along with my hide. In each case, we were able to track the situation through the use of the audit trails and determine that it was a human problem or failure. After about seven or eight incidents, the number of repeat visits decreased drastically. At the present time, we see about one physician a week with an obvious mistake fervently believed to be our error, and nearly always it is not. We have been very aggressive in refuting these challenges directly and without delay. The entire staff must learn to trust the system and its ability to produce accurate data. This challenge mechanism is, of course, the ultimate test of the system.

Reverse Education

In trying to handle the education of our enormous community of 1800 people, it soon became apparent that the whole process was doomed to failure because of the inability to communicate among services. There was a great deal of difficulty in getting the attention and interest of the nursing staff in the use of the terminal and the coordination of laboratory services. In the same context, we repeatedly attempted to reach the physicians, interns, and residents without success. Because of this, a new form of education was instituted which we call "reverse education."

Using this new technique, one sends out information adequate for the educational process, but anticipates that no one will read it. We only do this to have documentation that we have tried. Our secret weapon is the medical student. We made a special point of going to the students before they were put on hospital rotation. An entire day was spent showing them our videotapes, terminals, and all of our documentation. We gave them detailed instructions on how the floors ought to operate, how the terminal should work, and how the doctors can interface to the system. We then told them they were the only individuals in the hospital that were in a position to educate the physicians and clerks, and counseled them to do a patient but thorough job. The first group of medical students that hit the system in January 1976 were ideal teachers and instructors. What a potent weapon!

The students arrived on the wards and proceeded to get the data into the system with relative ease. The clerks watched and immediately began to put up territorial barriers around the system. We suddenly

experienced a reverse effect in which the clerks and nurses now wanted their terminals back. In the same manner, the students arrived on the floors with something the interns and residents did not know—how to get patient data out of the system. They were able to obtain doctor number reports and individual lab work back on all their patients faster than the residents and more expeditiously than the interns. To anyone acquainted with the medical community, this is the greatest stimulus to learn. In a matter of one week, the interns and residents were using the doctor inquiry function, patient inquiry function, and all the host of peripheral capabilities. We were getting calls from chief residents regarding ward reports for rounds, and the specimens started to arrive in good shape with the proper information attached. Our secret weapon worked, and we continue to use this mechanism as each new class is put into the hospital environment.

HOUSE STAFF ORIENTATION

When new house staff members arrive at the hospital, it is extremely important that they be thoroughly versed in the operation of the system, its restraints and constraints, and the ways to get their job done conveniently. We developed a videotape program along with a house-staff training manual, and through the use of medical students, trained faculty, and staff, we are able to integrate these new people.

INSERVICE EDUCATION

After our initial crisis-oriented program, the nurses and clerks in the hospital now receive in-service training on the system before they are placed on the floors. We are currently making progress in developing a strong liaison between the department and the other subservices in the hospital. Such ties are extremely important since both exist in concert for the betterment of the patient and the expeditious use of hospital facilities for efficient care.

27

Future Plans

INTRODUCTION

After reading our hair-raising story, one should ask, "Why become involved with such a program in the first place?" It is quite apparent to me, three years later, that our problems resulted from being the first ones into this area, and having to feel our way along from beginning to end. Since our vendor, or any other vendor for that matter, had virtually no experience in developing a minicomputer-based laboratory-information system, the unique problems we faced within the lab, and between the lab and the hospital, had not been totally elucidated prior to starting. We hope that through this book, we can provide some insight into the obvious systems problems that exist among the elements of this complicated set of environments. Our hope is to help future designers and builders through the rough stages into the smoother and gentler mode of operation which we now experience. All of our original problems have been resolved through the use of the communications system. It is delightful to sit in the laboratory and watch our phone lines on a high volume morning light up with personal calls and virtually no inquiries for laboratory data. All of our initial objectives have been

reached, and we are now in the position of looking toward the future and raising our sights a bit higher for additional development.

ADDITIONAL HORSEPOWER

Obviously, the system is totally saturated at this point, and we are still growing as a hospital and a department. After extensive discussions with our vendor about expanding the size of the system, we now have a program under way to double its current communication capability. This will allow additional peripheral areas that have not had a communication terminal for ordering, and will provide CRTs for doctors to inquire at remote sites. The current stress and overloading of the floor terminals can be eliminated, and the laboratory operation expanded to include an outpatient facility with additional peripheral terminals for data entry.

ON-LINE VERSUS OFF-LINE

In the design and specification of our system, we looked very carefully at the requirements for on-line operation. We have attempted to optimize those items that the physicians and floors need for daily service through the use of the on-line communication terminals in their area. In like manner, not much has been invested in fancy frills or gadgets for the communication computer. This choice allows us to optimize the use of the CPU in time sharing. One computer can only do so much in a certain length of time, and it is either handling floor problems or doing some of the more sophisticated reports requested of laboratory systems. We have elected to batch-process such things as quality control, epidemiologic reports, and certain administrative documents through the use of magnetic tapes. Since alternate batch systems are very reasonable and voluminous around the country, this kind of information can be handled conveniently in bulk form and be totally removed from the hospital communication system. The additional in-house computer power required to allow this to be done while the communication system is running is probably not justifiable when looked at in terms of the necessity of the reports requested.

LIBRARY CAPABILITY

Those who have watched the data processing market have noticed a drastic decrease in the cost of mass storage. This fact has serious

implications for medicine, since it offers the possibility of maintaining large on-line real-time library systems to be used through a communication medium. We are currently in the developmental stage of building an on-line real-time library of clinical pathology to be added to an additional library for anatomic and surgical pathology. These libraries we hope will spearhead the development of an ultimate real-time practice-oriented Library of Medicine optimized for patient care.

"NORMAL VALUE" STATISTICS

The communications system and its archive retrieval programs offer some very unique capabilities for research and study of the data that is presented to us every day by our many testing instruments. We utilize this information very poorly at the present time and do not have the time or the capability to sift through this data and really decipher the significance of it, except on a momentary basis for a single patient. To solve this problem, the department has integrated statistics within our systems group to offer us a new dimension in mathematical skills and capability. Biostatistics is tasked with the establishment of a new set of normal values, development of diagnostic routines based on data held within the system, and the use of the data base to support a diagnostic library as previously described using multivariate techniques for trend analysis, tracking, and monitoring programs [33]. It is far beyond the scope of this particular document to deal with these areas, but suffice it to say that the data base is there to support just these sorts of ventures without any additional input, and that the system some day may be in a position to learn as well as emulate.

TERMINALS

We have obviously learned our lesson on terminals, and are in the process of designing a new nursing station terminal as previously described. The major factors of noise and convenience cannot be underestimated and will have to be looked at very carefully when new terminals are proposed for various areas. The redundancy, service, and malleability of these units are primary concerns when major dollars are expended for hospital systems.

In like manner, specifications and criteria are needed to delineate the requirements of a nursing station, a laboratory, and other areas of the hospital with respect to noise, power protection, communication lines,

and the architectural design required to support communication systems. We are continuing to build hospitals in the traditional mold and need architects who are informed of the technology and requirements for modern communication systems. Until this is accomplished, we will forever need to rebuild hospitals and work in less than optimal environments. This is an expensive process, and certainly does not represent our best effort in coordinating concrete and medical technology.

WHAT HAS BEEN ACCOMPLISHED?

Our current system represents the amalgamation of the nursing station, admissions, and a complete pathology package. The ability to process this diversified information within one minicomputer has required a major investment of both personal and corporate time. The fact is that this module now exists as a parent to a family of systems which can be configured and established at the financial and administrative pace of an individual hospital.

Since the total system is far from complete, many additional hours of energy will be required to define the remaining subsystems. This remains a challenge to our staff, since our approach employs a completely compartmentalized configuration.

As a laboratorian, the success of our current package can only be measured by the total silence of my phone. After the difficulties of the early months such silence is a reward in and of itself [34]. We feel assured that those who choose a similar path drawing upon the experience of others, will find the next generation of systems more flexible and productive, such that the success of the venture will never be in doubt.

28

Comparative Systems

Hundreds of articles have been written about laboratory systems since their inception in the early sixties. Dr. A. E. Rappaport has a fine collection of bibliographic citations which can be used for reference [35]. J. Lloyd Johnson has reviewed the field of laboratory computers since 1971 and has followed the development of commercial systems and their performance [36].

In all these reports, the reader is cautioned about making absolute judgments based on the published information. Corporations and systems described here and elsewhere change as rapidly as the technology of electronics. It is currently possible to resurrect an entirely malfunctioning system in a matter of hours by the use of the proper materials, software, or philosophy. After being involved in the laboratory data-processing industry for ten years, I find that each year it becomes harder categorically to define any single corporate position in the field. Companies rise and fall almost overnight depending upon the capital backing their venture, and the management that heads design and marketing. One must be very cautious of overselling, underselling, and misinterpretation. To directly sidestep the comparison of our program with other vendors, Table 8 lists the current capabilities of our communica-

tion system as of January 1978. Even after reading the most current articles, it is impossible for us to determine whether other vendors can achieve the same measure of overall performance. We have reviewed the literature that is provided by competitive groups, and find it very difficult even to compare system features on an individual basis.

As a final note of caution, we would have to agree on one point with the J. Lloyd Johnson report: Caveat Emptor!

Table 8

On-Line Functions Available on the Shands LIS[a]

Nursing Terminal Functions
1. Laboratory orders (all areas)
2. Doctor number update (up to five doctors per patient)
3. Unable to draw (morning blood drawing exceptions)
4. Send message (to any terminal)
5. Inquiry by doctor (current doctor census)
6. Inquiry by specimen number (list all current orders)
7. Inquiry by patient (LIFO, FIFO, ward report, unfinished test)
8. Census report (by room, by ward)
9. Ward report (by doctor number)
10. Archive inquiry (index to previous laboratory data held on microfilm)

Admissions, Outpatient, and Emergency-Room Terminal Functions
1. Inpatient admit
2. Outpatient admit
3. Transfer
4. Discharge
5. Correct patient identification
6. Complete nursing station functions

Special Laboratory Processing Functions
1. Census search by name (exact spelling not necessary)
2. Inquiry by specimen number (special display for order processing)
3. Inquiry by medical record number (special display for order processing)
4. Confirmation of specimen (call special labels, date and time specimen, special date and time correction routine)
5. Test comment (special input for result reporting)
6. Comment paragraph (extended special comment input for result reporting)

Internal Laboratory Functions
1. Abnormal result report (by wards)
2. Billing report (to magnetic tape and also to the printer)
3. Chart reports (daily, new and repeat, complete, or by wards)
4. Chart reports (7-day, new and repeat, complete, or by wards)
5. Copy drum (magnetic tape/disc cartridge)
6. Delete/modify results

(continued)

Table 8—*continued*

7. Lab usage report (new and repeat)
8. Master worksheets (hematology, chemistry, immunology, blood bank, microscopy)
9. Patient summaries
10. Quality control report
11. Run summaries for the Coulter-S
12. SMAC tape (loading and printing procedure, plus verify)
13. SMAC worksheets
14. Specimen collection list (labels)
15. Specimen collection list (tubes)
16. Unfinished test report (all areas, by single labs)
17. Ward report by doctor number
18. Worksheets (hematology, chemistry, immunology, microscopy, by area and sub area, New and Repeat)
19. Room file update
20. Test file update
21. Expanded test file update
22. Terminal message file update
23. Message file update
24. Census report
25. Enter time/date (system)
26. Clear files
27. Enter message and print message
28. Differential result entry
29. Enter limits for files
30. Read cards (orders, results)
31. Read tapes
32. Load/verify drum
33. Mark-sense card batch review
34. Archive entry
35. Archive delete
36. Archive merge
37. Archive copy
38. Archive print
39. ADTL report (admit, discharge, transfer, listing)
40. Preparation summary listing (specimen splitting)
41. Print purge
42. Divert equipment (move output functions among peripherals)
43. Specimen number reset

Special Software Functions
1. Ability to collapse the system to one CPU if a single processor should fail.

---

^a The Shands LIS has functions for the nursing station, admissions, outpatient, emergency room, central laboratory, and central computer room areas. Special software exists to allow the contraction of the system to one central processing unit. Functions available as of January, 1978.

Bibliography

1. Gall, J. E., Norwood, D. D., Cook, M., Fleming, J., Rydell, R., and Watson, R. J., "Demonstration and Evaluation of a Total Hospital Information System. Final Project Report." Contract No. HSM 110-71-128, Department of Health, Education, and Welfare Health, Resources Administration, National Center for Health Services Research, NTIS Publication No. 262106, December 1975.
2. Hall, P. F. L., "Current Status of the Karolinska Hospital Computer System (Stockholm)." *In* Collen, M. F. (Ed.): *Hospital Computer Systems.* Wiley, New York, 1974, pp. 546–597.
3. Wasserman, A. I., "Minicomputers may maximize data processing," *Hospitals* **51**, 119–132 (1977).
4. Johnson, J. L., "Achieving the Optimum Information System Update 1976: The Laboratory." J. L. Lloyd Johnson Associates, Northfield, Illinois, 1976.
5. Grams, R. R., "The Current Status and Future Prospects for Computers in Hospitals," *Hospitals* **51**, 187–193 (1977).
6. White, R. L., and Meindl, J. D., "The impact of integrated electronics in medicine," *Science* **195**, 1119–1124 (1977).
7. Vallbona, C., and Spencer, W. A., "Texas Institute for Research and Rehabilitation Hospital Computer System (Houston)." *In* Collen, M. F. (Ed.): *Hospital Computer Systems.* Wiley, New York, 1974, pp. 662–700.
8. Watson, R. J., "A Large-Scale Professionally-Oriented Medical Information System—Five Years Later," *J. Med. Systems* **1**, 3–21 (1977).
9. Collen, M. F. (Ed.), *Hospital Computer Systems.* Wiley, New York, 1974.

247

10. Giordmaine, J. A., "Solid-State Electronics: Scientific Basis for Future Advances," *Science* **195**, 1235–1240 (1977).

11. Finley, P. R., Anderson, R., and Neese, R., "Electronic Data Processing in a Private Hospital Laboratory," *Am. J. Clin. Path.* **48**, 575 (1967).

12. Pribor, H. C., Kifkham, W. R., and Hoyt, R. S., "Small Computer Does a Big Job in This Hospital Laboratory," *Mod. Hosp.* **110**, 104 (1968).

13. Krieg, A. F., Johnson, T. J., McDonald, C., and Cotlove, E., *Clinical Laboratory Computerization*. University Park Press, Baltimore, 1971.

14. Henry, J. B., and Pruitt, C. T., "This Report System Reduces Lab Errors," *Mod. Hosp.* **104**, 118 (1964).

15. Grams, R. R., *Problem Solving System Analysis and Medicine*. Charles C Thomas, Springfield, Illinois, 1972.

16. Grams, R. R., *System-Analysis Workbook*. Charles C Thomas, Springfield, Illinois, 1972.

17. Grams, R. R., and Pastor, E. J., "New Concepts in the Design of a Clinical Laboratory Information System (LIS)," *Am. J. Clin. Path.* **65**, 662–674 (1976).

18. Brooks, A. H., "Training and Organization of Hospital Personnel for a Hospital Communication System." *In* Shires, D. B., Wolf, H. (Eds.): *Medinfo 77*, North-Holland Publishing Company, New York, 1977, pp. 989–992.

19. Schmitz, H. H., "The Anatomy of a Successful System Implementation," *Hospitals* **51**, 105 (1977).

20. Watson, R. J., "Medical Staff Response to a Computerized Medical Information System with Direct Physician Interface." *In* Anderson, J. and Forsythe, J. M., *Proceedings of the First World Conference on Medical Informatics*, Cotab, Stockholm, Sweden, pp. 299–302.

21. Grams, R. R., "The Systems Approach to Medical Problems." *In* Jenkin, M. A. (Ed.): *A Manual of Computers in Medical Practice*, The Society for Computer Medicine, Edina, Minnesota, 1977, pp. 17–26.

22. Boulding, K. E., "General Systems Theory—the Skeleton of Science," *Management Sci.* **2**, 197–209 (1956).

23. Barnett, G. O., and Zielstorff, R. D., "Data Systems Can Enhance or Hinder Medical Nursing Activities," *Hospitals* **51**, 157–161 (1977).

24. Virts, S. S., "Introducing the Hospital-Wide Information System to Hospital and Medical Staffs." *In* Shires, D. B., and Wolf, H. (Eds.): *Medinfo 77*, North-Holland Publishing Company, New York, 1977, pp. 993–998.

25. Caraway, W. T., "Sources of Error in Clinical Chemistry." *In* Meites, S. (Ed.): *Standard Methods of Clinical Chemistry*, Vol. 5, Academic Press, New York, 1965, pp. 19–30.

26. Statland, B. E., Winkel, P., and Bakeland, H., "Factors Contributing to Intraindividual Variation of Serum Constituents. 1. Within-Day Variation of Serum Constituents in Healthy Subjects," *Clin. Chem.* **19**, 1374–1379 (1973).

27. Sellers, D. E., and Grams, R. R., "Noise Specifications for a Hospital Communication System—a proposal," *J. Med. Systems* **1**, 63–64 (1977).

28. Sellers, D. E., and Grams, R. R., "Case Report—Documentation of Hospital Communication Noise Levels," *J. Med. Systems* 89–97 (1977).

29. Grams, R. R., and Lezotte, D., "The Laboratory Audit—PSRO for Pathology," *J. Med. Systems* **3**, 307–314 (1978).

30. Gudat, J. D., "Interfacing the Sequential Multiple Analyzer-Computer with a Laboratory Information System in a Teaching Hospital." *In* Shires, D. B., and Wolf, H. (Eds.): *Medinfo 77*, North-Holland Publishing Company, New York, 1977, p. 1074.

31. Litzkow, L., Ingram, W., and Lezotte, D., "The Evaluation of a Functional real-time Laboratory Records Retrieval and Archival System," *J. Med. Systems* **1**, 177–186 (1977).

32. Grams, R. R., and Thomas, R. G., "Cost Analysis of a Laboratory Information System (LIS)," *J. Med. Systems* **1**, 27–36 (1977).

33. Grams, R. R., Johnson, E., and Benson, E. S., "Laboratory Data Analysis System. Section I. Introduction and Overview," *Am. J. Clin. Path.* **55**, 177–181 (1972).

34. Grams, R. R., "Progress towards a Second Generation Laboratory Information System (LIS)," *J. Med. Systems* **3**, 263–274 (1978).

35. Rappaport, A. E., "Computers, Information, Retrieval, and Data Storage." *In* Race, J. R. (Ed.): *Laboratory Medicine*, Harper and Row, Hagerstown, Maryland, Volume 4, Chapter 23, 1977.

36. Johnson, J. L., *Achieving the Optimum Information System—the Laboratory*. J. Lloyd Johnson Associates, Northfield, Illinois, 1975.

APPENDIX *I*

The System Contract

INTRODUCTION

A properly signed and executed contract embodies the rules by which a hospital and vendor are expected to interact. Both parties need the assistance of legal counsel to protect their specific rights and assure that all obligations are mutually enforced. Special wording and descriptions were developed during our contract period which might be helpful to other institutions.

LEASE AGREEMENT

This AGREEMENT is made and entered into this __ day of ____, in the year 19__, by and between _____ (hereinafter referred to as ____), whose mailing address is _____, and _____ (hereinafter referred to as LESSEE), whose mailing address is _____. For and in consideration of the mutual covenants and conditions hereinafter stated, the LESSEE agrees to lease from __ and __ agrees to lease to the LESSEE a turnkey Uni-Lab System. The exact parameters of such a system are defined in

250

EXHIBIT A, attached hereto entitled ADDENDUM SYSTEM SPECIFICATION MANUAL for (ERLS) Laboratory Information for _____ (herein referred to as SPECIFICATION NUMBER 1403 ADDENDUM), dated ____, updated ____, which EXHIBIT A is embodied as a part of this AGREEMENT. The system includes both equipment and programming factors. The lease is based upon the terms and conditions as set forth in this AGREEMENT.

1. Definition of Dates and Terms.

(a) *Delivery Date.* The Delivery Date is defined as that date when the system equipment is physically transferred to the LESSEE's premises.

(b) *Scheduled Delivery Date.* The Scheduled Delivery Date is defined as that date upon which delivery of the equipment is scheduled to take place. This date may or may not be the same as the actual "Delivery Date."

(c) *Installation Date.* The Installation Date is defined as that date when _____ demonstrates that the System operates in accordance with Specifications (EXHIBIT A), and notifies the LESSEE in writing that the system is ready for use.

(d) *Acceptance Date.* The Acceptance Date is defined as that date following the completion of the successful performance period when the LESSEE determines the system operates in accordance with the specifications (EXHIBIT A), and State Standard of performance as set forth in Article 10(b) and notifies _____ in writing that the system is acceptable to LESSEE.

2. Period of Agreement.

This AGREEMENT shall become effective upon the date accepted and signed by LESSEE, and shall continue for __ years or longer if extended as set forth in Article 14(e) from the first day of the successful performance period as defined in Article 10(b) below and shall thereafter remain in effect unless terminated as provided in Article (14) Termination.

3. Shipment.

_____ shall arrange for transportation, rigging, drayage, and handling of the equipment in this system. Shipper shall invoice the LESSEE

directly for these services. LESSEE agrees to pay all such transportation charges both from and to _____'s place of manufacture.

4. Taxes.

THE LESSEE is an agency of the _____ and is presently a tax immune sovereign under the existing laws and is exempt from the payment of all taxes of any kind levied upon this System or measured by such price or on this AGREEMENT unless and until the ____ Legislature passes legislation allowing and permitting payment of taxes by the LESSEE herein.

5. Monthly Lease Charge.

The system items, as described in EXHIBIT A, are as of the date of this AGREEMENT, hereby leased to LESSEE, and for said items, LESSEE agrees to pay __ as sum of $__ monthly.

The lease price shall be paid as set forth in Article 6 of the AGREEMENT. The value of the system leased by ____ to LESSEE is $____.

6. Invoice and Charges.

(a) Charges shall be invoiced to the LESSEE monthly commencing on the first day of the month after successful completion of either the initial standard of performance period (the first __ days after installation) or a subsequent standard of performance period, if required. In any event, lease payment is payable on the first of the month for the previous month's lease charges or portion thereof, such portion based upon a 30-day month. Lease payments shall be due and payable __ days after date of invoice.

(b) Charges for fractional parts of a calender month shall be computed at the rate of 1/30th of the monthly rate for each day on and after the Acceptance Date.

7. Risk of Loss or Damage.

THE LESSEE shall be relieved from all risks of physical loss or damage to the equipment up to the time of delivery to the LESSEE's

installation site. Thereafter, the LESSEE assumes all risk of physical loss or damage to the equipment resulting from negligence of LESSEE. LESSEE shall at its own expense provide and maintain insurance in the amount of the equipment value specified herein to cover all risks of loss of the equipment. The insurance shall be subject to the approval of _____, which approval shall not be unreasonably withheld, and shall provide for payment in the event of loss to _____ as its interest may appear. LESSEE agrees to provide evidence of such insurance coverage and to notify _____ before cancellation of any such policy.

8.   Reservation of Title.

Title to the equipment (including all spare or maintenance parts, test equipment, and maintenance tools delivered by __) is and at all times shall remain in ____.

9.   Installation.

Equipment leased under this AGREEMENT will be installed by _____ and made ready for use by the LESSEE. The LESSEE shall, at its expense, have the site prepared in accordance with _____'s written specification __ days before the "Scheduled Delivery Date." _____ will notify LESSEE of this date by written notice.

10.   Standard of Performance.

(a)   _____ shall certify in writing to the LESSEE when the System is installed and ready for use. The performance period (a period of __ consecutive calendar days) shall commence on the first State workday following certification, at which time operational control becomes the responsibility of the LESSEE. It is not required that one thirty-day period expires in order for another performance period to begin.

(b)   If the System operates at an average level of effectiveness of 90 per cent or more for a period of thirty (30) consecutive days from the commencement date of the performance period, it shall be deemed to have met the LESSEE's standard of performance and shall constitute a successful performance period. The average effectiveness level is a

percentage figure, determined by dividing the total operational use time of the system by total operational use time of the system plus associated equipment failure downtime. Associated equipment failure due to malfunctions that:

  i.   do not result in a loss of any of the system functions, or
  ii. are covered by redundant equipment or system backup procedure,

is not considered in arriving at the calculation of average effectiveness level called for herein. In addition, the equipment shall operate in substantial conformance with _____'s published specifications applicable to such equipment on the date of this AGREEMENT. _____'s documents will contain performance characteristics applicable to each machine.

(c)   Equipment to the contract by amendment shall operate in conformance with _____'s published specifications applicable to such equipment at the time of such amendment.

(d)   _____, without charge to LESSEE, shall train not more than 12 of the LESSEE'S initial operating personnel at LESSEE's location or as mutually agreed upon at any other location.

11.   System Maintainability.

(a)   System shall not be accepted by the LESSEE and charges will not be paid by the LESSEE until the standard of performance is met.

(b)   Immediately upon successful completion of the performance period, LESSEE shall notify _____ in writing of acceptance of the system and authorize the lease charges to begin on the first day of the successful performance period.

(c)   If successful completion of the performance period is not attained on or before __, __, 19__, LESSEE shall have the option of terminating the contract, or continuing the performance tests. LESSEE's option to terminate the contract shall remain in effect until such time as a successful completion of the performance period is attained.

12.   Maintenance Service and Warranty.

(a)   _____ warrants for a period of one (1) year from the first day of the successful performance period that the equipment supplied hereunder will be free from defects in material and workmanship.

_____'s obligation for any breach of warranty shall be limited to repair or replacement of the defective unit at no charge to the LESSEE.

(b) _____ shall have no obligation other than as set out in paragraph 12(a) above, under this article to provide maintenance or make repairs or replacements required through normal wear and tear (except via agreement for equipment maintenance) or necessitated in whole or in part by catastrophic causes, fault or negligence of the user, or by cause external to the equipment, such as, but not limited to, power failure or excessive environmental factors. Parts removed and replaced become the property of _____.

(c) Programs furnished and operated in accord with EXHIBIT A herein, are warranted for a period of one (1) year following the first day of the successful performance period. Such warranty includes logical defects and performance as set forth in the Specifications, EXHIBIT A. Such defective programs shall be corrected or replaced. Programming modification performed by persons other than _____, without _____'s approval (written), shall void this warranty.

(d) The LESSEE agrees to execute an agreement for equipment maintenance with _____ at the date of execution of this AGREEMENT, upon terms, prices, and conditions as set forth in the Maintenance Agreement attached hereto. The LESSEE further agrees to renew the Maintenance Agreement at a monthly charge to be negotiated between the parties on a yearly basis to provide coverage for the entire lease period.

(e) In the event the parties are unable to reach agreement to renew the maintenance agreement referred to herein, the LESSEE shall have the option to and hereby agrees to obtain, and keep in full force and effect throughout the term of this lease, including all extensions thereof, a Maintenance contract with a Maintenance organization or persons acceptable to _____ (which acceptance shall not be unreasonably withheld) covering all periods of use with cost of said Maintenance contract to be borne in full by LESSEE. The Maintenance Agreement obtained in accordance with the provisions of this paragraph 12 (e) shall satisfy the obligations of the LESSEE under paragraph 12 (d), *supra*.

13. Liability.

The LESSEE assumes all risks of any loss, expense, or injury incurred by an employee, customer, or invitee of the LESSEE or any other person or party (except agents or employees of _____) to the extent of

liability insurance carried by the LESSEE for such purposes, provided said injury, loss, expense, or damage is not caused in any manner by negligence of ____.

14.   Termination.

(a)   Except as provided below, this AGREEMENT shall not be subject to termination in whole or in part by either party until the expiration of __ years (or longer if extended) from the first day of the successful performance period. At any time after the expiration of this period and upon receipt of at least __ days written notice by either party, which notice may be given during said period, either party may terminate this AGREEMENT. The LESSEE's obligation to pay all lease and other charges which shall have accrued up to and including the termination date shall survive any termination of this AGREE-MENT.

(b)   The performance by the LESSEE of any of its obligation under this AGREEMENT shall be subject to and contingent upon the availability of monies lawfully appropriated and applicable for such purposes. If the LESSEE deems at anytime during the term of this AGREEMENT, that monies applicable to this AGREEMENT shall not be available for the remainder of the terms, the LESSEE shall promptly so notify _____ whereupon the obligations of the parties herein shall end upon the giving of such notice and this AGREEMENT shall be considered as canceled by mutual consent as provided herein-after.

(c)   LESSEE shall have the right to terminate this AGREEMENT as to all or as to any specific item(s) of equipment included hereunder:

   i.   upon mutual consent of both parties,
   ii.   on the first anniversary date provided __ days prior written notice has been provided, or,
   iii.   after the first anniversary date provided the __ days prior written notice has been provided. LESSEE shall be liable only for accumulated payments due prior to the effective date of such notice.

(d)   LESSEE shall have the right to terminate this AGREEMENT as to all or as to any specific item(s) of equipment included hereunder for failure of _____ to substantially comply with contractural commitments contained herein.

(e)   _____ grants to the LESSEE the option to extend the term of this lease, at a monthly charge to be negotiated and under the same

terms and conditions stated herein. This option shall be deemed exercised by the LESSEE upon written notice to _____ at any time prior to __ days before the end of the term of this LEASE AGREEMENT. The lease extension period may be canceled by either the LESSEE or _____ by giving __ days prior written notice one to the other.

15.   General Provisions.

(a)   Neither party shall have the right to assign its right or obligations under this AGREEMENT without the written consent of the other party provided, however, the successor in interest by merger, consolidation, operation of law, assignment, purchase, or otherwise of the entire business of either party shall acquire all interest of such party hereunder. _____ shall be entitled to assign all or part of the payment or payments under this AGREEMENT.

(b)   The LESSEE agrees not to employ or use additional attachments, features, or devices on the equipment or make changes or alterations to the equipment covered hereby without the written consent of _____ in each case. The LESSEE will, however, provide _____ adequate opportunity to make any changes or alterations which _____ deems necessary or desirable.

(c)   The LESSEE agrees not to remove the equipment from the location in which it is installed, except in an emergency, without the prior written consent of _____.

(d)   This AGREEMENT shall be governed by the laws of the State of ____ and there are no understandings, agreements, or representations express or implied not specified herein.

(e)   The foregoing terms and conditions shall prevail notwithstanding any variance with the terms and conditions of any purchase order submitted by the LESSEE. This AGREEMENT shall not be deemed or construed to be modified, amended, rescinded, canceled, or waived in whole or part except by written amendment mutually agreed to and executed by the parties hereto.

(f)   LESSEE shall furnish all consumables, such as paper forms and printer ribbons, and storage media, such as magnetic tape or disc cartridges.

(g)   _____ shall substantially comply with the contents of their ADDENDUM SYSTEM SPECIFICATION MANUAL for (ERLS) Laboratory Information System for _____ (herein referred to as SPECIFICATION NUMBER 1403 ADDENDUM, dated ____, 19__,

updated ____, 19__,) which is EXHIBIT A, and is embodied as a part of this AGREEMENT. In the event of a conflict between ADDENDUM SPECIFICATION MANUAL FOR (ERLS) Laboratory Information System for ____ (herein referred to as SPECIFICATION NUMBER 1403 ADDENDUM, dated ____, 19__, updated ____, 19__,) which is EXHIBIT A, and this AGREEMENT, this AGREEMENT will take precedence.

File Building Procedure

INTRODUCTION

Each laboratory must describe every procedure performed in detail. A general form was created and used to collect file building elements. Special messages are derived from these forms to denote specimen processing instructions to be housed and communicated by the system. The actual collection and verification of this information is a time consuming process and should be the responsibility of a senior technologist or pathologist.

LABORATORY PROCEDURE DOCUMENTATION

A. GENERAL
1. Full test name:
2. Abbreviated name (16 characters)
3. Abbreviated name (5 characters)
4. Test number:
5. Lab area performed:

B. DESCRIPTORS
  1. Is test a titer? Y N
  2. Is this a battery? Y N
     a. What are the tests included?:
C. PATIENT SAMPLE
  1. Sample tube type:
  2. Sample Tube volume (1/4):
D. TESTING SAMPLE
  1. Type of specimen:
  2. Volume of specimen:
  3. Specimen type:
E. RESULTS
  1. Unit of result:
  2. Digits to the right of the decimal place:
  3. High normal limit
  4. Low normal limit
  5. Reject High value
  6. Reject low value
  7. Tabulated age sex normals is needed:
F. BUSINESS FACTORS
  1. Work unit from CAP:
  2. Billing code number:
  3. Hospital cost:
  4. Professional fee:
G. ORDER PARAMETERS
  1. Is quantity factor required? Y N
     a. What word is used?
     b. Minimum quantity allowed:
     c. Maximum quantity allowed:
  2. Is a source message needed? Y N
  3. Is a time location message needed? Y N
     a. Where is message sent?

4.	Order Message Segment Generator

	STAT ORDER	ROUTINE ORDER

Test available: High staff
              Low staff
Can specimen be held?

Special processing
instructions: (refrig, container,
    transport, etc.)

Patient instructions:
(NPO, diet, injections, etc.)

Nursing instructions:
(scheduling, who to call,
    labels, etc.)

Who acquires specimen?
   High staff:
   Low staff:
Mark time of day for
lab or ward acquisition.

Actual order
Message: Leave Blank

H. SPECIAL ANALYSIS FACTORS
   1. Is this a charge only test? Y N
   2. Worksheet requirements:
      a. Should this test be grouped with others on a worksheet? Y N
         1) How?
      b. Are any calculations required on the worksheet? Y N
         1) What are they?
      c. Lay out your worksheet page for recording machine data and calculating test results. This should be a bench-type design for ease of calculation.

The Shands System Flowcharts

INTRODUCTION

Flowcharting is the means by which one can accurately describe an operating system within a hospital. By employing the tools of description, investigation, research, creativity, and good judgment, the process of a system study is accomplished. The system study or final product is a collection of the vital information needed to enable one to understand what has taken place, what is taking place at the present, and what should occur in the future. The operational system analysis can only be accomplished by providing a problem statement, listing the goals and objectives, and recording the steps involved through the use of flowcharts and operational statements.

The problem statement which appears at the beginning of the document is an accumulation of the ideas and concepts relevant to a particular problem. This is written in as brief and concise a format as possible while still stating the complete problem.

The next emphasis is placed on listing the goals and objectives set

forth in the study. These are ranked according to their importance to the document, the first objective being the most important and the last being the least significant. Each objective is as short and concise as possible.

The flowcharting process involves a number of basic components: overview flowchart, systems flowcharts, operational statements, and exhibits. The overview flowchart accomplishes two basic objectives: it provides an index to the systems flowcharting, while at the same time providing the reader an opportunity to understand the complete system in its very broadest sense. From the overview flowchart, the document proceeds to the specific system documentation. This documentation is best accomplished through the use of graphic symbols that accurately and intelligibly allow the reader to progress through the natural flow of the study. Each step in the process should be carefully described so that the reader has no difficulty in following the proper flow of work from page to page. This section includes all the minutia of specific flowchart details. Each major section may contain many subsections, but these are written in such a manner that, if desired, one could connect all the major and subsystem flowcharts to produce one large document showing all the steps involved in the total process.

Operational statements accompany each page of the total document. Each flowchart is matched with an operational statement page. Each operational statement page contains a narrative of statements that concisely describe what is happening in the flowcharts.

Operational statements also link the flowcharts and those parts of the document called exhibits. These are usually paper documents which add meaning to the process. They may be paper reports, such as forms used for daily operations, or may include the computer-generated copies of worksheets, laboratory reports, and so on. All exhibits in the study should be numbered according to their flowchart designation.

By employing the tools of graphics and verbal description, one can create a document which provides continuity and intelligent management of the large body of information that may be necessary to understand a particular problem or system.

SYSTEM SYMBOLS

	Symbol	Name	Description

Process symbols — This rectangle or square shows that some operation is being done or performed.

Offpage connector — This symbol tells the reader that the system continues on another page. The area above the line designated where it is continued "from", and the area below the line tells where it is going to.

Manual input — This represents some type of manual input, such as keyboard entry.

Decision — The diamond is used to indicate to the reader that a decision has to be made: yes or no.

Document — This symbol represents a paper document, created either by an input or output, line printer or typewriter.

Online file — This symbol represents any data which is stored in a computer and can be reached immediately upon request.

Offline file — This symbol represents an offline storage file, ex., metal file cabinet.

Disk — This symbol represents a disk used to store large amounts of readily available information in a computer.

Drum — This symbol represents a drum used to store large amounts of readily available information in a computer.

Terminal — This represents the beginning or end of a system, a halt, or an interruption in the flowchart process.

Paper tape — This is employed whenever paper tape is used as an input or output to a system.

This document also contains a number of other symbols such as specimen tubes, slides, etc. which are self explanatory as the reader progresses through the document.

THE PROBLEM STATEMENT

How to provide a prompt, accurate, reliable pathology information system in a 500-bed, state-supported, acute-care, general hospital with associated Emergency Room and Outpatient Clinics. Integral services to be optimized include test ordering, specimen acquisition and delivery, specimen processing, specimen testing, result recording, information transmission, quality control, and complete system audit for management.

OVERVIEW FLOWCHART I   Level 1

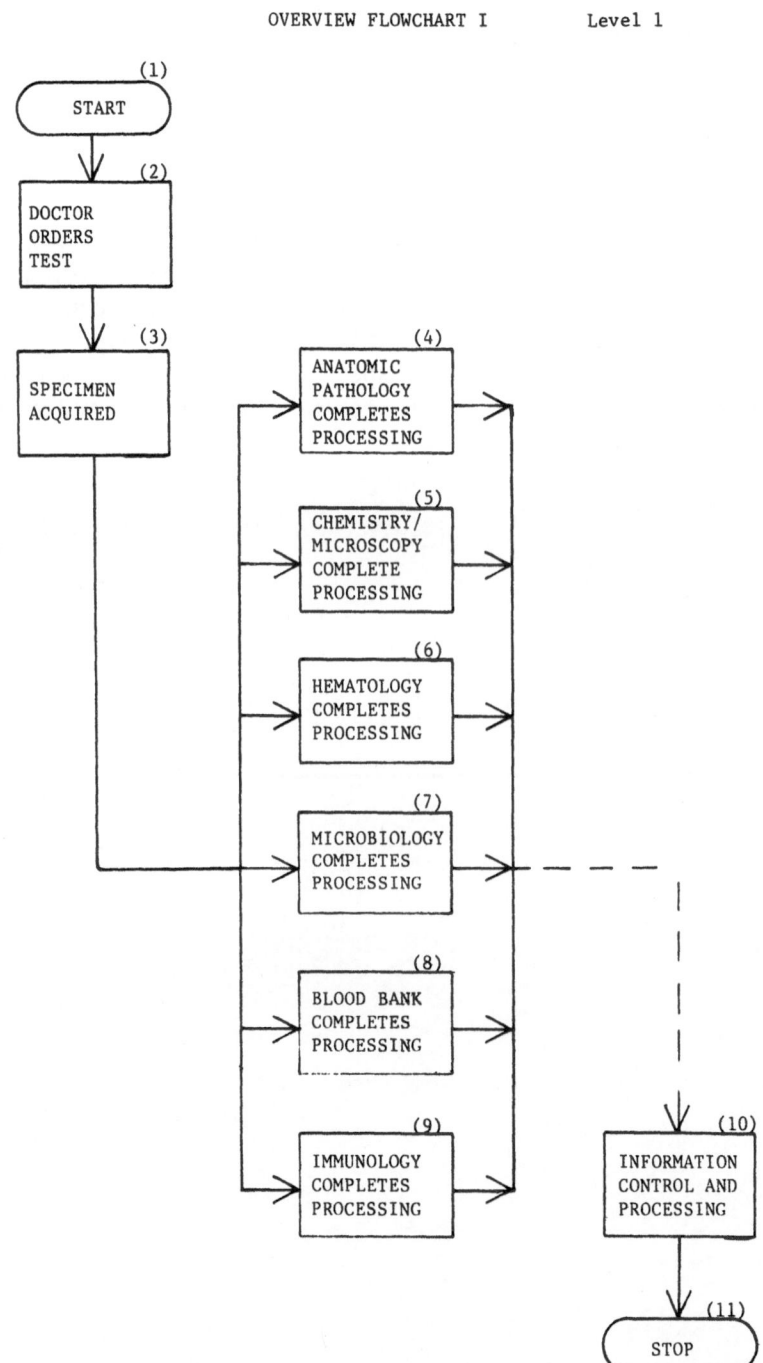

OPERATIONS STATEMENTS

Overview Flowchart I: Level 1

1.   Terminal symbol indicates the starting point of the University of Florida Pathology Services system.

2.   The first basic step in pursuing pathology services is for the doctor to initiate an order in either the Outpatient or Inpatient care centers. Connect to operation (3).

3.   The specimen is acquired by the various laboratory services to produce a quantitative or qualitative result. Connect to any or all of operations (4), (5), (6), (7), (8), (9).

4.   Anatomic Pathology processes the specimen and completes a report for physician review. Connect to operation (10).

5.   Chemistry and Microscopy complete processing of a specimen for physician review. Connect to operation (10).

6.   Hematology completes processing of a specimen for physician review. Connect to operation (10).

7.   Microbiology completes processing of a patient specimen for physician review. Connect to operation (10).

8.   Blood Bank receives a specimen and follows the instruction for set-up of Blood Bank products to be administered to the patient. Connect to operation (10).

9.   Immunology receives a specimen and completes a result for physician review. Connect to operation (10).

10.   Laboratory test data from all areas are processed through the computer and a number of reports are generated. A sequence of online and off-line functions are performed. Connect to operation (11).

11.   Termination of the University of Florida Pathology Services system.

FLOWCHART IIA   Level 2
DOCTOR ORDERS TEST

Flowchart II A: Level 2

Doctor Orders Test

1. Off-page connector: From—location unspecified. To—operation (2).
2. There are a number of different areas in the hospital from which doctors' orders can originate. Connect to operations (3), (5), (6), (8), (9), (11), (12).
3. Off-page connector: From—operation (3). To—Flowchart II B1.
4. Decision: A—proceed to hospital admissions. B—proceed to Inpatient. C—proceed to next decision block.
5. Off-page connector: From—operation (5). To—Flowchart II D1.
6. Off-page connector: from—operation (6). To—Flowchart II F1.
7. Decision: A—proceed to Emergency Room. B—proceed to Dialysis. C—Proceed to next decision block.
8. Off-page connector: From—operation (8). To—Flowchart II H1.
9. Off-page connector: From—operation (9). To—Flowchart II I1.
10. Decision: A—proceed to Obstetrics. B—proceed to Outpatient Clinics.
11. Off-page connector: From—operation (11). To—Flowchart II K1.

FLOWCHART IIB   Level 2

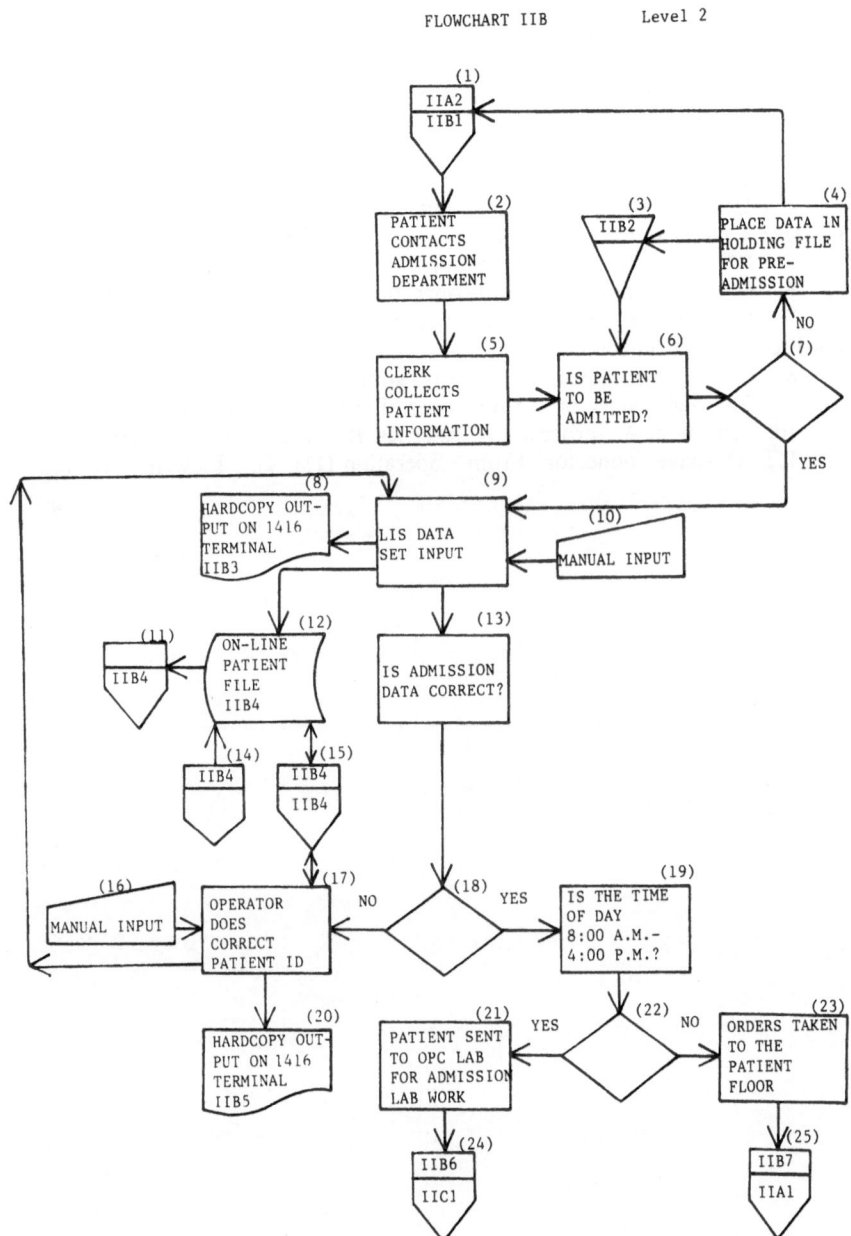

Flowcharts II B: Level 2

1. Off-page connector: From—Flowchart II A2. To—operation (2).

2. Patient contacts Admissions Department for admission to the hospital. Connect to operation (5).

3. This is an off-line file cabinet in which patient admission information is kept. Connect to operations (4), (6).

4. Patient admission information may be gathered ahead of time and kept in a holding file until the patient enters the hospital. Connect to operation (3).

5. A hospital interviewer collects all pertinent patient admission information. Connect to operation (6).

6. Is patient admitted to the hospital? Connect to operation (7).

7. Decision: A—No, connect to operation (4). B—Yes, connect to operation (9).

8. See Exhibit II B3. This shows the admission hardcopy output of the 1416 terminal. Connect to operation (9).

9. Patient admission information is entered into the computer. This information includes medical record number, name, age, sex, problem, doctor number, room number, and admission number. Connect to operation (13).

10. Admission information is manually entered into the system. Connect to operation (9).

11. This symbol indicates that information may be called forth from the patient on-line file. Connect to operation (12).

12. On-line patient file exists which shows all patients in the hospital which require lab work. Connect to operation (9).

13. Is the admission information gathered on the patient accurate? Connect to operation (18).

14. This symbol indicates that information on the patient may be entered into or called forth from the on-line file. Connect to operation (12).

15. This symbol indicates that admission information may be entered into or called forth from the on-line file. Connect to operation (12).

16. Correct patient information is manually put into the system. Connect to operation (17).

17. Operator does a correct patient ID in which updated information is added or wrong information corrected, such as name, medical record number, age, sex, problem, doctor number, room number, and admission number. Connect to operations (9), (12).

18. Decision: A—No, connect to operation (17). B—Yes, connect to operation (19).

19. Is the time of day between 8:00 AM and 4:00 PM? Connect to operation (22).

20. See Exhibit II B5. This shows the hardcopy output on the 1416 terminal of the correct patient ID. Connect to operation (17).

21. Patients are sent to Outpatient lab for the admission lab work. Connect to operation (24).

22. Decision: A—Yes, connect to operation (21). B—No, connect to operation (23).

23. Patient's orders are taken to the patient's floor. Connect to operation (25).

24. Off-page connector: From—operation (24). To—Flowchart II C1.

25. Off-page connector: From—operation (25). To—Flowchart II A1.

Exhibit II B3

```
**READY
GENRL ADMIT, USER ID:        02, 10:08       03/21/77      STATION 18



    MR#  285801
    NAME: FXXX, LINDA G  OK?  Y
    SEX:  F OK?  Y
    AGE?  17Y  OK?  Y
    PROBLEM: STATUS ASTHMA    OK?  Y
    DR#:  924
    WXXXXX, H  OK?  Y
    ROOM:  A232A  OK?  Y
    ADMIS#:  1832789  OK?  Y
    PROT#:  00  OK?  Y
    ENTRY OK?  Y


            -- -- ----
    10:09  ENTRY ACCEPTED
    MR#  011581
    NAME:  WXXXXXXX, HAYWOOD   OK?  Y
    SEX:  M  OK?  Y
    AGE:  73Y  OK?  Y
    PROBLEM: LIVER MALIGNANCY  OK? ·Y
    DR#:  537
    MXXXX, T  OK?  Y
    ROOM:  H472C  OK?  Y
    ADMIS#:  1833485  OK?  Y
    PROT#:  00  OK?  Y
    ENTRY OK?  Y
```

Exhibit II B5

```
**READY
CORRECT PT ID, USER ID:   87,  20:01   04/12/77,    STATION 13


MR#  294873    OK?  Y XXXXXXX, MXX  02M  F  H476B  OK?  Y
MR#:  OK?  Y
NAME:  XXXXXXX, MXX   OK?  Y
SEX:  02M  F  OK?  Y
AGE:  02M  F  OK?  Y
PROBLEM:  NOT EATING  OK?  Y
ADMIS#:  1473847  OK?  N
ADMIS#:  1473874  OK?  Y
PROT#:  00  OK?  Y
ENTRY OK?  Y

               ---------------------20:02  ENTRY ACCEPTED
```

FLOWCHART IIC   Level 2

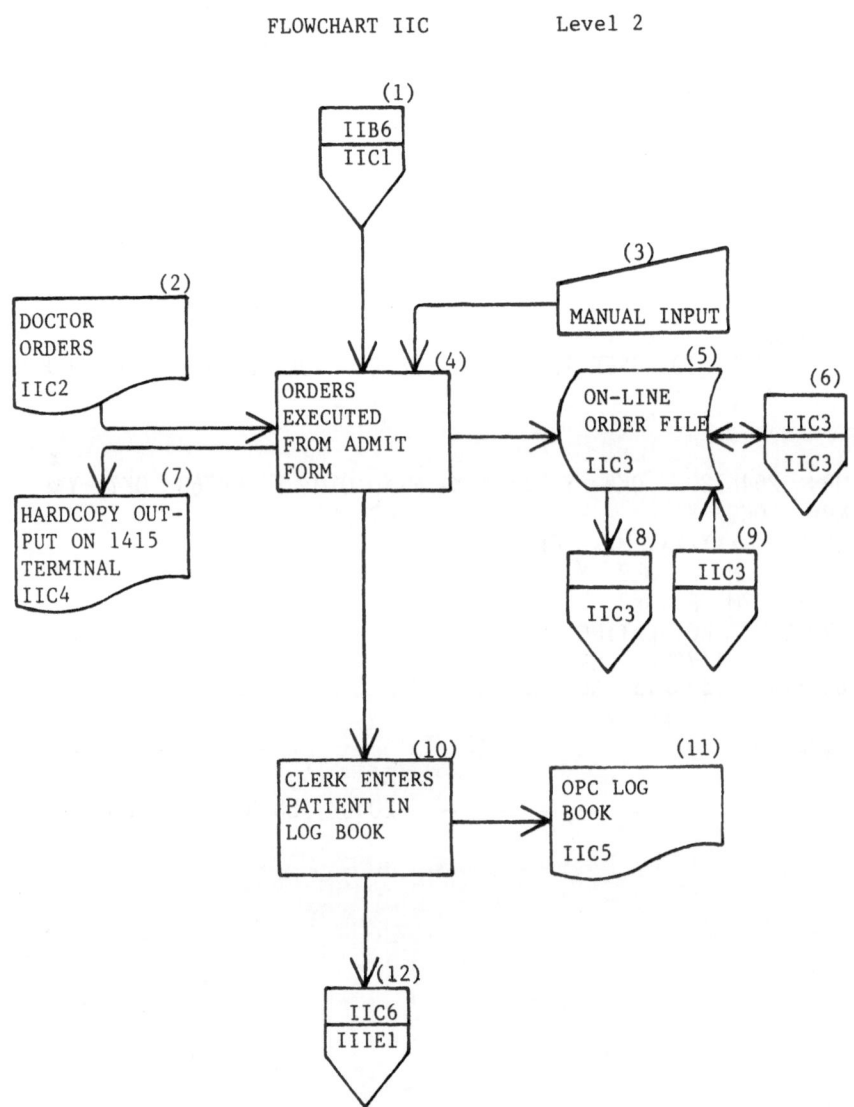

Flowchart II C: Level 2

1. Off-page connector: From—Flowchart II B6. To—operation (4).

2. See Exhibit II C2. This is the form used by the doctor on the floor to enter orders. Connect to operation (4).

3. The patient orders are manually entered on the 1415 terminal by the operator. Connect to operation (4).

4. The patient's orders for work are executed from the admission form. Connect to operation (10).

5. An on-line order file exists which shows all lab orders. Connect to operation (4).

6. Laboratory orders may be placed in the file or called forth. Connect to operation (5).

7. See Exhibit II C4. This shows the hardcopy output of the patient lab orders on the 1451 terminal. Connect to operation (4).

8. Lab orders may be called from the on-line order file. Connect to operation (5).

9. Lab orders may be entered into the on-line order file. Connect to operation (5).

10. Clerks enter the patient name, date, and type of bloods needed for particular tests into the log book before drawing the specimens. Connect to operation (12).

11. See Exhibit II C5. A page from an outpatient log book. Connect to operation (10).

12. Off-page connector: From—operation (12). To—Flowchart III E1.

Exhibit II C2

PHYSICIAN'S ORDERS

HOSPITAL AND CLINICS
UNIVERSITY OF FLORIDA

"Generic Equivalent permitted
un₁ess this square is initialed
bv Physician"

Date	Doctor's Orders	Doctor's Signature	Hour Comp.	Nurse's Signature	

Exhibit II C4

**READY
LAB ORDER, USER ID: 09, 22:35   03/05/77,   STATION 18

MR# 296413   OK? Y
NAME: DXXXX, OTIS G H584A 09 , 22:36 03/05/77 OK? Y
DR#: 751
PROBLEM: PL EFFUSSION OK? Y
T# 095 ADLT LYTS BUN CR OK? Y STAT: N EXP# Y
ENTRY OK? Y
T# 130 AMYLASE IU/L OK? Y STAT: N EXP# Y
ENTRY OK? Y
T# 001 HEMOGRAM OK? Y STAT: N EXP# Y
ENTRY OK? Y
T#

FLOWCHART IID   Level 2

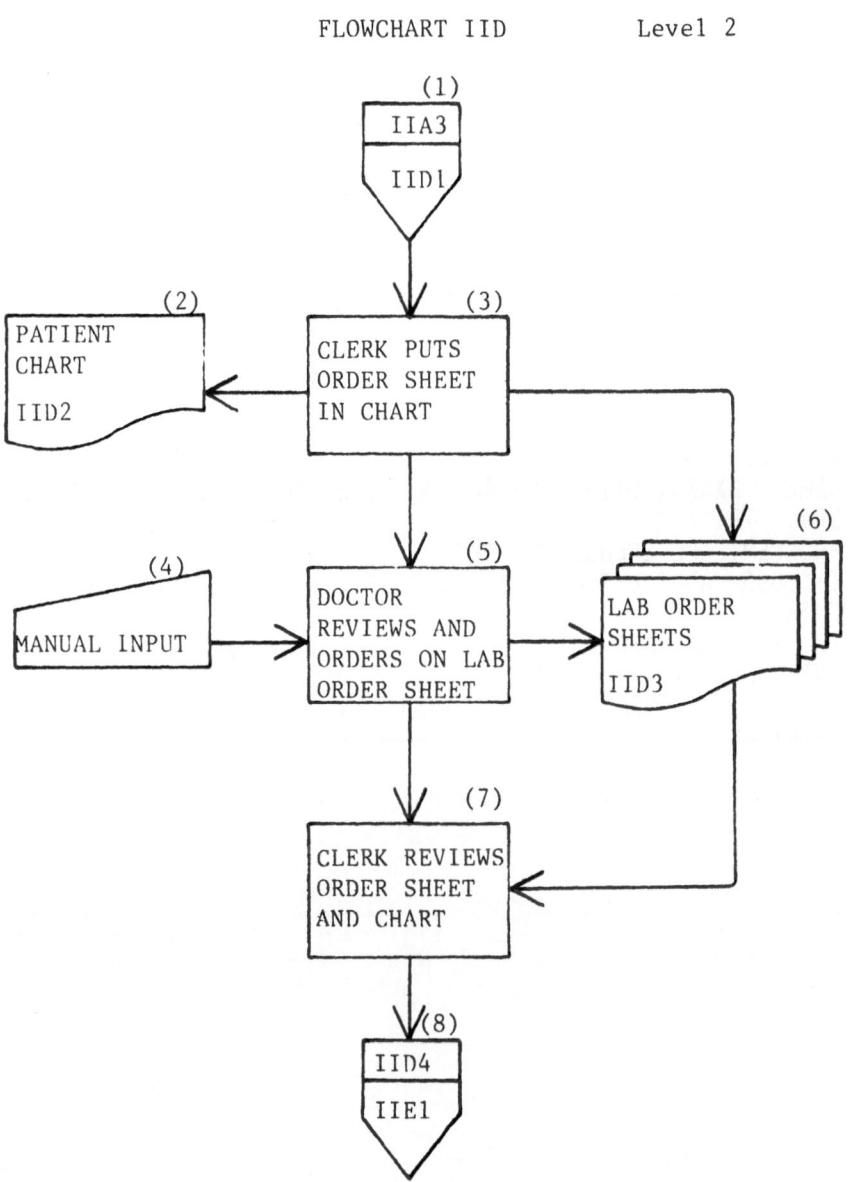

(1)
IIA3
IID1

(2)
PATIENT
CHART
IID2

(3)
CLERK PUTS
ORDER SHEET
IN CHART

(4)
MANUAL INPUT

(5)
DOCTOR
REVIEWS AND
ORDERS ON LAB
ORDER SHEET

(6)
LAB ORDER
SHEETS
IID3

(7)
CLERK REVIEWS
ORDER SHEET
AND CHART

(8)
IID4
IIE1

Flowchart II D: Level 2

1. Off-page connector: From—Flowchart II A3. To—operation (3).
2. See Exhibit II D2. A sample copy of the patient's chart. Connect to operation (3).
3. The clerk places an order sheet in the patient's chart. Connect to operation (5).
4. The doctor manually enters the orders on the laboratory sheet. Connect to operation (5).
5. The doctor reviews the patient's chart and then orders laboratory work on laboratory order sheets. Connect to operation (7).
6. See Exhibit II D3. Primary laboratory order sheets. Pink: (Hematology, Blood Bank, Microscopy; Blue: Chemistry; Green: Immunology, Microbiology; White: general short order from which includes all the above plus Anatomic Pathology. Connect to operations (5), (7).
7. The clerk reviews the order sheet and charts for accuracy and enters information where needed. Connect to operation (8).
8. Off-page connector: From—operation (8). To—Flowchart II E1.

Exhibit II C5

NAME   BLOODS DRAWN   DATE _____

	7 R	15 R	7 G HEP	V	3 GR	BB	PT	

Exhibit II D2

TEACHING HOSPITAL AND CLINICS
UNIVERSITY OF FLORIDA

FOLDER

I II III IV V
OF
1 2 3 4 5

RECORDS MUST BE AVAILABLE FOR
PATIENT CARE AT ALL TIMES

PLEASE OBSERVE THE FOLLOWING:

1 RECORDS MAY NOT BE REMOVED FROM THE HOSPITAL

2 RETURN RECORDS PROMPTLY TO THE MEDICAL RECORD DEPT.

3 WHEN OBTAINING RECORD GIVE RECORD ROOM FULL IDENTIFICA-
TION (NAME & LOCATION) OF PERSON WHO WILL HAVE POSSESSION

4 RECORDS MUST BE VISIBLY AVAILABLE AT ALL TIMES DO NOT LEAVE
RECORDS IN DRAWERS, CABINETS, BRIEFCASES, ETC.

5 WHEN RECORD IS SENT ELSEWHERE THAN TO RECORD ROOM, SEND
TRANSFER SLIP TO MEDICAL RECORD ROOM IMMEDIATELY.

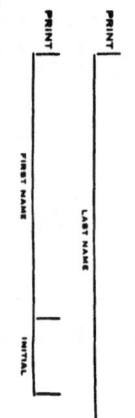

PRINT   PRINT

FIRST NAME   LAST NAME

INITIAL

INFORMATION IN THIS RECORD IS CONFIDENTIAL

refer inquiries for medical information to
Medical Record Administrators

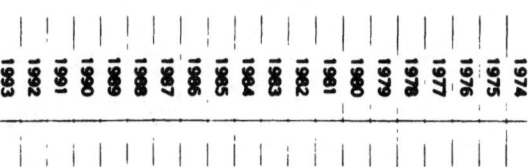

1993 1992 1991 1990 1989 1988 1987 1986 1985 1984 1983 1982 1981 1980 1979 1978 1977 1976 1975 1974

Exhibit II D3
**INPATIENT
LABORATORY ORDER
GENERAL SHORT FORM**

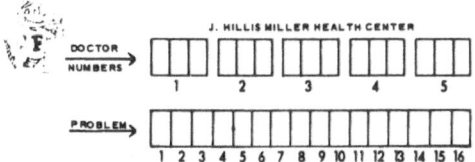

DOCTOR NUMBERS →   J. HILLIS MILLER HEALTH CENTER

1   2   3   4   5

PROBLEM →

1 2 3 4 5 6 7 8 9 10 11 12 13 14 15 16

PERTINENT HISTORY OR MESSAGE TO LAB AREA:**

PROVISIONAL DIAGNOSIS:**

CIRCLE TEST NUMBER FOR ROUTINE ORDER
(X) BOX IF STAT[1] OR EXPEDITE[2]

TEST #	ST	•	EXP	TEST NAME	RESULT	TEST #	ST	•	EXP	TEST NAME	RESULT	TEST #	ST	••	EXP	TEST NAME
				CHEMISTRY						**MICROSCOPY**						**ANATOMIC**
095	R			Adult Lytes, BUN, Crea.		400		U		Urinalysis						**PATHOLOGY**
075	R			Sodium (NA)		444		U		Qualitative HCG		513		••		Routine Surg Path
076	R			Potassium (K)		448		U		Addis Count						SOURCE:
077	R			Chloride (Cl)		469		U		Calculi Analysis		507		••		Pathology Consult
078	R			Carbon Dioxide (CO₂)		401		U		Creatinine Clearance		508		••		PAP. Smears-Gyn
079	R			BUN		426		U		17-Ketosteroids				LMP		**HORMONES** IUD ?
080	R			Creatinine		425		U		17-Hydroxy Steroids		509		••		Cytology non-Gyn
272	R			Metabolic Profile		668		S		Semen Analysis						SOURCE:
081	R			Uric Acid		412		U		Urine Calcium – 24 Hr.		521				Cell Block
083	R			Phosphorus (PO₄)		402		U		Urine Creatinine – 24 Hr.						
084	R			Glucose		418		U		24-Hour Protein – 24 Hr.						**BLOOD BANK #UNITS**
274	R			Liver/Enzyme Profile		423		U		VMA		351	R			AHG (Factor VIII)
085	R			T. Protein						**IMMUNOLOGY &**		381	R			Cryoprecipitate
086	R			Albumin						**SEROLOGY**		364	R			DAG (Direct Coombs)
089	R			T. Bilirubin		288		R		Immunoglob Serum		370	R			Fresh Frozen Plasma
090	R			D. Bilirubin						IgC, IgA, IgM		354	R			Ind. Coombs (Antibody Screen)
091	R			Alk. Phosphatase		290		R		IgE, RIA		367	R			Packed Red Cells
092	R			LDH		301		R		Insulin, RIA		371	R			Platelet Concent.
093	R			SGOT		275		R		Anti-Nuclear Ab.		369	R			Stored Frozen Plasma
094	R			SGPT		295		R		Anti-Streptolysin O		352	R			Type & Hold
						292		R		VDRL – Serum		373	R			WBC Poor Pkd. Cells
						293		R		FTA-ABS Serum		365	R			Whole Blood
125	R			Acetone		280		R		Mono Spot test						Mssg.
129	R			Ac-d Phosphatase		294		R		Rubella Antibody						
142	R			Alcohol		278		R		Rheumatoid Factor						
130	R			Amylase		302		R		T4, RIA						
143	R			Barbiturate		321		R.		T₃, RIA						
082	R			Calcium (CA)		284		R		AUST. Ag: (HBs Ag.)						**MICROBIOLOGY**
169	R			CPK		276		R		C'3 Complement						**SOURCE/SPECIMEN**
117	GY			Glucose, 2Hr PC		277		R		C'4 Complement		603				Urine Cult
111	R			Magnesium MG.)		298		R		Digoxin, RIA		598				Blood Cult
109	R			Osmolality						**HEMATOLOGY**						
145	R			Salicylate		001		V		Hemogram		576				AFB Culture
087	R			Cholesterol		005		V		WBC		583				AFB Stain
118	GY			GTT, 3Hr		002		V		HGB		590				B-Strep Screen
157	R			Iron Profile		003		V		HCT		575				Fungus Cult
137	R			Lipo. Electro, (Trig Chol.)		004		V		RBC		591				GC Culture
140	R			Protein Electro, (T. Protein)		006		V		Differential (Order Separately)		584				Gram Stain
086	R			Triglyceride		010		V		Platelet Count		579				Ova & Parasites
				MICROSCOPY		011		V		ESR		577				Occult Blood
459	C			CSF Profile		012		V		Retic, Count		658				PKU
				(Gluc, Prot, Count		022		V		Sickle Screen						
				& D.ff)		020		V		HGB Electro.						
467	S			Body Fluid Cells		007		B		PT						ORDERED AT ADMISSION ONLY
				SOURCE		008		B		PTT		699				Admission Screen (400, 001, 284, 292)
						009		B		TT						

[1]SPECIMEN LEGEND   GN-GREEN TOP   V-PURPLE TOP   S-SPECIAL   BT-BULLET   R-15-RED
B-BLUE TOP   R-RED TOP (7 ml)   U-URINE   D-DIRECT   C-CSF   TOP (15ml)
GY-GREY TOP   •
1. STAT-USUALLY LESS THAN ONE HOUR   2. EXPEDITE-USUALLY 2-6 HOURS ON SELECTED PROCEDURES

REVISED 7/76   15-1400-1

INPATIENT
LABORATORY ORDER

Exhibit II D3   HEMATOLOGY · BLOOD BANK · MICROSCOPY

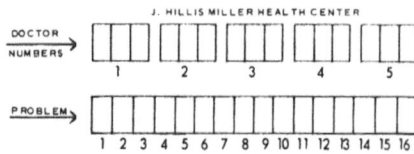

J. HILLIS MILLER HEALTH CENTER

DOCTOR NUMBERS →

1   2   3   4   5

PROBLEM →

1 2 3 4 5 6 7 8 9 10 11 12 13 14 15 16

MESSAGE:

CIRCLE TEST NUMBER FOR ROUTINE ORDER
(X) - BOX IF STAT¹ OR EXPEDITE²

TEST#	ST	·	EXP	TEST NAME	RESULT	TEST#	ST	·	EXP	TEST NAME	#UNITS	TEST#	ST	·	TEST NAME	RESULT
				HEMATOLOGY		373	R			WBC Poor Pkd Cells					**RANDOM URINE CHEMISTRY**	
001	V			Hemogram:		374	R			Isohemagglutinin		422		U	Amylase	
005	V			WBC		358	R			Prenatal Evaluation		411		U	Chloride (CL)	
002	V			HGB		376	R			Peds Walking Donor		451		U	Myoglobin	
003	V			HCT								478		U	Osmolality	
004	V			RBC						**MICROSCOPY**	RESULT	453		U	Porphyrin Screen	
006	V			Differential (Order Separately)		444		U		Qualitative HCG		409		U	Potassium (K)	
007	B			PT		400		U		Urinalysis		407		U	Sodium (NA)	
008	B			PTT		487		U		Urine Pr. Electrophoresis		443		U	Urobilinogen Screen	
009	B			TT								455		U	Amino Acid Screen	
010	V			Platelet Count						**24 HR URINE CHEMISTRY**		413		U	Calcium (CA)	
011				ESR		448		U		Addis Count		402		U	Creatinine	
012				Retic Count		435		U		Aldosterone		421		U	Glucose, Peds Screen	
022	V			Sickle Screen		456		U		Amino Acid Chrom.		454		U	Hemosiderin	
013	V			EOS Count		437		U		Amino Acid Nitrogen		450		U	Homogentisic Acid	
014				Bleeding Time		412		U		Calcium (CA)		452		U	Melanogens	
015				Clotting Time		427		U		Catecholamines		457		U	Phenothiazine	
370	V			HGB Electro		410		U		Chloride (CL)		415		U	Phosphorus PO₄	
21	V			Fetal HGB's		402		U		Creatinine		419		U	Protein	
321				Cryoglobulin		438		U		Copper		405		U	Urea	
024				Cryofibrinogen		401		U		Creatinine Clearance		417		U	Uric Acid	
025	V			WBC Alk Ptase		482		U		Delta-Amino Lev Acid					**CSF ANALYSIS**	
026				OS Fragility		434		U		Estriol Pregnancy		459		C	CSF Profile: (Gluc, Prot,	
029				Sperm: Stain, Nasal, etc.		433		U		Estrogens					Count & Diff.)	
						420		U		Glucose		447		C	CSF Cell Count & Diff	
				BLOOD BANK	#UNITS	432		U		Gonadotropin (HCG)		467		C	CSF Electrolytes:	
150		B		Rhogam		424		U		5 HIAA					NA K CL:	
151				AHG Factor VIII)		429		U		Homovanillic Acid		465		C	CSF Chloride	
156				ABO Grp Rh Genotype		436		U		Hydroxyproline		461		C	CSF Glucose	
155		B		Antibody Ident.		425		U		17 Hydroxysteroids		466		C	CSF LDH	
141		B		Indirect Combs		426		U		17-Ketosteroids		463		C	CSF Potassium	
142		B		Antibody Titer		479		U		Magnesium MG		460		C	CSF Protein	
				Negative Eval		149		U		Metals (HG, PB, AS		464		C	CSF Sodium	
9				Platelet &		428		U		Metanephrines		488		C	CSF Electrophoresis	
160				Sperm Antibody		475		U		Oxalate						
164				Cell Counts		414		U		Phosphorus PO₄					**BODY FLUIDS**	SOURCE
6				Therapeutic Phlebotomy		441		U		Porphyrin PBG CP UP		474		S	Amylase	
9				Therapeutic Plasmapheresis								467		S	Count & Diff	
				Type & Crossmatch:		408		U		Potassium K		483		S	Electrolytes	
61				Whole Blood		430		U		Pregnanediol		47		S	Glucose	
52				Packed Red Cells		431		U		Pregnanetriol		440		S	LDH	
				Packed Red Cells		17				Protein		47		S		
				Fresh Frozen		50				Sodium NA						
						11				Amino Creatinine					**OTHER**	
						11										

Exhibit II D3
INPATIENT
LABORATORY ORDER
IMMUNO & MICROBIOLOGY

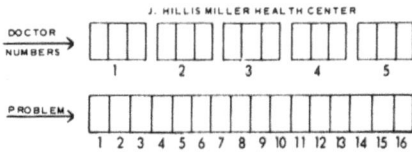

J. HILLIS MILLER HEALTH CENTER

DOCTOR NUMBERS

1   2   3   4   5

PROBLEM

1 2 3 4 5 6 7 8 9 10 11 12 13 14 15 16

NOTE: Microbiology Specimens must be clearly labeled to show Source & Specimen location.

CIRCLE TEST NUMBER FOR ROUTINE ORDER
X) - BOX IF STAT[1] OR EXPEDITE[2]

TEST#	ST	•	EXP.	TEST NAME	RESULT	TEST#	ST	•	EXP.	TEST NAME	RESULTS	TEST#	ST	•	TEST NAME	SOURCE
				CLINICAL		323		R		E. Histolytica Ab.		591			G.C. Culture	
				IMMUMOLOGY								658			Guthrie Test PKU	
275		R		Anti-Nuclear Ab		308		S		Tissue Typing		628			Hemovac Culture	
276		R		C 3 Complement		330		S		HLA 27 Typing		582			India Ink	
277		R		C 4 Complement								632			Joint Fluid Culture	
339		R		C3 Proactivator								587			KOH PREP	
278		R		Rheumatoid Factor								594			Listeria Culture	
279		U		Ig. Light Chains								588			Malaria Smear	
280		R		Mono Spot Test								646			Motem Plac Culture	
383		R		EB Virus, AB. Titre								649			Misc. Routine Culture	
384		R		Aust. Ag. HBsAg						MICROBIOLOGY	SOURCE	612			Nasopharyngeal Cult	
385		R		Alpha-1 Antitrypsin		635				Abdominal Wall Culture		610			Nose Culture Routine	
788		R		Immunoglob Serum		636				Abscess Culture		577			Occult Blood	
				IgG, IgA, IgM,		596				Actinomyces Culture		579			Ova & Parasites	
289		R		Immunoglobulin-D		576				AFB Culture		644			Pelvic Absc. Culture	
290		R		IgE, RIA		583				AFB Stain		629			Penrose Culture	
291		C		Immunoglob CFS		645				Amniotic FL Culture		620			Periton Dial Cath	
				IgG-CSF, IgA-CSF,		581				Amoeba Culture		621			Periton Dial Fluid	
				IgM-CSF.		663				Anaerobic Culture		634			Periton Absc. Culture	
292		R		VDRL- Serum		653				Antibiotic Level		633			Periton Exud Culture	
293		R		FTA-ABS Serum		632				Antibiotic Sens Tube D		593			Pertussis Culture	
340		C		VDRL, CSF		590				B Strep Screen		586			Pinworm Slide	
294		R		Rubella Antibody		650				Biopsy Culture		631			Pleural Cavity Asp	
295		R		Anti-Streptolysin O		598				Blood Culture		651			Quantitative Culture	
796		R		C Reactive Protein		600				Blood, Post Bypass		622			Skin Culture Axilla	
297		R		Febrile Agg. Titre		599				Blood, Pre Bypass		673			Skin Culture Groin	
298		R		Digoxin, RIA		616				Branch Brush BX		627			Skin Graft Culture	
299		S		Renin R A		615				Branch Wash Culture		613			Sputum Culture	
309		R		Human Growth Hor, RIA		595				Brucella Culture		609			Stool Culture	
101		R		Insulin, R-A		626				Burn Quan Culture BX		580			Stool Screen	
192		R		T3 RIA		625				Burn Wound Culture		597			T. Vaginalis Culture	
52		R		T7 RIA		592				C Diphtheriae Culture		589			T. Vaginalis Wet Mount	
31		R		T3 Resin Uptake		618				Cath Site Culture		659			Testurio Culture	
		R		PB		619				Cath Tip Culture		611			Throat Culture	
133		R		T4 Unbound		641				Cervical Culture		614			Tracheal Culture	
18		R		TSH		630				Chest Tube Culture		617			Trans Trach Asp	

Exhibit II D3

INPATIENT
LABORATORY ORDER
CHEMISTRY

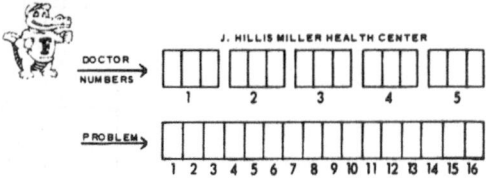

J. HILLIS MILLER HEALTH CENTER

DOCTOR NUMBERS

1   2   3   4   5

PROBLEM

1 2 3 4 5 6 7 8 9 10 11 12 13 14 15 16

MESSAGE:

CIRCLE TEST NUMBER FOR ROUTINE ORDER
(X) - BOX IF STAT[1] OR EXPEDITE[2]

TEST #	ST	•	EXP	TEST NAME	RESULT	TEST #	ST	•	EXP	TEST NAME	RESULT	TEST #	ST	•	EXP	TEST NAME	RESULT
						082			R	Calcium (CA)		'121			GY	Lactose Tol Test:	
095	R			Adult Lytes, BUN, Crea.		169			R	CPK						FBS 15, 30, 45, 60,	
075	R			Sodium (NA)		152			GN	Fibrinogen						90 Min	
076	R			Potassium (K)		117			GY	Glucose, 2Hr PC		122			GY	Insulin Tol Test:	
077	R			Chloride (CL)		151			GY	Lactic Acid						Preinjection, 30, 45	
078	R			Carbon Dioxide (CO₂)		159			R	Lithium						60, 90 Min	
079	R			BUN		111			R	Magnesium (MG)		123			GY	3Hr Tolbutamide T.T.	
080	R			Creatinine		109			R	Osmolality						Preinjection,2,5,10,	
272	R			Metabolic Profile		145			R	Salicylate						20,40,60,90,120	
081	R			Uric Acid												150, 180 Min	
083	R			Phosphorus (PO₄)		170			R	Aldolase		124			GY	1Hr Tolbutamide T.T.	
084	R			Glucose		161			S	Amniotic Fl Creatinine						Preinjection, 2, 5, 10,	
274	R			Liver Enzyme Profile		267			S	Amniotic Fl Gluc						20,40,60 Min	
085	R			T. Protein		149			R	Carotene							
086	P			Albumin		132			R	Ceruloplasmin							
089	R			T. Bilirubin		067			R	Cholesterol					—REFERRAL LAB TESTS-AUDITED—	
090	R			D. Bilirubin		134			R	Cholinesterase					INITIAL ENDOCRINOLOGY CONSULT REQUIRED	
091	R			Alk. Phosphatase		156			R-15	Cortisol		099			GN	ACTH	
092	R			LDH		197			R	CPK-MB		171			GN	Aldosterone	
093	R			SGOT		195			R	Gamma GT		112			GN	Calcitonin	
094	R			SGPT		135			V	G6PD (Red Cell)		179			R	Parathyroid Hormone	
						127			R	HBDH		201			V	Serotonin	
						153			GN	Hemoglobin, Plasma							
			PEDIATRIC PROCEDURES			158			R	Iron (FE)							
102	BT			Peds Lytes, BUN, Crea.		157			R	Iron Profile					—PLEASE LIMIT ORDERS-AUDITED—	
103	BT			Sodium (NA)						(Iron, TIBC,% Sat)							
104	BT			Potassium (K)		136			R	LAP		268			R	Alpha-Fetoprotein	
105	BT			Chloride (CL)		131			R	Lipase		133			R-45	Copper	
106	BT			Carbon Dioxide (CO₂)		137			R	Lipo. Electro. (Chol & Trig.)		163			R	Creatine	
107	BT			BUN		198			R	LDH-isoenzymes		113			R-15	Estradiol	
108	BT			Creatinine		154			GN	Oxygen Sat. (Art.)		173			R	FSH	
116	BT			Peds Glucose		155			GN	Oxygen Sat. (Ven.)		166			R	Gastrin	
						140			R	Protein Electro. (T. Prot.)		175			R	HCG (Quantitative)	
						160			S	Sweat Chloride		164			R	Haptoglobin	
						088			R	Triglyceride		167			GY	Histamine	
												144			GY	Lead	
												172			R	Luteinizing Hormone	
125	R			Acetone								178			R	Lysozyme	
129	R			Acid Phosphatase						TOLERANCE TESTS		168			R-45	Quinidine	
142	R			Alcohol		118			GY	3Hr Gluc Tol Test:		176			R	Testosterone	
146	GN			Ammonia						FBS, ½, 1,2,3 Hr		202			R	Thiocyanate	
162	S			Amniotic Fl Scan		119			GY	5Hr Gluc Tol Test:		150			R-15	Vitamin A	
115	R			Amylase						FBS,½, 1,2,3,4, 5 Hr		100			R-45	Vitamin C	
141	R			Barbiturate		120			CV	Rapid IV GTT		203			R	Vitamin E	
147	R			Bromide						Preinjection, 10, 20							
148	R			BSP						30,40,50,60 Min							

SPECIMEN LEGEND
R-RED TOP   GN-GREEN TOP   V-PURPLE TOP   S-SPECIAL   BT-BULLET   R-15-RED TOP 15ml
P-RED TOP 7ml   U-URINE   D-DIRECT   C-CSF

[1] STAT IS ALWAYS LESS THAN ONE HOUR   [2] EXPEDITE USUALLY 2-6 HOURS ON SELECTED PROCEDURES   REVISED 7 76   18-1402-1

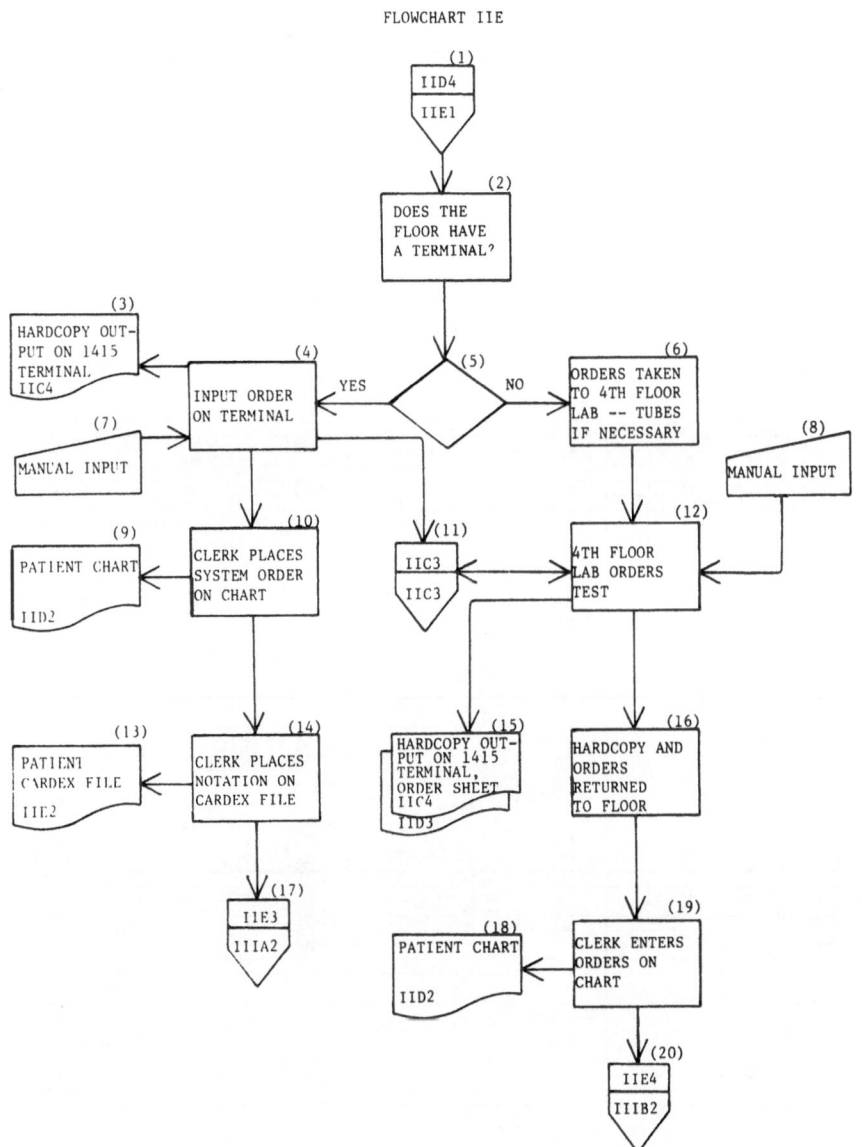

FLOWCHART IIE

Flowchart II E

1. Off-page connector: From—Flowchart II D4. To—operation (2).
2. Does the floor have a terminal? Connect to operation (5).
3. Hardcopy of laboratory order. See Exhibit II C4.
4. The clerk orders lab work on the terminal. Connect to operation (10).
5. Decision: A—Yes, connect to operation (4). B—No, connect to operation (6).
6. The lab orders and specimen tubes (if necessary) are hand carried to the 4th floor lab area for processing. Connect to operation (12).
7. The orders are manually entered on the terminal. Connect to operation (4).
8. The computer operator manually orders on the terminal. Connect to operation (12).
9. Patient chart. See Exhibit II D2.
10. Clerk places orders in the patient's chart. Connect to operation (14).
11. The on-line order file shows all lab orders. Connect to operations (4), (12).
12. The floor does not have its own terminal so the 4th floor lab places the order. Connect to operation (16).
13. See Exhibit II E2. The patient cardex file shows all available information on the patient: admission information, medication, nursing and doctor orders, notes, etc. Connect to operation (14).
14. Clerk places order information on cardex file. Connect to operation (17).
15. Hardcopy output of orders and order sheet. See Exhibits II C4 and II D3.
16. Once the lab work is ordered in the lab, the hardcopy of the order and original orders are returned to the floor. Connect to operation (19).
17. Off-page connector: From—operation (17). To—Flowchart III A2.
18. Patient chart. See Exhibit II D2.
19. The clerk places the order hardcopy on the patient's chart. Connect to operation (20).
20. Off-page connector: From—operation (20). To—Flowchart III B2.

Exhibit II E2

ADMISSION   DATA

#15 0794 0

NAME

ADDRESS   SERV. CE

OCCUPATION

PHYSICIAN   PHONE

ROLE IN FAMILY   FIN CODE   HOSP NUMBER

RELIGION   DATE OF BIRTH   AGE

LANGUAGE SPOKEN

ADMISSION NOTE

ALLERGIES

PROSTHESES

SPECIAL CONSIDERATIONS

POST DISCHARGE PLANNING

DISPOSITION   ESTIMATED DATE OF DISCHARGE

HEALTH TEAM MEMBERS

OUTPATIENT THERAPIES

REFERRALS

EQUIPMENT SUPPLIES MEDICATIONS DIET

INSTRUCTION FOR PATIENT & FAMILY

SHANDS TEACHING HOSPITAL · GAINESVILLE FLORIDA

Exhibit II E2

MEDICATION LABEL

CIRCLE DOSAGE HOURS

DATE	TIME	DRUG NAME	DOSAGE													
NURSE'S SIGNATURE		FREQUENCY	ROUTE	7	8	9	10	11	12	13	14	15	16	17	18
PATIENT NAME		NUMBER	DOCTOR	19	20	21	22	23	24	1	2	3	4	5	6
DATE	TIME	DRUG NAME	DOSAGE													
NURSE'S SIGNATURE		FREQUENCY	ROUTE	7	8	9	10	11	12	13	14	15	16	17	18
PATIENT NAME		NUMBER	DOCTOR	19	20	21	22	23	24	1	2	3	4	5	6
DATE	TIME	DRUG NAME	DOSAGE													
NURSE'S SIGNATURE		FREQUENCY	ROUTE	7	8	9	10	11	12	13	14	15	16	17	18
PATIENT NAME		NUMBER	DOCTOR	19	20	21	22	23	24	1	2	3	4	5	6
DATE	TIME	DRUG NAME	DOSAGE													
NURSE'S SIGNATURE		FREQUENCY	ROUTE	7	8	9	10	11	12	13	14	15	16	17	18
PATIENT NAME		NUMBER	DOCTOR	19	20	21	22	23	24	1	2	3	4	5	6

CLERK

Exhibit II E2

#138344-8061

DATE	TREATMENTS	DATE	TREATMENTS

Exhibit II 1.2

DIET	URINE		ACTIVITIES		DATE ORD	SPECIMEN COLLECTION 15-0793-0	DATE SENT
		SP G	B R			URINE	
		S & A	BRP				
		STRAIN	CHAIR				
		FRACTIONAL	AMB				
SNACK		FOLEY	HEAD OF BED				
			TRANSPORT				
	DRAINS		PROTECTIVE MEASURES				
FLUIDS		LEVINE / NG					
		CHEST	SIDE RAILS			STOOL	
		WOUND	RESTRAINTS				
		OTHER	BATH				
DIETARY ASSISTANCE	VITAL SIGNS		COMPLETE				
FEED PT		TPR	PARTIAL				
PREPARE FOOD			SELF				
		BP	SHOWER			SPUTUM	
INTAKE		CUP	VENTILATION				
OUTPUT		BM S	O₂				
		WTS	T C D R				
		SEIZURE PREC	IPPB				
PATIENT CARE INDEX			PD				
I	II	III					

FLOWCHART IIF   Level 2

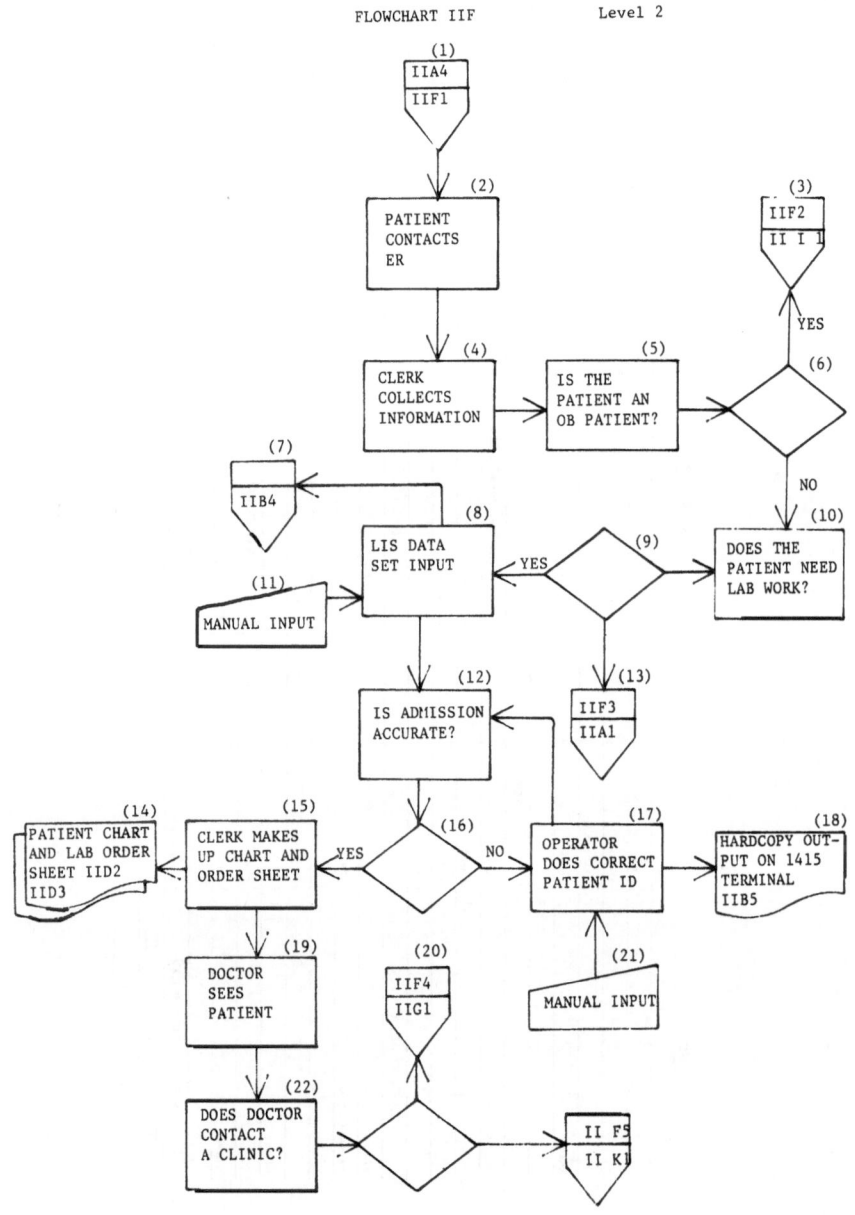

Flowchart II F

1. Off-page connector: From—Flowchart II A4. To—operation (2).
2. The patient contacts the Emergency Room for treatment. Connect to operation (4).
3. Off-page connector: From—operation (3). To—Flowchart II I1.
4. A clerk collects all pertinent patient information. Connect to operation (5).
5. Is the patient an Obstetrics patient? Connect to operation (6).
6. Decision: A—Yes, connect to operation (3). B—No, connect to operation (10).
7. On-line patient file. Connect to operation (8).
8. Patient admission information is entered into the computer. Connect to operation (12).
9. Decision: A—Yes, connect to operation (8). B—No, connect to Flowchart II A1.
10. Does the patient need lab work? Connect to operation (9).
11. Emergency Room admission information is manually entered into the LIS system. Connect to operation (8).
12. Is admission information gathered on the patient accurate? Connect to operation (16).
13. Off-page connector: From—operation (13). To—Flowchart II A1.
14. Patient chart and lab orders. See Exhibit II D2 and II D3.
15. Clerk makes out a chart and order sheet which contains all information on a patient that the doctor will need. Connect to operation (19).
16. Decision: A—Yes, connect to operation (15). B—No, connect to operation (17).
17. Clerk does a correct patient ID in which updated information is added or wrong informations corrected. Connect to operations (12) and (18).
18. Hardcopy of correct patient ID. See Exhibit II B5.
19. Doctor examines the patient. Connect to operation (22).
20. Off-page connector: From—operation (20). To—Flowchart II G1.
21. Correct patient information is manually put into the system. Connect to operation (17).
22. Does doctor contact a clinic? Connect to operation (23).
23. Decision: A—Yes, connect to operation (24). B—No, connect to operation (20).
24. Off-page connector: From—operation (24). To—Flowchart II K1.

FLOWCHART IIG

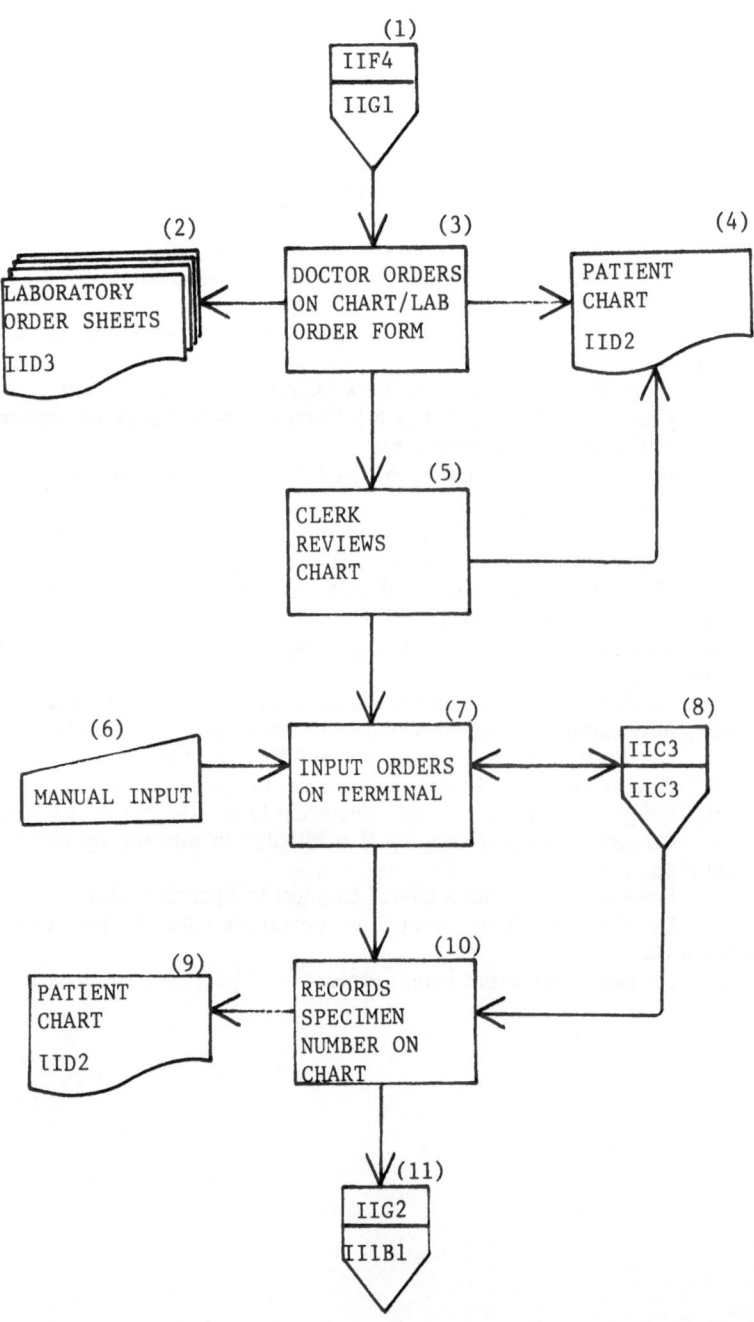

Flowchart II G

1. Off-page connector: From—Flowchart II F4. To—operation (3).

2. Laboratory order sheets. See Exhibit II D3.

3. Doctor enters orders on the patient's chart and the lab order forms. Connect to operation (5).

4. Patient chart. See Exhibit II D2.

5. Clerk reviews the chart to make sure the doctor orders are written on the chart. Connect to operations (4), (7).

6. The doctor's orders are manually entered. Connect to operation (7).

7. The orders are entered into the file structure. Connect to operation (10).

8. The on-line order file shows all lab orders. Connect to operations (7), (10).

9. Patient chart. See Exhibit II D2.

10. The clerk records the specimen number assigned by the terminal on the patient's chart. Connect to operation (11).

11. Off-page connector: From—operation (11). To—Flowchart III B1.

FLOWCHART IIH

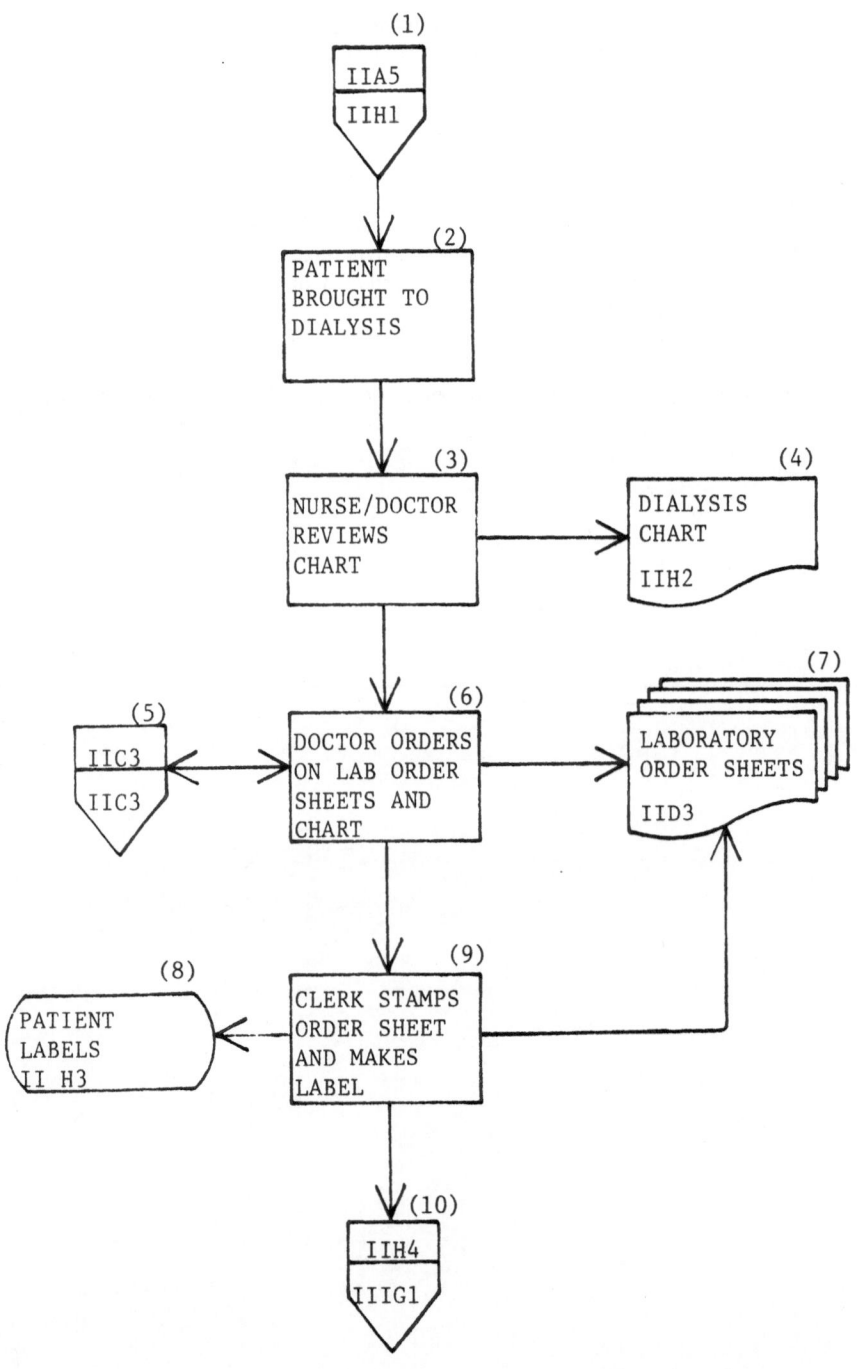

Flowchart II H

1. Off-page connector: From—Flowchart II A5. To—operation (2).
2. Patient is brought to Dialysis for treatment. Connect to operation (3).
3. Nurse and doctor review the patient's chart. Connect to operation (6).
4. See Exhibit II H2. Dialysis chart is maintained which shows all pertinent information on the patient. Connect to operation (3).
5. On-line order file which shows all lab orders. Connect to operation (6).
6. Doctor orders lab work on order sheet and records information on the patient's chart. Connect to operation (9).
7. Laboratory order sheets. See Exhibit II D3.
8. See Exhibit II H3. Labels are made for the patient which show medical record number, name, and date of birth. Connect to operation (9).
9. The clerk stamps the order sheets and makes the label for patient. Connect to operation (10).
10. Off-page connector: From—operation (10). To—Flowchart III G1.

Exhibit II H2

Name _____ Date _____ Dialyzer-Use _____

Hosp. No. _____ Time On _____ Time Off _____

Blood Access _____ Total Heparin _____ Total IV Fluids _____

Estimated Dry Wt. _____ TMP _____ Previous HCT/Date _____(pre dialysis)

Present HCT/Date _____(pre-dialysis)

	Apical		Temp	Previous Wt.	Today's Wt.	Previous B/P	Today's B/P
Pre							
Post							

Time	B/P	Pump Speed	Drip Pressure	Neg. Pressure	Medications	IV Fluids (N/S, Blood, etc.

Blood Work:

Nurse's Notes:

Exhibit II H2

MACHINE CHECKLIST

Machine No. _____

Blood Pump No. _____

Blood Lines _____

Dialysate Lines _____

Conductivity _____

Dialysate Meter _____

Temperature _____

Drip Chamber _____

Negative Pressure _____

Blood Leak _____

Clinitest _____.

Green Lights On _____

Alarm Lights Off __ _____

Signature _____

Exhibit II H3

2299   P   31-34-05
    DXXX, MARY A
    103 JUNE ST
    MARIETTA, GEORGIA 31635
MC 8690439   09/16/76 S

FLOWCHART II I

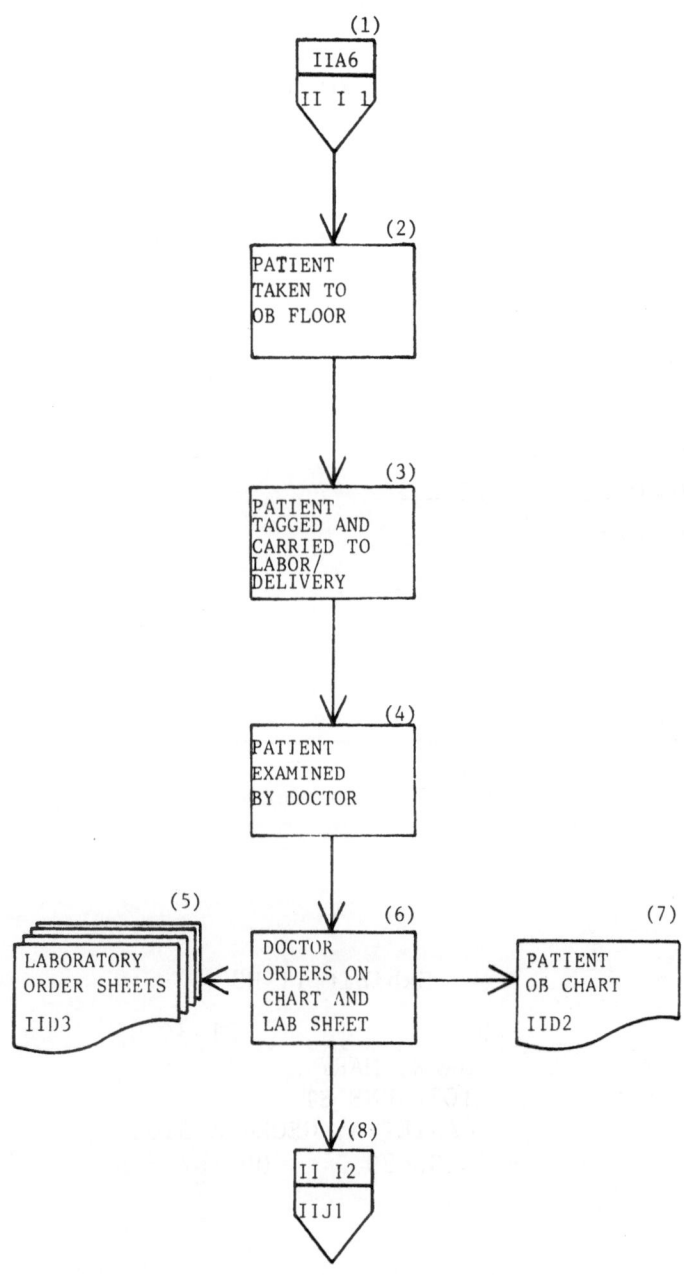

Flowchart II I

    1. Off-page connector: From—Flowchart II A6. To—operation (2).

    2. Patient is taken to the Obstetrics floor for examination by the doctor. Connect to operation (3).

    3. Patient is tagged with identification bracelet and carried to the labor/delivery room. Connect to operation (4).

    4. Patient is examined by the doctor. Connect to operation (6).

    5. Laboratory order sheet. See Exhibit II D3.

    6. Doctor orders lab work on lab sheets and records orders on the chart. Connect to operation (8).

    7. Patient OB chart. See Exhibit II D2. Laboratory orders are entered on the patient's OB chart which contains all pertinent information on the patient. Connect to operation (6).

    8. Off-page connector: From—operation (8). To—Flowchart II J1.

FLOWCHART IIJ

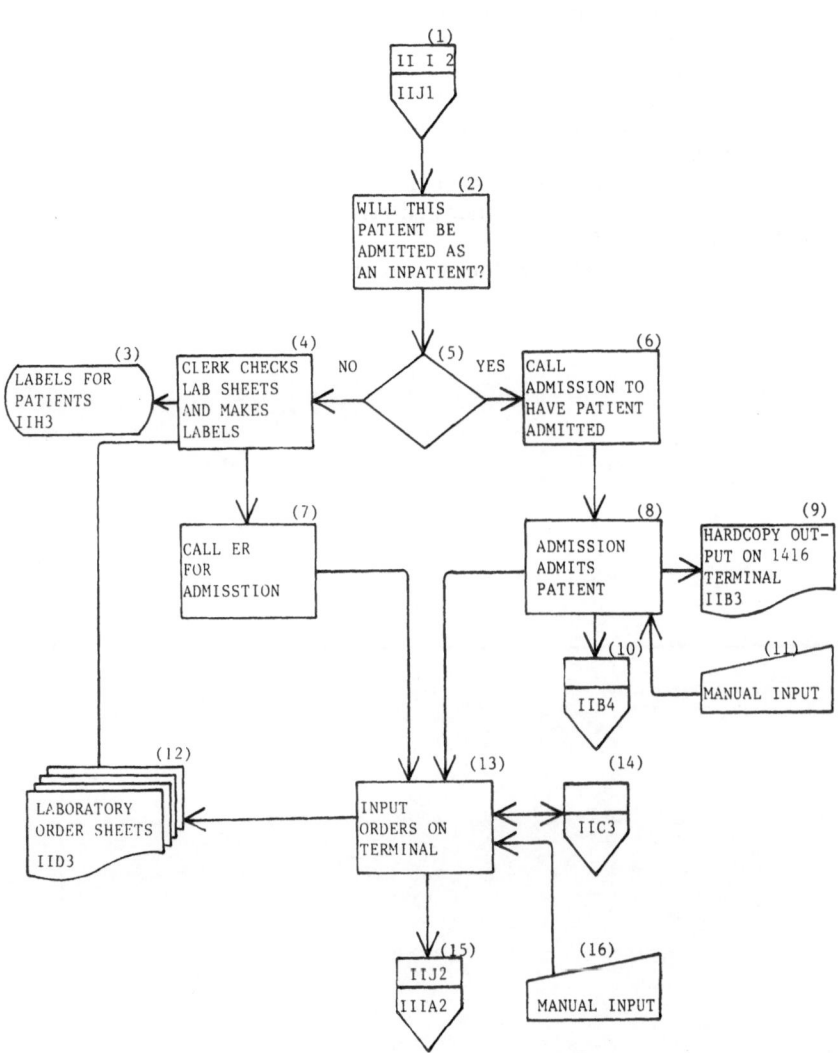

Flowchart II J

1. Off-page connector: From—Flowchart II I3. To—operation (2).

2. Will this patient be admitted as an Inpatient? Connect to operation (5).

3. Labels for patient. See Exhibit II H3.

4. Clerk checks the lab sheets for accuracy and makes labels which show patient name, medical record number, and tests ordered. Connect to operation (7).

5. Decision: A—Yes, connect to operation (6). B—No, connect to operation (4).

6. The OB floor calls the Admission Department to have the patient admitted as an Inpatient. Connect to operation (8).

7. The OB floor calls Emergency Room to have the patient admitted as an Outpatient. Connect to operation (13).

8. Admissions admits the patient as an Inpatient. Connect to operation (13).

9. Hardcopy of the patient's admission to the hospital. See Exhibit II B3.

10. An on-line patient file exists which shows all patients in the hospital who require lab work. Connect to operation (8).

11. Admission information is manually entered into the system. Connect to operation (8).

12. Laboratory order sheets. See Exhibit II D3.

13. The clerk orders the lab work on the terminal. Connect to operation (15).

14. The on-line order file contains all laboratory work ordered. Connect to operation (13).

15. Off-page connector: From—operation (15). To—Flowchart III A2.

16. The laboratory orders are manually entered into the system. Connect to operation (13).

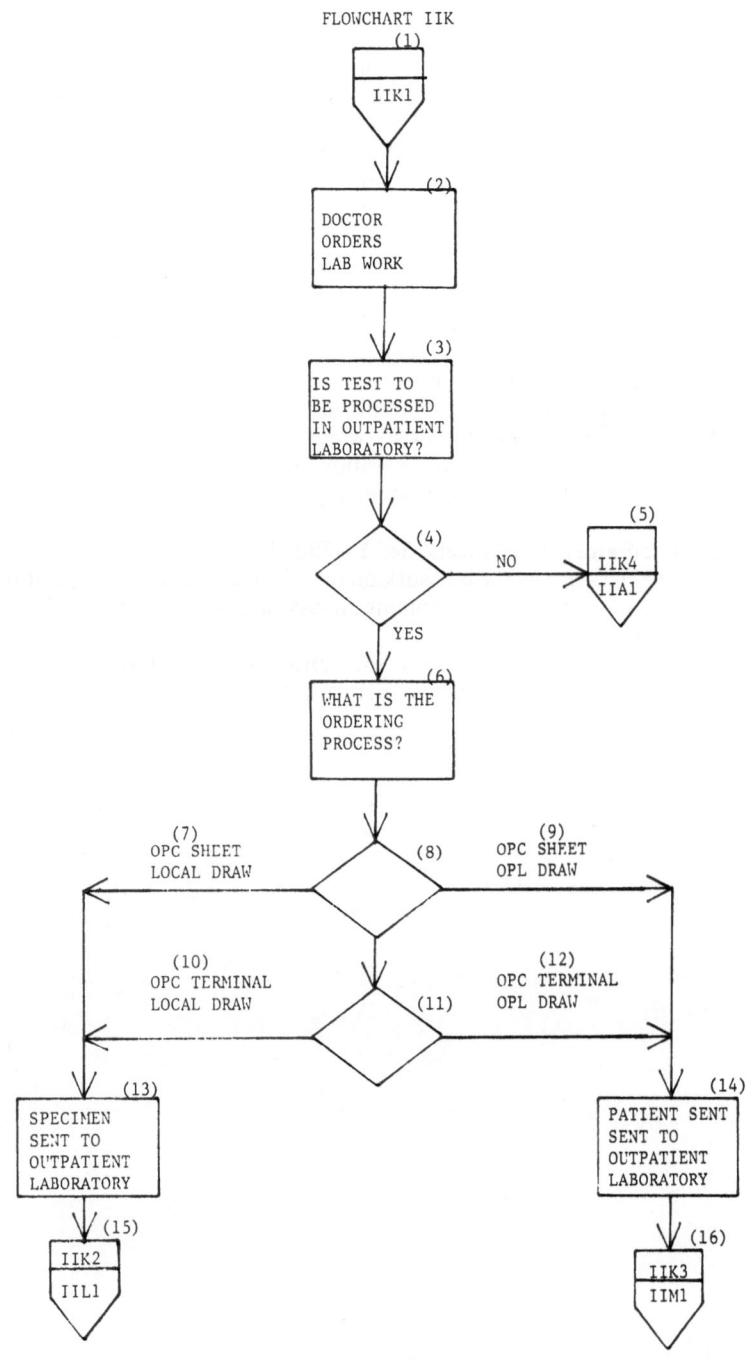

Flowchart II K

Outpatient Clinics

1. Off-page connector: From—Flowchart II A7. To—operation (2).
2. The doctor orders lab work. Connect to operation (3).
3. Is the test to be processed in the Outpatient laboratory? Connect to operation (4).
4. Decision: A—Yes, connect to operation (6). B—No, connect to operation (5).
5. The tests are not to be performed in the Outpatient lab and the process is halted.
6. What is the ordering process? Connect to operation (8).
7. The Outpatient Clinic draws its own specimens and orders on an order sheet. Connect to operation (13).
8. Decision: A—the Outpatient Clinic draws its own specimens and orders on an order sheet. Connect to operation (13). B—the Outpatient Clinic orders on an order sheet and sends the patient to the Outpatient lab to be drawn. C—Proceed to next decision block.
9. The Outpatient Clinic orders on an order sheet and sends the patient to the outpatient lab to be drawn. Connect to operation (14).
10. The Outpatient Clinic has its own terminal for entering orders and draws their own specimens. Connect to operation (13).
11. Decision: A—the outpatient Clinic has its own terminal for entering orders and draws its own specimens. Connect to operation (13). B—the Outpatient Clinic has a terminal for entering orders but sends the patient to the Outpatient lab to be drawn. Connect to operation (14).
12. The Outpatient Clinic has a terminal for entering orders but sends the patient to the Outpatient lab to be drawn. Connect to operation (14).
13. The specimen that is drawn in the clinics is sent to the Outpatient laboratory to be processed. Connect to operation (14).
14. The patients are sent to the Outpatient laboratory to have specimens drawn. Connect to operation (16).
15. Off-page connector: From—operation (15). To—Flowchart II L1.
16. Off-page connector: From—operation (16). To—Flowchart II M1.

FLOWCHART IIL

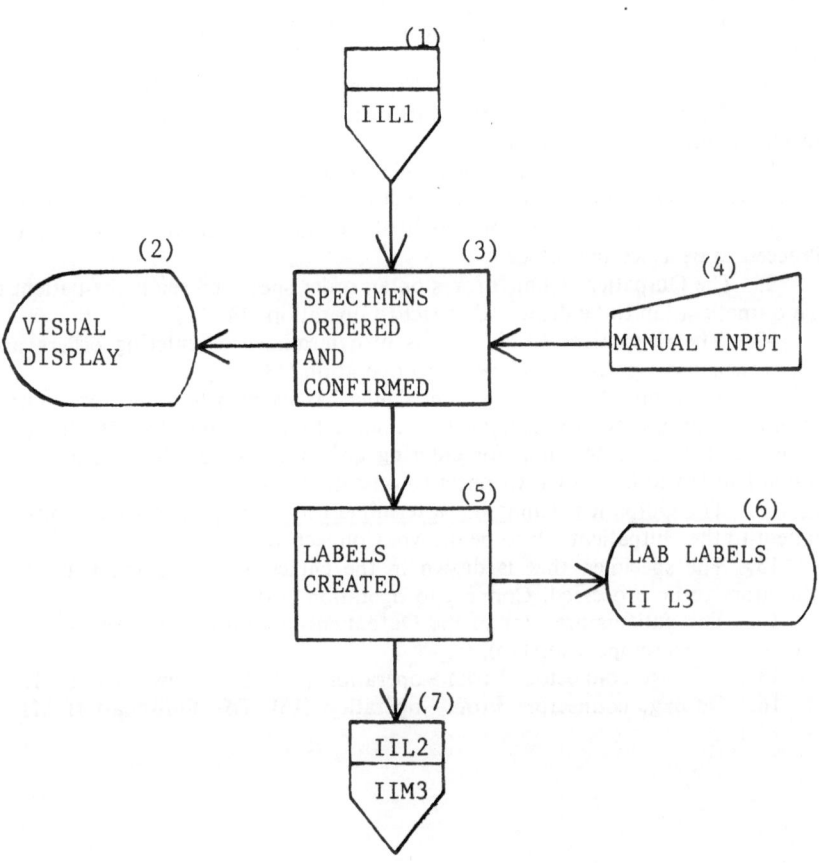

Flowchart II L

1. Off-page connector: From—location unspecified. To—operation (3).
2. Visual displays or orders on the terminal.
3. The patient specimens are ordered on the terminal if not previously ordered in the clinics and then confirmed. Connect to operation (5).
4. The process of ordering and confirming is a manual input. Connect to operation (3).
5. The labels are created when the order is confirmed. Connect to operation (7).
6. See Exhibit II L3. Lab labels are ordered for every laboratory test ordered.
7. Off-page connector: From—operation (7). To—Flowchart II M3.

Exhibit II L3

2319
284 AUSTRALIA ANTIG
DXXXXX, EARSULA T
A633A   1834185
08:30 04/06/76 282812

2319
284 AUSTRALIA ANTIG
DXXXXX, EARSULA T
A633A   1834185
08:30 04/06/76 282812

FLOWCHART IIM

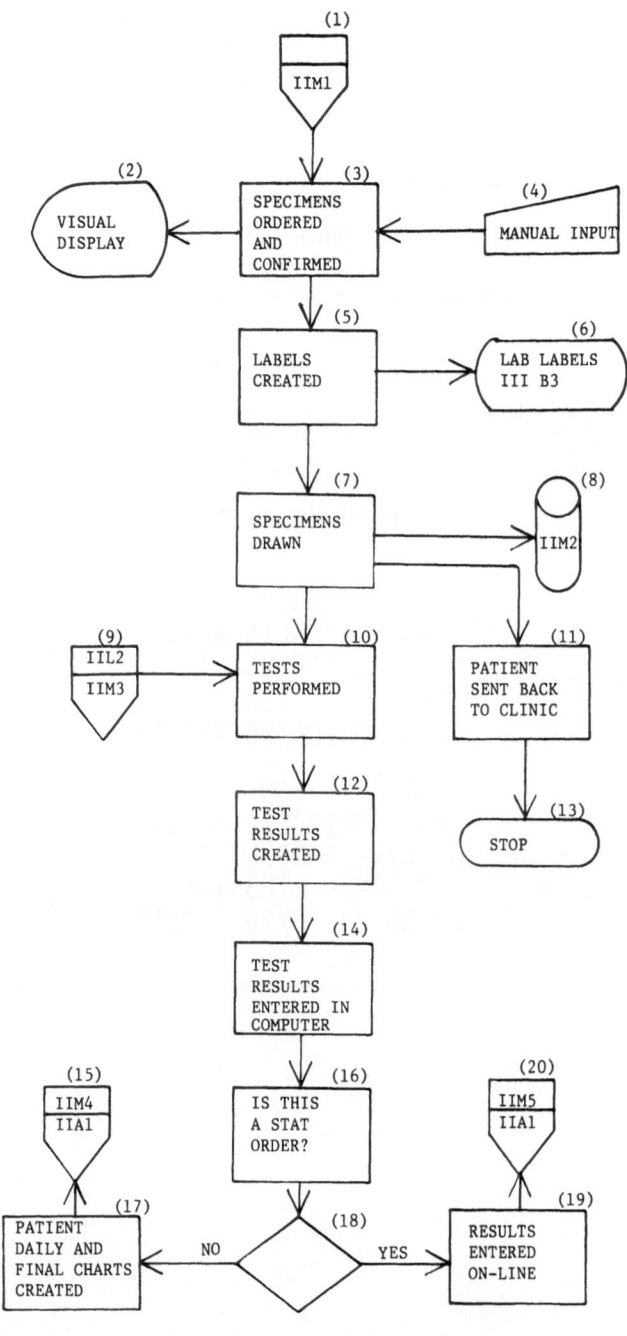

Flowchart II M

1. Off-page connector: From—location unspecified. To—operation (3).
2. Visual display of orders on the terminal.
3. The patient's specimens are ordered on the terminal if not previously ordered in the clinics and then confirmed. Connect to operation (5).
4. The process of ordering and confirming is a manual process. Connect to operation (3).
5. The labels are created when the order is confirmed. Connect to operation (7).
6. Lab labels. See Exhibit III B3.
7. The specimens are drawn. Connect to operations (10), (11).
8. Specimen tube.
9. Off-page connector: From—Flowchart II L2. To—operation (10).
10. The tests are performed. Connect to operation (12).
11. The patient is sent back to the clinic. Connect to operation (13).
12. The test results are created. Connect to operation (14).
13. When the patient returns to the clinic, the process is complete.
14. The test results are entered into the computer. Connect to operation (16).
15. Once the patient's daily and final charts are created, the processing of that particular specimen is complete.
16. Is this a stat order? Connect to operation (18).
17. The patient's daily and final charts are created. Connect to operation (15).
18. Decision: A—Yes, connect to operation (19). B—No, connect to operation (17).
19. The test results are entered on-line and may be called forth in the clinic area on a terminal. Connect to operation (20).
20. Once the results are on-line and may be retrieved, the processing of that particular specimen is complete.

FLOWCHART IIIA   Level 2
SPECIMEN ACQUIRED

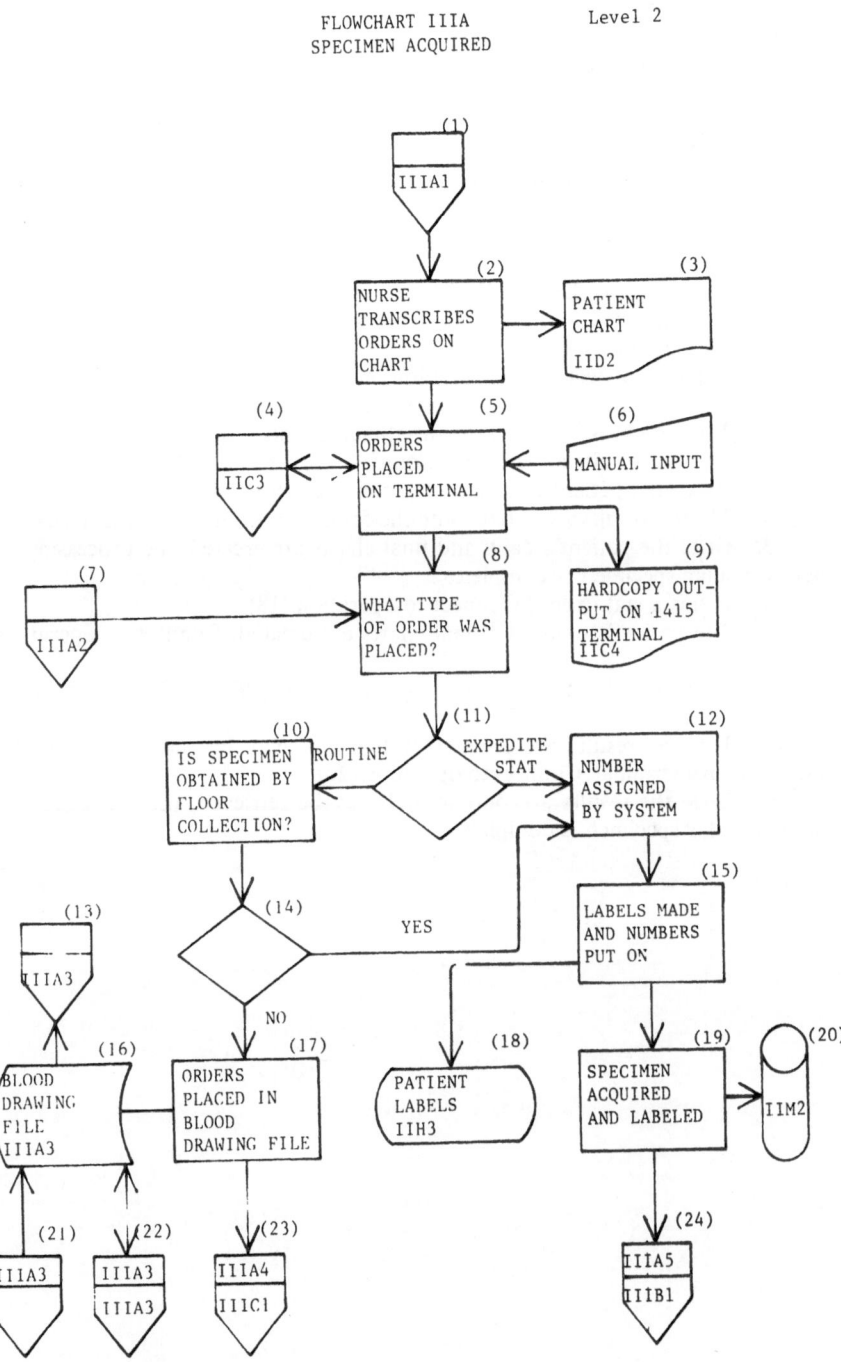

Flowchart III A

Specimen Acquired

1. Off-page connector: From—location unspecified. To—operation (2).
2. The nurse transcribes the doctor's orders on the chart. Connect to operation (5).
3. Patient chart. See Exhibit II D2.
4. On-line order file which contains all ordered laboratory work. Connect to operation (5).
5. The laboratory orders are entered on the system. Connect to operation (8).
6. The laboratory orders are manually entered into the system. Connect to operation (5).
7. All orders which have already been ordered and placed on the patient chart enter here. Connect to operation (8).
8. What type of order is placed? Connect to operation (11).
9. Hardcopy of laboratory orders. Connect to operation (5).
10. Is specimen obtained by floor collection? Connect to operation (14).
11. Decision: A—Routine, connect to operation (10). B—Expedite or STAT, connect to operation (12).
12. Once the order is placed, the system assigns a number to that particular test. Connect to operation (15).
13. Information may be called forth from the on-line blood drawing file. Connect to operation (16).
14. Decision: A—Yes, connect to operation (12). B—No, connect to operation (17).
15. Labels are made for the patients by an addressograph plate and the numbers assigned by the system are handwritten on the labels. Connect to operation (19).
16. The computer-based blood-drawing file contains all the patients in the hospital for morning blood collection. Connect to operation (17).
17. Orders are placed in the blood drawing file. Connect to operation (23).
18. Patient labels. See Exhibit II H3.
19. The specimen is acquired and labeled, showing patient name, medical record number, and tests ordered. Connect to operation (24).
20. Specimen tubes. Connect to operation (19).
21. Information may be entered into the blood drawing file. Connect to operation (16).
22. Information may be called forth or entered into the blood drawing file. Connect to operation (16).
23. Off-page connector: From—operation (23). To—Flowchart III C1.
24. Off-page connector: From—operation (24). To—Flowchart III B1.

FLOWCHART IIIB   Level 2

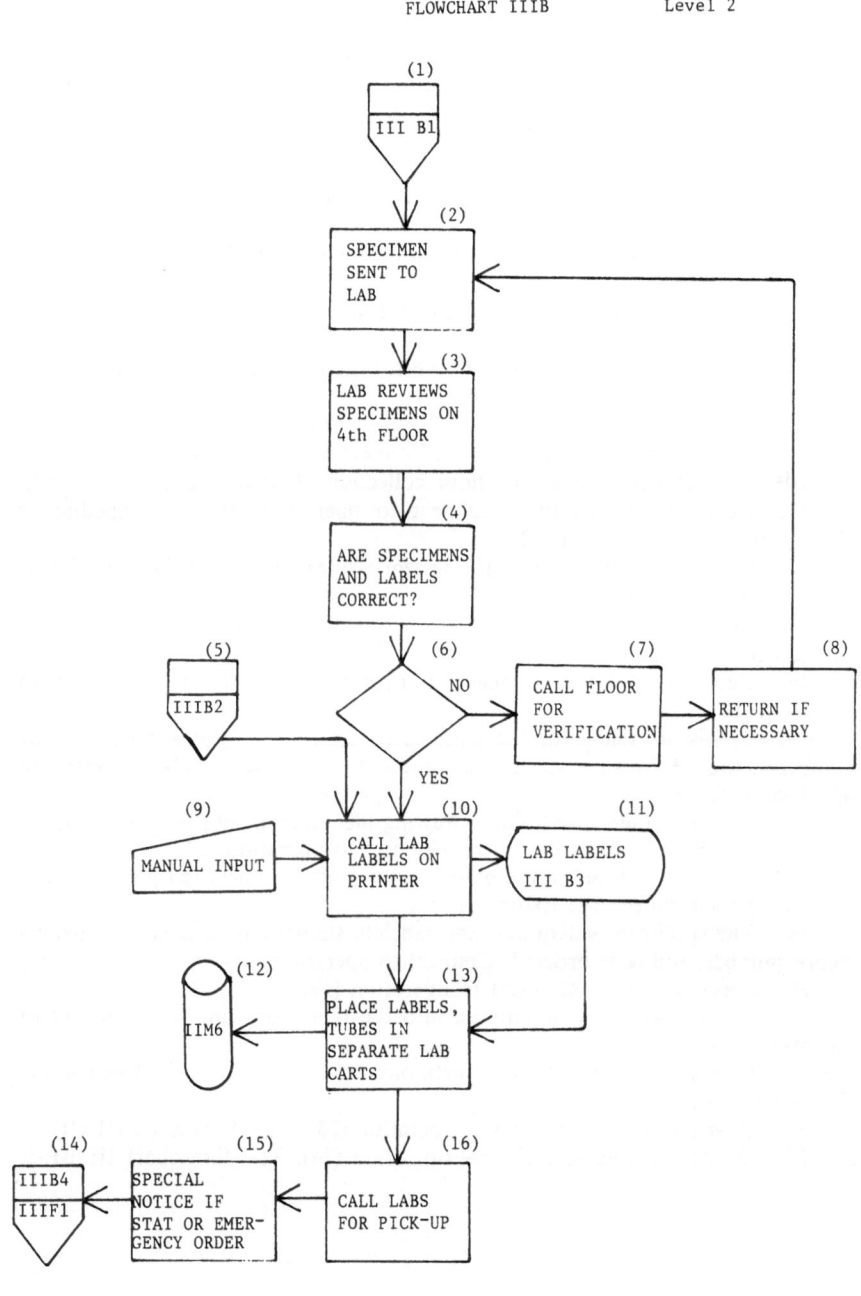

Flowchart III B

1.   Off-page connector: From—location unspecified. To—operation (2).
2.   Specimen is sent to the laboratory. Connect to operation (3).
3.   The 4th floor laboratory reviews specimens for correct information. Connect to operation (4).
4.   Are the specimens and labels correct? Connect to operation (6).
5.   The 4th floor laboratory orders the test labels for the Outpatient specimens and the hand-carried specimens at this time. Connect to operation (10).
6.   Decision: A—Yes, connect to operation (10). B—No, connect to operation (7).
7.   Call the floors for verification if something is wrong with the specimen or labels. Connect to operation (8).
8.   The specimen and labels are returned to the floor if they cannot be corrected by phone. Connect to operation (2).
9.   The labels are manually ordered on the label printer. Connect to operation (10).
10.   The computer operator checks the specimen number by inquiry and orders all lab labels on the label printer. Connect to operation (13).
11.   Lab labels. See Exhibit II L3. Connect to operations (10), (13).
12.   Specimen tubes. Connect to operation (13).
13.   The labels and tubes are placed in the separate lab carts to await pickup or delivery. Connect to operation (16).
14.   Off-page connector: From—operation (14). To—Flowchart III F1.
15.   If the order is stat or emergency, the individual lab is called immediately, otherwise they are held until there are multiple specimens before calling. Connect to operation (14).
16.   The individual labs are called regarding specimens or the operators deliver from the computer room. Connect to operation (15).

FLOWCHART IIIC   Level 2

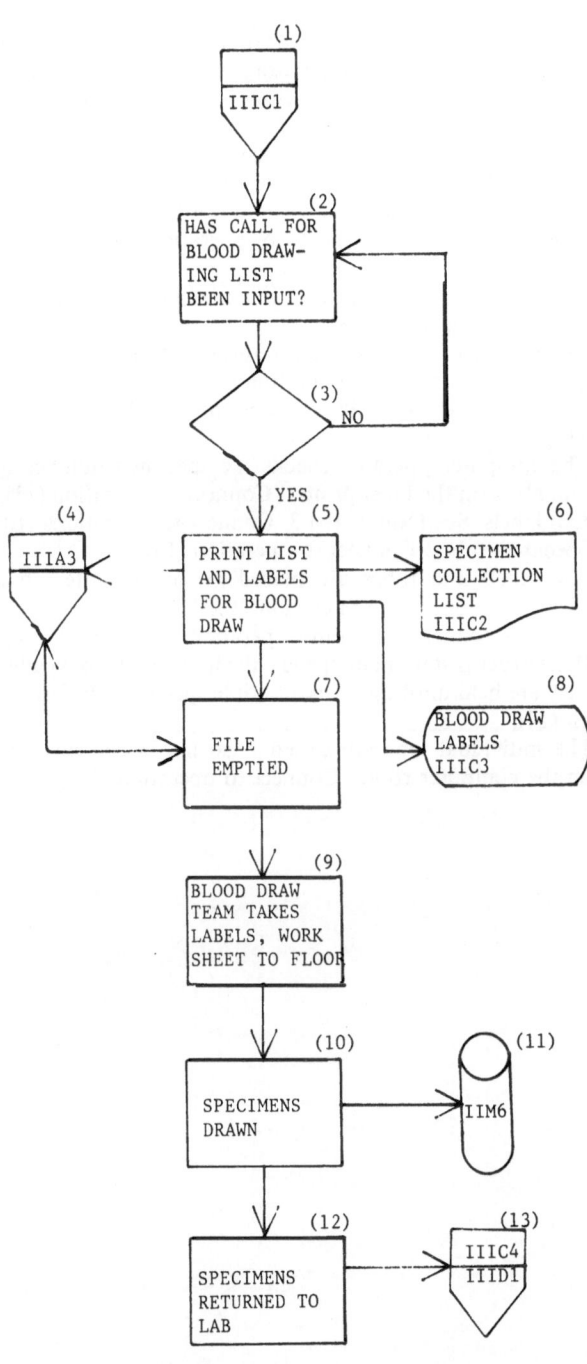

Flowchart III C

1. Off-page connector: From—location unspecified. To—operation (2).
2. Has the call for the blood drawing list been input? Connect to operation (3).
3. Decision: A—No, connect to operation (2). B—Yes, connect to operation (5).
4. This is an on-line blood drawing file. Connect to operations (5) and (7).
5. Computer gives a print-out list of patients to be drawn and labels needed for the individual blood tubes. Connect to operation (7).
6. See Exhibit III C2. Specimen collection list is a list of the patients from which blood is to be drawn by the blood drawing team. It gives the patient's name, medical record number, room number, test, tubes, and specimen number. Connect to operation (5).
7. Once the file is printed, the file is emptied until the following day. Connect to operations (4) and (9).
8. See Exhibit III C3. Blood draw labels contain the same information as the specimen collection list. Connect to operation (5).
9. Blood draw team picks up the labels and work sheets at 6:15 AM and takes them to the floor for blood draws. Connect to operation (10).
10. The specimens are drawn. Connect to operation (12).
11. Specimen tubes. Connect to operation (10).
12. Specimens are taken to the laboratory for processing. Connect to operation (13).
13. Off-stage connector: From—operation (13). To—Flowchart III D1.

Exhibit III C2

OB/GYN ROOM	SPEC NAME	COLLECT LIST	TUBE SPEC	06·17 TEST	09/13/76	REPEAT TUBES
H381B	NXXXXXXXX, DAISY V		1036	HEMOGRAM		1 PURPLE
	1939068	71Y F 312343				
H382A	HXXX, VICTORIA E		1038	HEMOGRAM		1 PURPLE
	1934724	61Y F 296907				
H383A	CXXXX, WINNIE B		1039	GLUCOSE MG/DL		1 RED-7
	1938681	27Y F 302994		ADLT LYTS BUN CR		
H385A	CXXXX, HILDA F		1041	HCT		1 PURPLE
	1938681	27Y F 161692				
H367A	NXXXXX, ETHEL M		1042	HEMOGRAM		1 RED-7
	1923110	62Y F 302887		SGPT IU/L		1 PURPLE
				SGOT IU/L		
				ALK PHOS IU/L		
				ADLT LYTS BUN CR		

Exhibit III C3

1036
NXXXXXXX, DAISY V
  H318B   1939068
06:17 09/13/76 PURPLE
       312343

1039
CXXX, WINNIE B.
  H383A   1938681
06:17 09/13/76 RED-7
       302994

1041
CXXXX, HILDA F
  H385A   1938681
06:17 09/13/76 PURPLE
       161692

1042
NXXXXX, ETHEL M.
  H367A   1923110
06:17 09/13/76 RED-7
       302887

FLOWCHART IIID

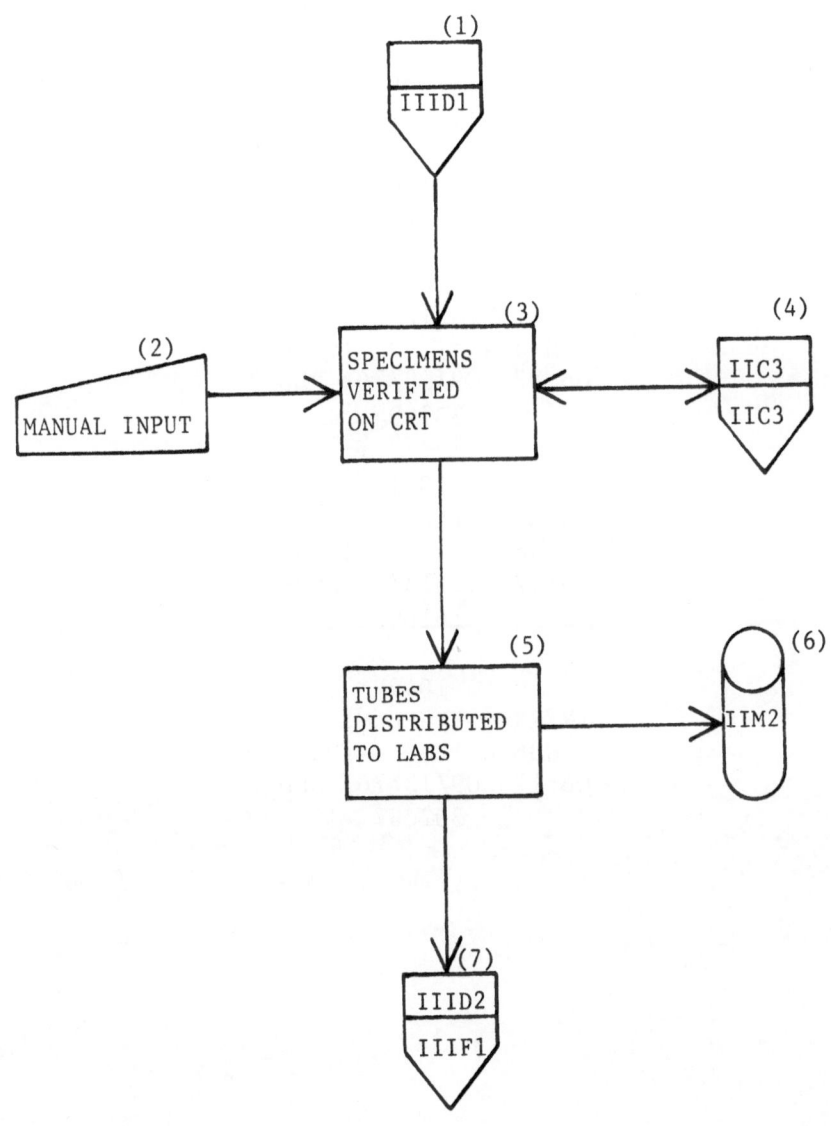

Flowchart III D

1. Off-page connector: From—location unspecified. To—operation (3).
2. Verification of specimen collection is manually entered into the system. Connect to operation (3).
3. Specimens are verified by ordering the labels for the individual labs. Connect to operation (5).
4. The on-line order file contains all laboratory work ordered in the hospital. Connect to operation (3).
5. The individual tubes are distributed to the labs. Connect to operation (7).
6. Specimen tubes. Connect to operation (5).
7. Off-page connector: From—operation (7). To—Flowchart III F1.

FLOWCHART IIIE   Level 2

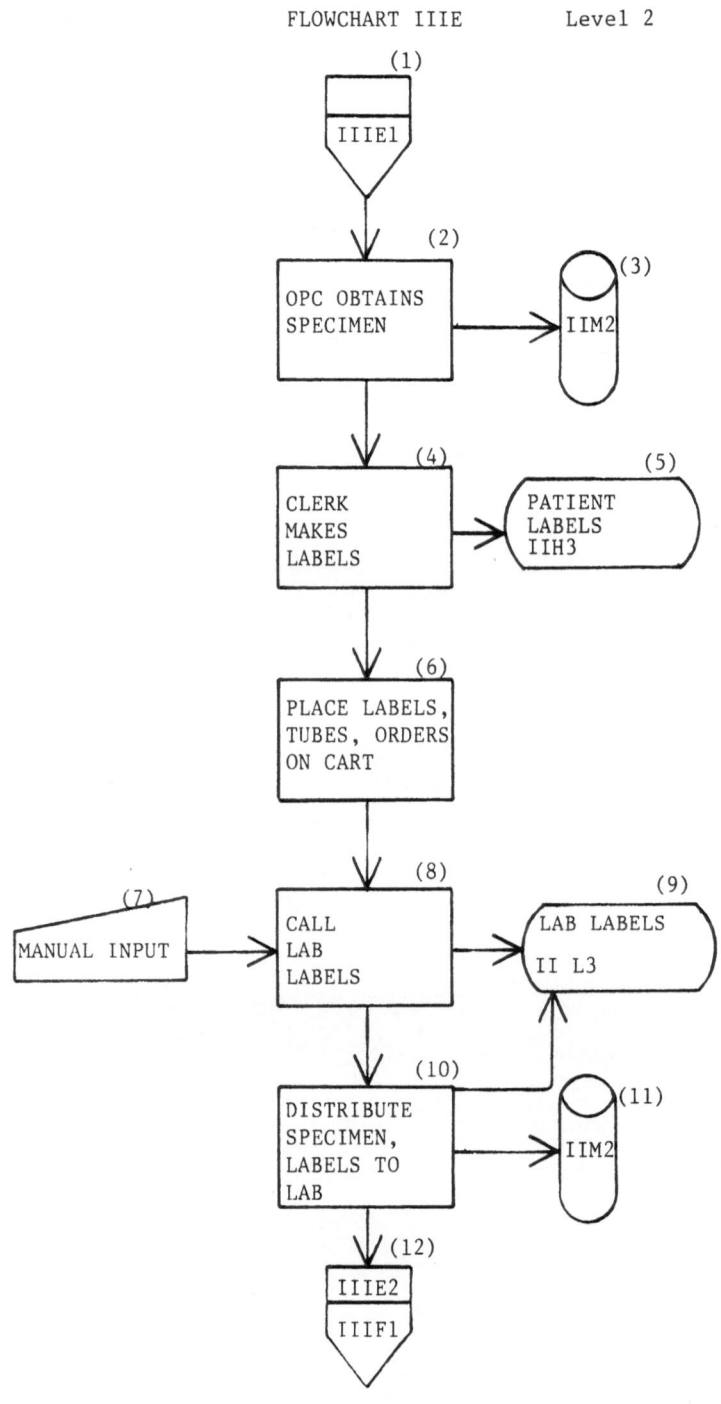

Flowchart III E

1. Off-page connector: From—location unspecified. To—operation (2).
2. Outpatient Clinic obtains the specimen. Connect to operation (4).
3. Specimen tube. Connect to operation (2).
4. The clerk makes out a label for each patient. Connect to operation (7).
5. Labels for patients. See Exhibit II H3.
6. Anatomic Pathology hand carries its specimens to the lab for processing (before 8 AM or after 5 PM only). The labels, tubes, and orders, if correct, are placed in the cart for processing. Connect to operation (7).
7. The patient's lab order, tubes, and labels are placed in the cart. Connect to operation (9).
8. The specimen lab labels are manually ordered on the system. Connect to operation (9).
9. The computer room orders the lab labels on the printer. This is also a confirmation of the order. Connect to operation (11).
10. Lab labels. See Exhibit II L3.
11. The specimens and labels are distributed to the individual labs. Connect to operation (13).
12. Specimen tube. Connect to operation (11).
13. Off-page connector: From—operation (13). To—Flowchart III F1.

FLOWCHART IIIF   Level 2

Flowchart III F

1. Off-page connector: From—location unspecified. To—operation (3).
2. Off-page connector: From—operation (2). To—Flowchart IV A1.
3. Decision: A—proceed to Anatomic Pathology. B—proceed to Chemistry/ Microscopy. C—proceed to next decision block.
4. Off-page connector: From—operation (4). To—Flowchart V A1.
5. Off-page connector: From—operation (5). To—Flowchart VI A1.
6. Decision: A—proceed to Hematology. B—proceed to Microbiology. C—proceed to next decision block.
7. Off-page connector: From—operation (7). To—Flowchart VII A1.
8. Off-page connector: From—operation (8). To—Flowchart VIII A1.
9. Decision: A—proceed to Blood Bank. B—proceed to Immunology.
10. Off-page connector: From—operation (10). To—Flowchart IX A1.

FLOWCHART IIIG   Level 2

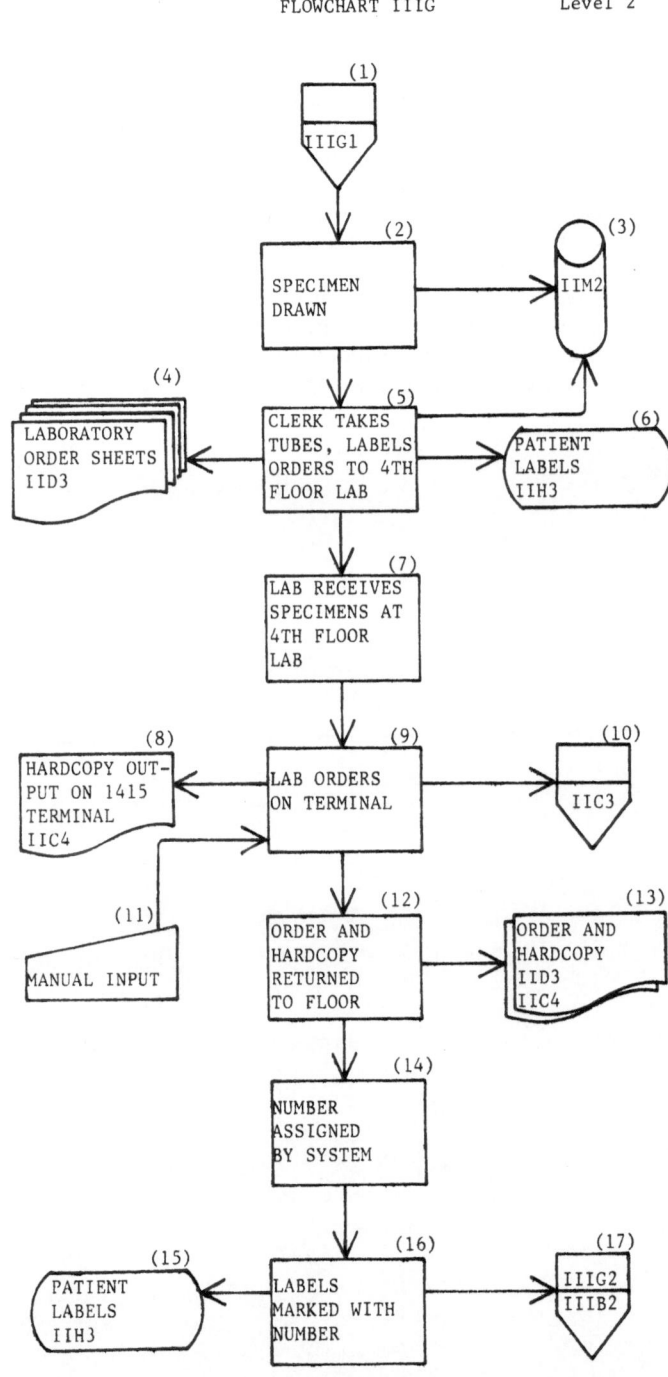

Flowchart III G: Level 2

1. Off-page connector: From—location unspecified. To—operation (2).
2. The specimen is drawn. Connect to operation (5).
3. Specimen tube. Connect to operations (2), (5).
4. Laboratory order sheet. See Exhibit II D3.
5. The clerk takes the tubes, labels, and order to the 4th floor lab. Connect to operation (7).
6. Patient labels. See Exhibit II H3.
7. The lab reviews the specimen at the 4th floor lab for accuracy. Connect to operation (9).
8. A hardcopy output of the patient's lab orders is printed on the 1415 terminal. Connect to operation (9).
9. Lab orders on the terminal. Connect to operation (12).
10. The on-line order file contains all lab orders. Connect to operation (9).
11. The orders are manually entered on the 1415 terminal. Connect to operation (9).
12. The original order and hardcopy print-out of the orders are returned to the floor for filing. Connect to operation (14).
13. Lab order and hardcopy print-out on the 1415 terminal. See Exhibits II D3 and II C4.
14. A specimen number is assigned by the system when the test is ordered. Connect to operation (16).
15. Patient labels. See Exhibit II H3.
16. The number assigned by the system is placed on the label. Connect to operation (17).
17. Off-page connector: From—operation (17). To—Flowchart III B2.

FLOWCHART IVA   Level 2
ANATOMIC PATHOLOGY

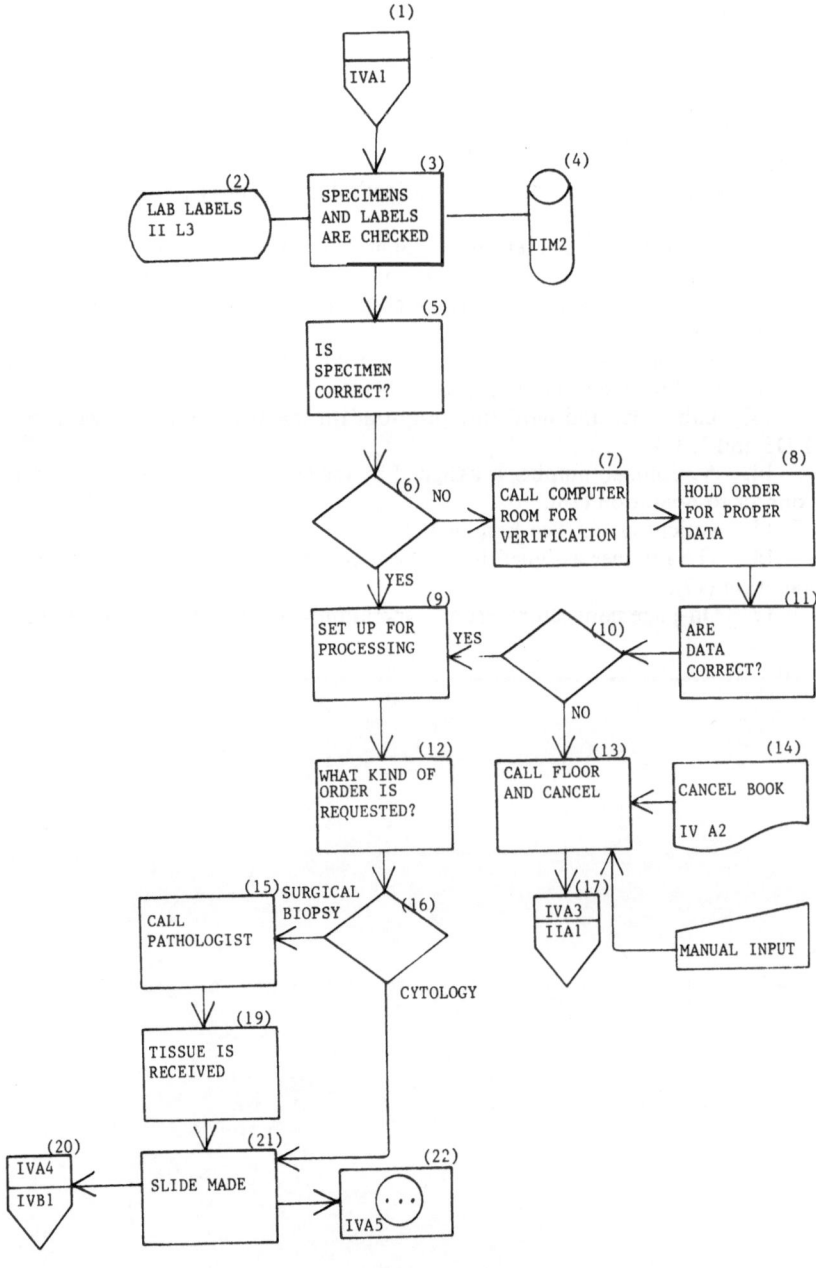

Flowchart IV A

Anatomic Pathology

1. Off-page connector: From—location unspecified. To—operation (3).
2. Lab labels. See Exhibit II L3.
3. Specimens and labels are checked for accuracy. Connect to operation (5).
4. Specimen tubes. Connect to operation (3).
5. Is the specimen correct? Connect to operation (6).
6. Decision: A—Yes, connect to operation (9). B—No, connect to operation (7).
7. The computer room is called for verification of order. Connect to operation (8).
8. The order is held for proper data. Connect to operation (11).
9. The specimen is set up for processing. Connect to operation (12).
10. Decision: A—Yes, connect to operation (9). B—No, connect to operation (13).
11. Are data correct? Connect to operation (10).
12. What kind of order is requested? Connect to operation (16).
13. The floor is called and the order canceled. Connect to operation (17).
14. See Exhibit IV A2. A book is kept in which all canceled lab orders are logged. Connect to operation (13).
15. The pathologist or resident is called to process the tissue. Connect to operation (19).
16. Decision: A—surgical biopsy, connect to operation (15). B—cytology, connect to operation (21).
17. Off-page connector: From—operation (17). To—Flowchart II A1.
18. The order is manually canceled on the system. Connect to operation (13).
19. The tissue is received. Connect to operation (21).
20. Off-page connector: From—operation (20). To—Flowchart IV B1.
21. A slide is made of the specimen. Connect to operation (20).
22. Specimen slide. Connect to operation (21).

Exhibit IV A2

"CANCEL LAB ORDER"

MEDICAL RECORD NO. _____

TEST NO. _____

SPEC. NO. _____

PERSON REQUESTING
CANCEL _____

OPERATORS
SIGNATURE _____

TIME _____

DATE _____

FLOOR _____

WHY _____

_____

"CANCEL LAB ORDER"

MEDICAL RECORD NO. _____

TEST NO. _____

SPEC. NO. _____

PERSON REQUESTING
CANCEL _____

OPERATORS
SIGNATURE _____

TIME _____

DATE _____

FLOOR _____

WHY _____

_____

The Cancel Lab Order is used by the laboratory technologist to document why a particular order was canceled. Some of the reasons for a cancelation are as follows:

1. Order placed—sample never received.
2. The specimen quantity received was not sufficient to run the test.
3. Duplicate specimen received.
4. Unsatisfactory specimen received.

FLOWCHART IVB

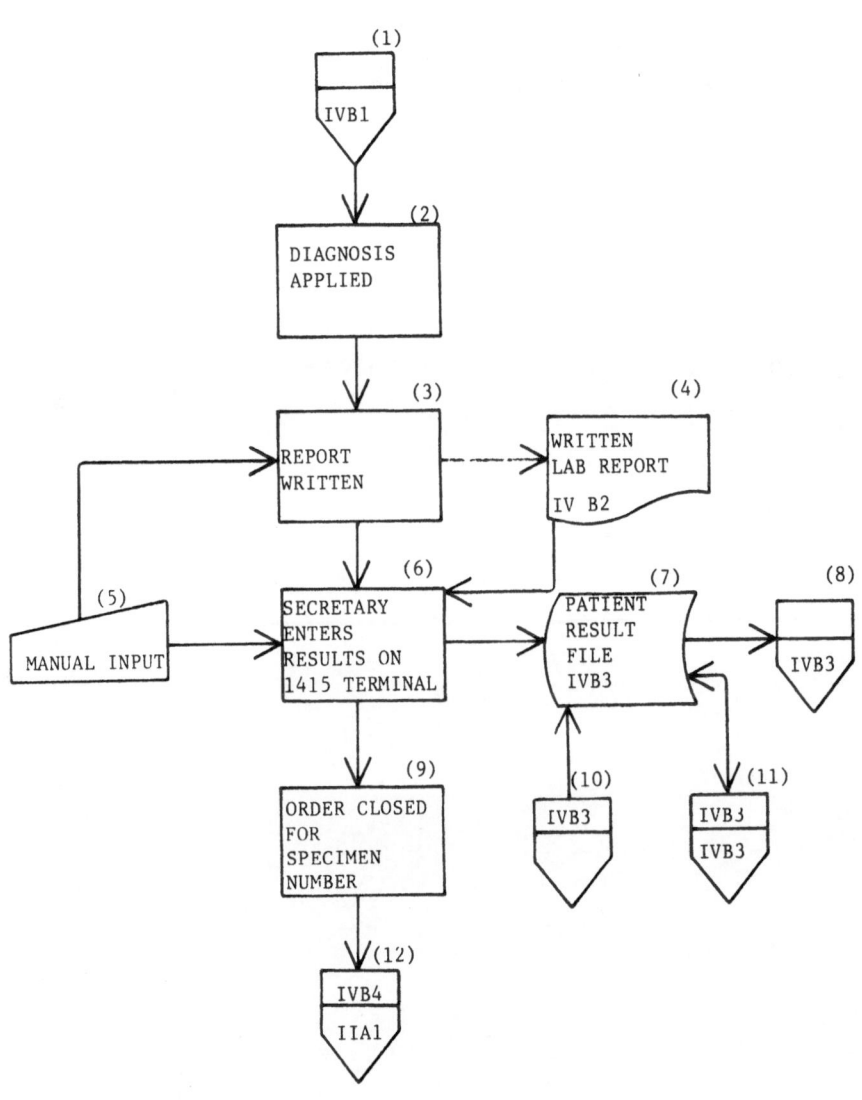

Flowchart IV B

1. Off-page connector: From—location unspecified. To—operation (2).
2. A diagnosis is applied to the specimen. Connect to operation (3).
3. A report is written on the specimen. Connect to operation (6).
4. See Exhibit IV B2. A written lab report of test findings. Connect to operations (3), (6).
5. The written report and entry on the 1415 terminal are both manual procedures. Connect to operations (3), (6).
6. The secretary enters the test results on the 1415 terminal. Connect to operation (9).
7. An on-line patient result file exists which contains all the test results on lab work. Connect to operation (6).
8. Test results may be called forth from the on-line file. Connect to operation (7).
9. The order cycle is complete. Connect to operation (12).
10. Test results may be entered into the on-line file. Connect to operation (7).
11. Test results may be called from the on-line file. Connect to operation (7).
12. Off-page connector: From—operation (12). To—Flowchart II A1.

Exhibit IV B2

SURGICAL PATHOLOGY REPORT

NAME _____   HOSPITAL NUMBER _____

DOCTOR _____   SURG. PATH NUMBER _____

DATE _____ AGE _____   ROOM NUMBER _____

SPECIMEN _____

CLINICAL DATA _____

GROSS DESCRIPTION:

Exhibit IV B2

4 XXXX	17	9/16	SXXXXXX, MXX	3XXXXXX	H 439	30	F	P
ADMISSION NO	REG	ADM DATE	PATIENT NAME	MED REC NO	FLOOR	AGE	SE/	FIN CODE

SEND TO

- [ ] BRACE SHOP
- [ ] CARDIOVASCULAR LAB
- [ ] CYTOLOGY
- [ ] ECG
- [ ] EEG
- [ ] INHALATION THERAPY
- [ ] NUCLEAR MEDICINE
- [ ] OCCUPATIONAL THERAPY
- [ ] PHYSICAL THERAPY
- [ ] SURG PATH
- [ ] X RAY
- [ ] BLOOD BANK
- [ ]

TREATMENT LOCATION [ ] WARD [ ] SERVICE DEPT TRANSPORT BY [ ] WHEEL CHAIR [ ] STRETCHER

05380-76

REQUEST

TREATMENT OBJECTIVES SPECIAL INSTRUCTIONS NATURE OF SPECIMEN

PROVISIONAL DIAGNOSIS

PERTINENT HISTORY

PRECAUTIONS (MEDICATIONS OR X RAY FINDINGS)

TIME OF COLLECTION HR [ ] AM [ ] PM DATE OF COLLECTION [ ] ISOLATION

LEWIS 70974 REQUESTED BY _____ MD SERVICE _____ DATE _____

CONSULTATION / SERVICE REQUEST
SHANDS TEACHING HOSPITAL AND CLINICS

GROSS DESCRIPTION:

The specimen comes in two parts:

#1 is labeled "right breast mass" and consists of a 3 x 3.5 x 3 cm.
well encapsulated, pinkish tan multilobulated mass with a small
amount of areolar fatty tissue on its surface. On cut section, the
tissue bulges from the cut surface and is a homogenous and tan in
character except for the most central portion which is more violeous
in color. There are no cystic spaces and again the well-defined
capsule is noted about the lesion. Representative sections will be
submitted.

#2 is labeled "left neck mass" and consists of 2 x 1.5 x 2 cm.
apparent lymph node whose external surface is rough and violeous
to dark pink in color. On cut surface the mass appears to be a
homogenous pink in texture with a very thin well-defined capsule.
The entire specimen will be submitted.
(TF Bunt, M.D./dh   9-17-76)

DIAGNOSIS: Right breast mass, excisional biopsy: Plasmacytoma.

            Left neck mass, excisional biopsy: Plasmacytoma.

FXXXXXXXX VXXXXXXX, M.D.
Pathologist

FLOWCHART VA   Level 2
CHEMISTRY/MICROSCOPY

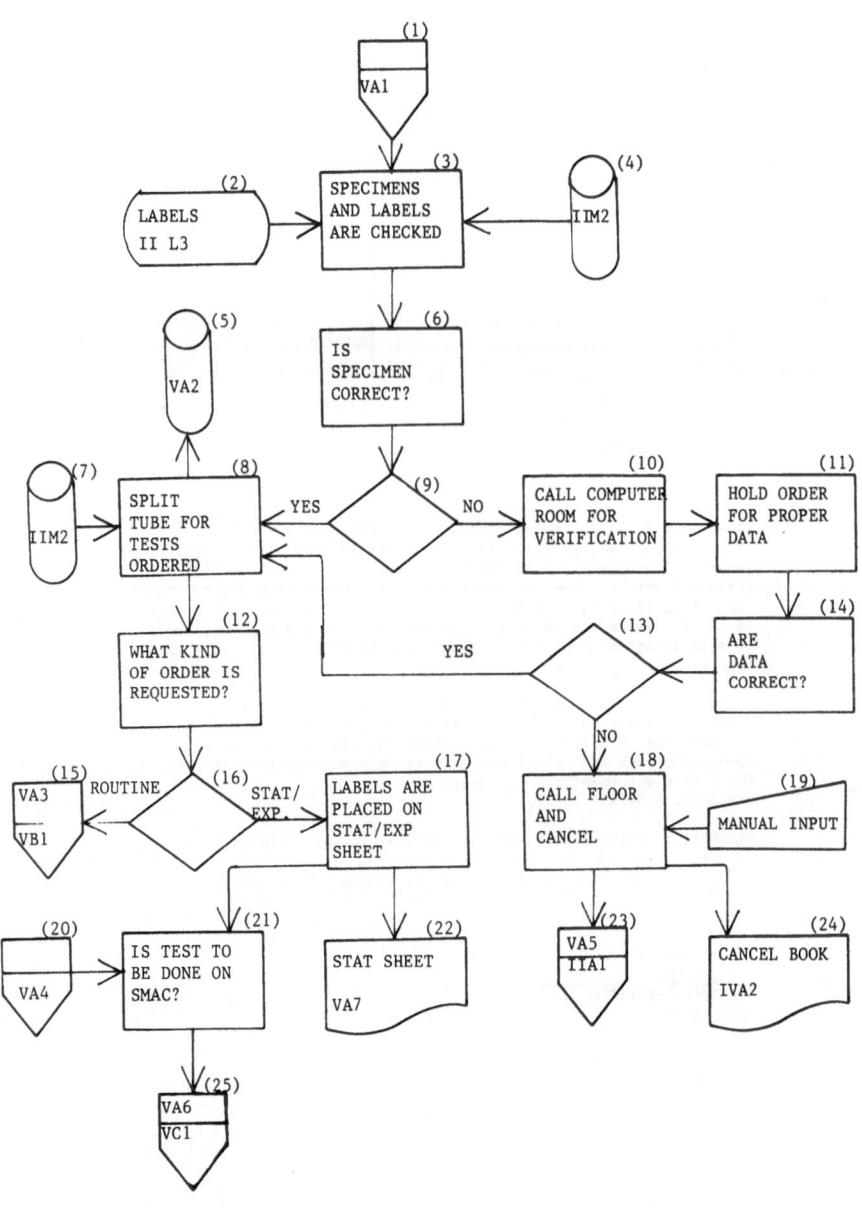

Flowchart V A

Chemistry Microscopy

1. Off-page connector: From—location unspecified. To—operation (3).
2. Lab labels. See Exhibit II L3.
3. Specimens and labels are checked for accuracy. Connect to operation (6).
4. Specimen tube. Connect to operation (3).
5. Serum tube. Connect to operation (8).
6. Is the specimen correct? Connect to operation (9).
7. Specimen tube. Connect to operation (8).
8. The tube is spun down and the serum or plasma is placed in a new tube. Connect to operation (12).
9. Decision: A—Yes, connect to operation (8). B—No, connect to operation (10).
10. The computer room is called for verification. Connect to operation (11).
11. The order is held until the specimen is corrected. Connect to operation (14).
12. What kind of order is requested? Connect to operation (16).
13. Decision: A—Yes, connect to operation (8). B—No, connect to operation (18).
14. Are data correct? Connect to operation (13).
15. Off-page connector: From—operation (15). To—Flowchart V B1.
16. Decision: A—Routine, connect to operation (15). B—Stat or expedite, connect to operation (17).
17. Labels are placed on the expedite/stat sheets. Connect to operation (21).
18. The floor is called and the test canceled. Connect to operation (23).
19. The order is manually canceled on the system. Connect to operation (18).
20. If the tests are prepared and the work sheets are obtained; enter here. Connect to operation (21).
21. Is test to be done on SMAC? Connect to operation (25).
22. See Exhibit V A7. Stat sheet is a listing of the names of persons and test results. Connect to operation (17).
23. Off-page connector: From—operation (23). To—Flowchart II A1.
24. Cancel book. See Exhibit IV A2.
25. Off-page connector: From—operation (25). To—Flowchart V C1.

CHEMISTRY STATS

Exhibit V A7

DATE

NAME	HOSP #	FL.. TIME	Na	K	Cl	CO$_2$	BUN	Creat	UA	PO$_4$	Glu	T.P.	Alb	T.bili	D.bili	Alk	LDH	OT	PT	Ca	Mg	Amy	Miscellaneous

The chemistry stat sheet is a manual system for recording laboratory results. This enables the technology to give results by phone to areas presently without terminals.

FLOWCHART VB

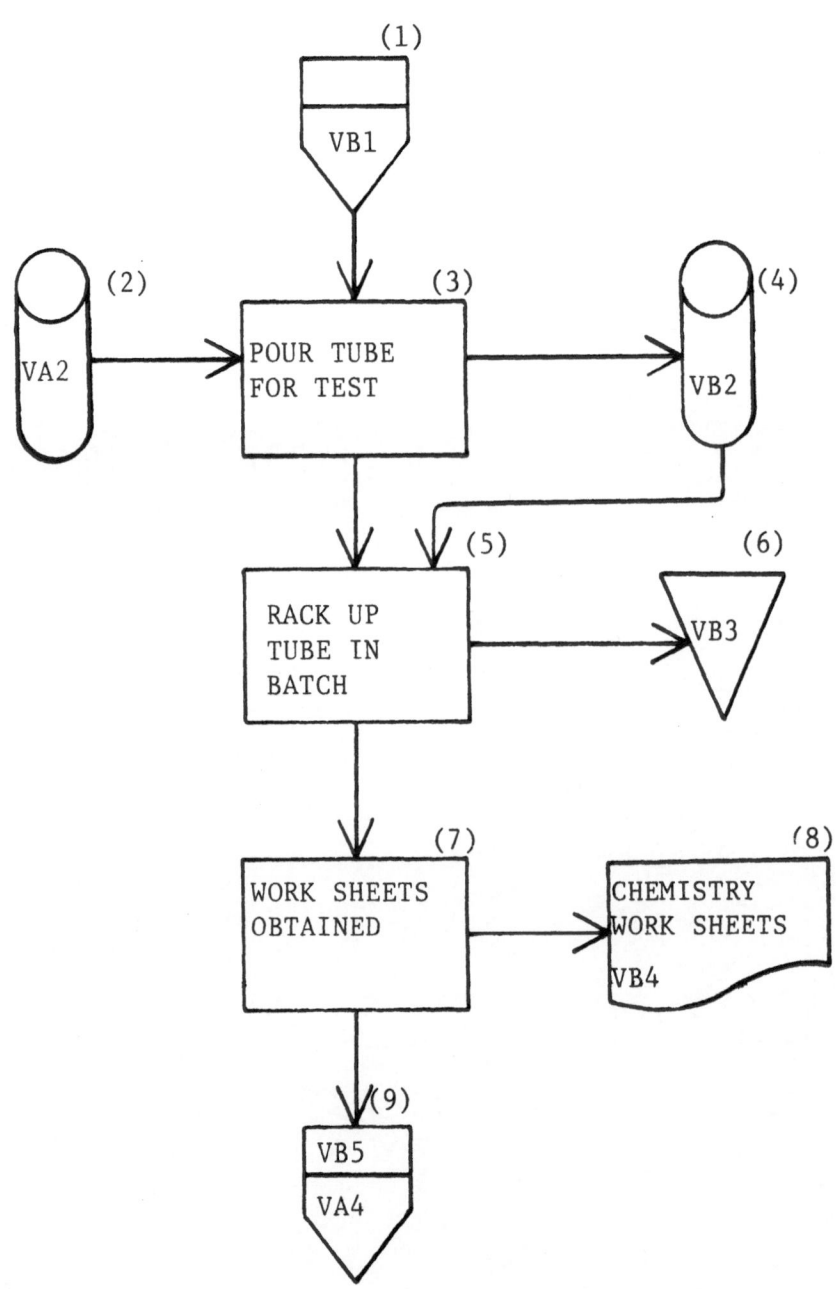

Flowchart V B

1. Off-page connector: From—location unspecified. To—operation (3).
2. Serum tube. Connect to operation (3).
3. The serum is poured into a special tube so it may be run on a test instrument. Connect to operation (5).
4. Serum tube. Connect to operations (3), (6).
5. A tube is put in the batch and is held briefly for other tubes before running the test. Connect to operation (7).
6. The batch is set aside until there are several tubes which can be run. Connect to operation (5).
7. The work sheets are obtained. Connect to operation (9).
8. See Exhibit V B3. Chemistry work sheets contain the patient name, specimen number, and a section to record test results. Connect to operation (7).
9. Off-page connector: From—operation (9). To—Flowchart V A4.

Exhibit V B4

09/06/76   SMAC GROUP 1   96   08:37

PATIENT NAME	SPEC NO.	NA (075)	K (076)	CL (077)	CO2 (078)	BUN (079)	CREAT (080)	UR AC (081)	TECH
MXXXX, NANCY P	1081	-----							----
BXXXXX, BETTY	1111	-----							----
FXXXXXX, ELMER	7174	-----							----
MXXXX, NANCY P	1081		-----						----
TXXXXX, SAM	1101		-----						----
BXXXXXX, BETTY	1111		-----						----
MXXXX, NANCY P	1081			-----					----
BXXXXX, BETTY	1111			-----					----
MXXXX, NANCY P	1081				-----				----
BXXXXXX, BETTY	1111				-----				----
PXXXXXX, THOMAS	0008					-----			----
AXXXXX, ROBERT	1057					-----			----
AXXXXXX, THOMA	1097					-----			----
BXXXXXX, BETTY	1111					-----			----
PXXXXX, THOMAS	0008						-----		----
BXXXX, MAGGIE	1051						-----		----
AXXXXX, ROBERT	1057						-----		----
EXXXXXX, VERNO	1059						-----		----
AXXXXXX, THOMA	1097						-----		----
WXXXXX, NANCY	1159							-----	----

Exhibit V B4

| 10/14/77 | | ATOMIC ABSOR | | | 110 | | 08:35 | |

PATIENT NAME	SPEC. NO.	CALC (082)	MG (111)	LITH (159)	COP (133)	LEAD (144)	TECH
GXXXX, ROLAND	0033	-----					----
AXXXXXX, MEREDI	2321	-----					----
CXXX, BELVA A	2417	-----					----
LXXXXX, GLENDA	3040	-----					----
BXXXXXX, SIDNEY	3043	-----					----
CXXXXX, PAULA	3047	-----					----
BXXXX, MYRTIE	3074	-----					----
AXXXX, CLARA M	3090	-----					----
KXXXXXXX, WILL	3106	-----					----
HXXXXX, CARL H	3117	-----					----
FXXXX, MARY N	0004	-----					----
MXXXXXX, GIRL	2321		-----				----
AXXXXXXX, MEREDI	3117		-----				----
FXXXX, MARY N	3043		-----				----
BXXXXX, SIDNEY				-----			----

Exhibit V B4

| 08/19/76 | | ACA | TESTS | | | | 123 | | 08:40 |

PATIENT NAME	SPEC NO.	AC PT (129)	CPK (169)	SAL (145)	HBDH (127)	LLDH (126)	LC AC (151)	ALC (142)	TECH
WXXXXX, ROBERT*	3050	-----							----
PXXXXX, COLLIE	3079	-----							----
MXXXXXXXX, BE	0036		-----						----
LXXXXX, AUSTIN	3030		-----						----
PXXXXX, ETHEL	3075		-----						----
LXXXXX, AUSTIN	0105		-----						----
JXXXXX, ANNA	3099		-----						----
BXXXXX, AMLIN	3121		-----						----
MXXXXXXXX, BE	3151				-----				----

Exhibit V B4

| 09/01/76 | | OSMOLALITY | | 109 | 8:38 |

PATIENT NAME	SPEC	RESULT		TECH
PXXXXXXX, ANGE	0097	------		----
HXXXX, SYBLE	0102	------		----
CXXXXX, CHERYL	0160	------		----

FLOWCHART VC

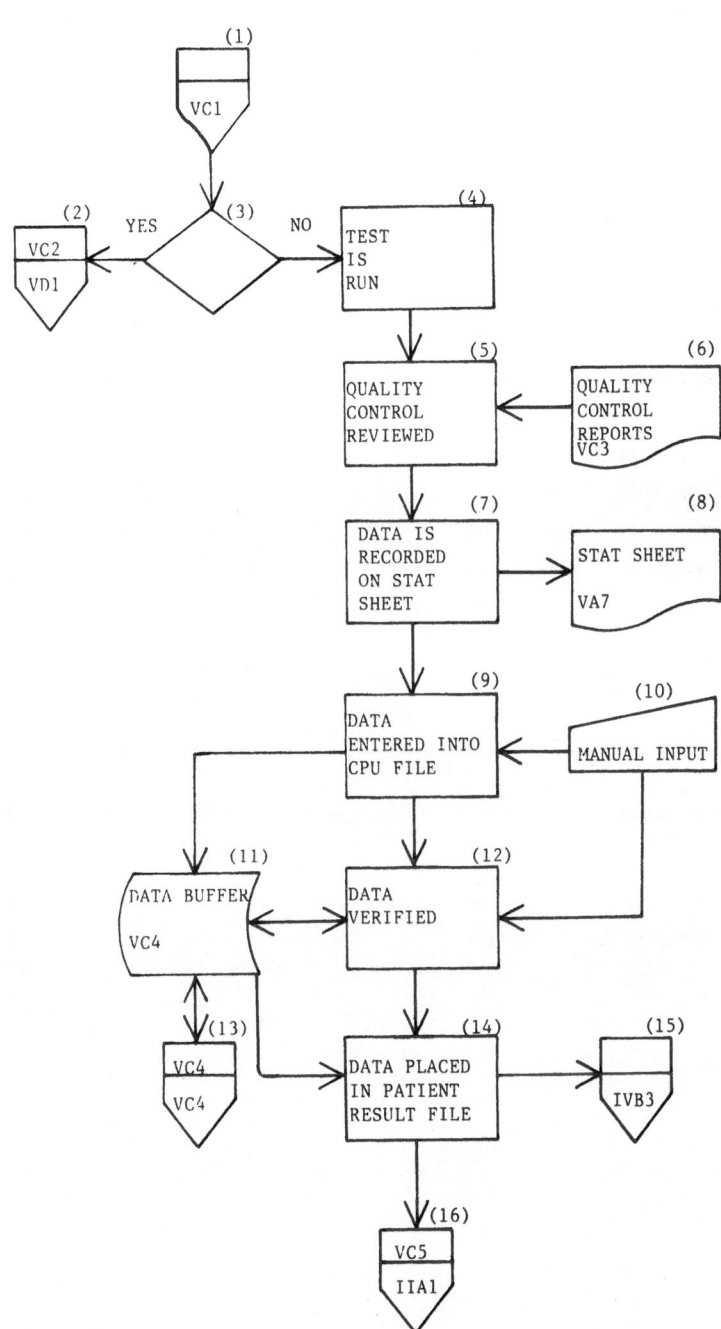

Flowchart V C

1. Off-page connector: From—location unspecified. To—operation (3).
2. Off-page connector: From—operation (2). To—Flowchart V D1.
3. Decision: A—Yes, connect to operation (2). B—No, connect to operation (4).
4. The test is run. Connect to operation (5).
5. The test result is recorded and reviewed against normal values. Connect to operation (7).
6. See Exhibit V C3. Quality control reports show the results and the mean of each test for a period of one month. Connect to operation (5).
7. The data is recorded on the stat sheet. Connect to operation (9).
8. Stat sheet. See exhibit V A7.
9. The data is entered into the CPU file. Connect to operation (12).
10. The test results are manually entered and verified on the system. Connect to operations (9), (12).
11. Once the test results are entered into the CPU file, they are stored in a buffer until verified. Connect to operations (9), (12), (14).
12. The test results are verified. Connect to operation (14).
13. Information may be entered into or called forth from the buffer. Connect to operation (14).
14. Once the test results are verified, they are placed in an on-line patient result file. Connect to operation (16).
15. Results that have been run and verified are entered in the patient result file. Connect to operation (14).
16. Off-page connector: From—operation (16). To—Flowchart II A1.

Exhibit V C3

QUALITY CONTROL PROBLEM SHEET

TEST _____ DATE _____ TECH _____

PROBLEM _____

SOLUTION _____

Exhibit V C3

Method ___ OSMO _____   Month __ Oct. 76 _____

Hyland I

Day	Readings →														
1	243	234													
2															
3	238														
4															
5															
6	257														
7															
8	235														
9	241	252													
10															
11	243														
12															
13															
14															
15															

Exhibit V C3

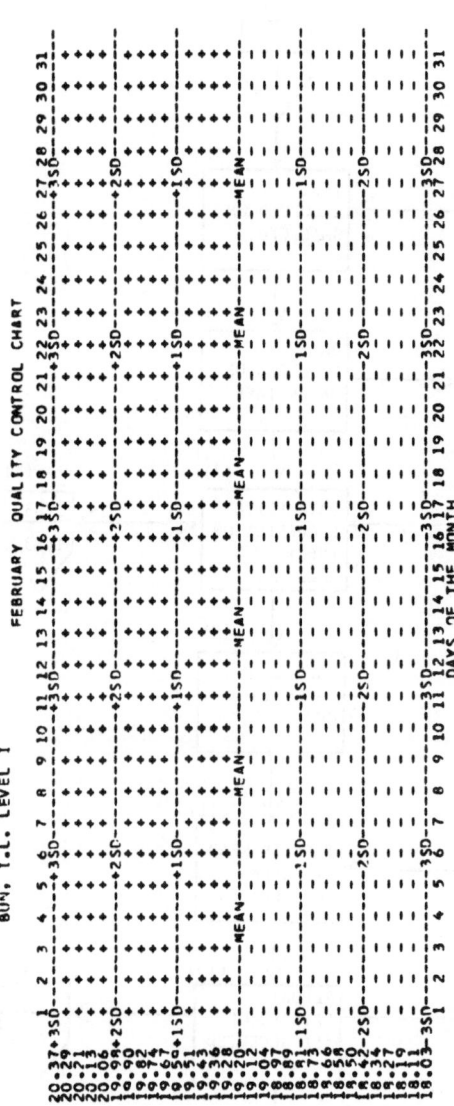

FEBRUARY QUALITY CONTROL CHART

BUN, I.L. LEVEL I

VARIANCE=   0.151   STANDARD DEVIATION=   0.389   COEFFICIENT OF VARIATION=   2.025   MEAN=   19.200   N=   65.

VARIANCE=   0.262   STANDARD DEVIATION=   0.512   COEFFICIENT OF VARIATION=   2.636   MEAN=   19.438   N=   16.

NUMBER OF MONTHS POOLED = 5

THE OBSERVED PATTERN OF VARIATION IS SAID TO BE UNNATURAL OR THE PROCESS IS SAID TO BE OUT OF CONTROL IF ANY ONE OR MORE OF THE FOLLOWING EVENTS OCCURS:

(1) A SINGLE POINT FALLS OUTSIDE OF THE CONTROL LIMIT;I.E., BEYOND + OR - 3SD

(2) TWO OUT OF THREE SUCCESSIVE POINTS FALL OUTSIDE OF + OR - 2SD

(3) FOUR OUT OF FIVE SUCCESSIVE POINTS FALL OUTSIDE OF + OR - 1SD

(4) EIGHT POINTS IN SUCCESSION FALL EITHER ABOVE OR BELOW THE MEAN

FLOWCHART VD

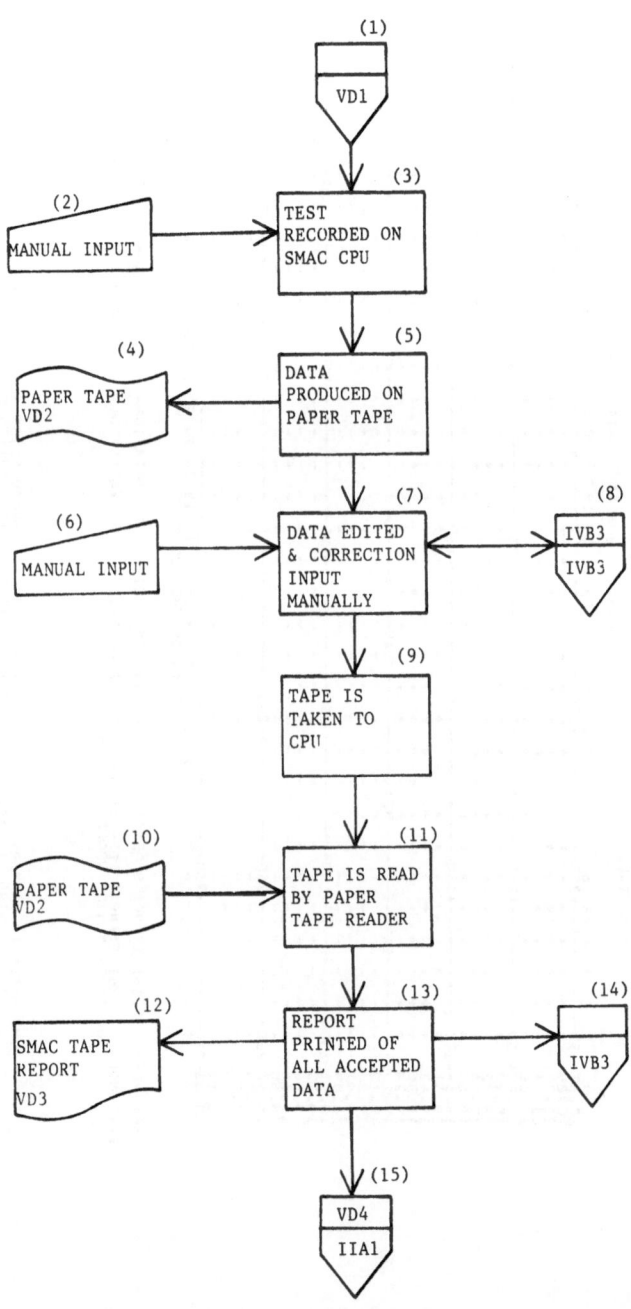

Flowchart V D

1. Off-page connector: From—location unspecified. To—operation (3).
2. The tests are manually entered into the SMAC central processing unit. Connect to operation (3).
3. The tests are recorded on the SMAC central processing unit. Connect to operation (5).
4. See Exhibit V D2. A paper tape is produced which contains all SMAC test results. Connect to operation (5).
5. The SMAC test results are printed out on a paper tape. Connect to operation (7).
6. The incorrect SMAC results are corrected manually on the Chemistry terminal. Connect to operation (7).
7. The SMAC results that are wrong are put in manually on the Chemistry terminal first, which automatically cancels the results of the SMAC tape. Connect to operation (9).
8. Results that have been entered and verified are maintained in a patient result file. Connect to operation (7).
9. The paper tape is taken to the CPU. Connect to operation (11).
10. Paper tape. Exhibit V D2 (not shown).
11. The tape is read by the paper tape reader and put on drum storage. Connect to operation (13).
12. See Exhibit V D3. SMAC tape report is a print-out of all SMAC results. Connect to operation (13).
13. A report is printed of all accepted data each time a SMAC paper tape is run through the central processing unit. Connect to operation (15).
14. An on-line patient result exists which contains all the test results on lab work. Connect to operation (13).
15. Off-page connector: From—operation (15). To—Flowchart II A1.

Exhibit V D3

```
               /-----STANDARD-----    /        /
                  LOT "     B7A001B6M979/0706771030
       /0037/   /    /    /    /    /    /    /     /    /    /    /    /    /    /
                 /    /    /    /    /    /    /    /


           CHECK IDEE              /0706771030
   ****77/0038/0144/0044/0106/0002/0020/0012/0053/----*0035/0097/0046/0028/
       ----*----*0018/0001/0103/0200/0030/0019*

    3024       /                    /    /
                                    /0706771031
   000034/0039/0147/0071/0118/0000*0054/0049/0085/----*0071/0271/0062/0039/
       ----*----*0076/0004/0223/0402/0065/0081/

    0049       /                    /    /
                                    /0706771031
   000035/0040/0133/0043/0095/0029/0025/0007/0022/----*0028/0188/0057/0033/
       ----*----*0008/0005/0293/0270/0150/0199/

    0046       /                    /  /0706771032
   000036/0041/0146/0036/0108/0031/0010/0006/0021/----*0024/0127/0062/0039/
       ----*----*0012/0003/0070/    G0060/0055/
```

FLOWCHART VIA   LEVEL 2
HEMATOLOGY

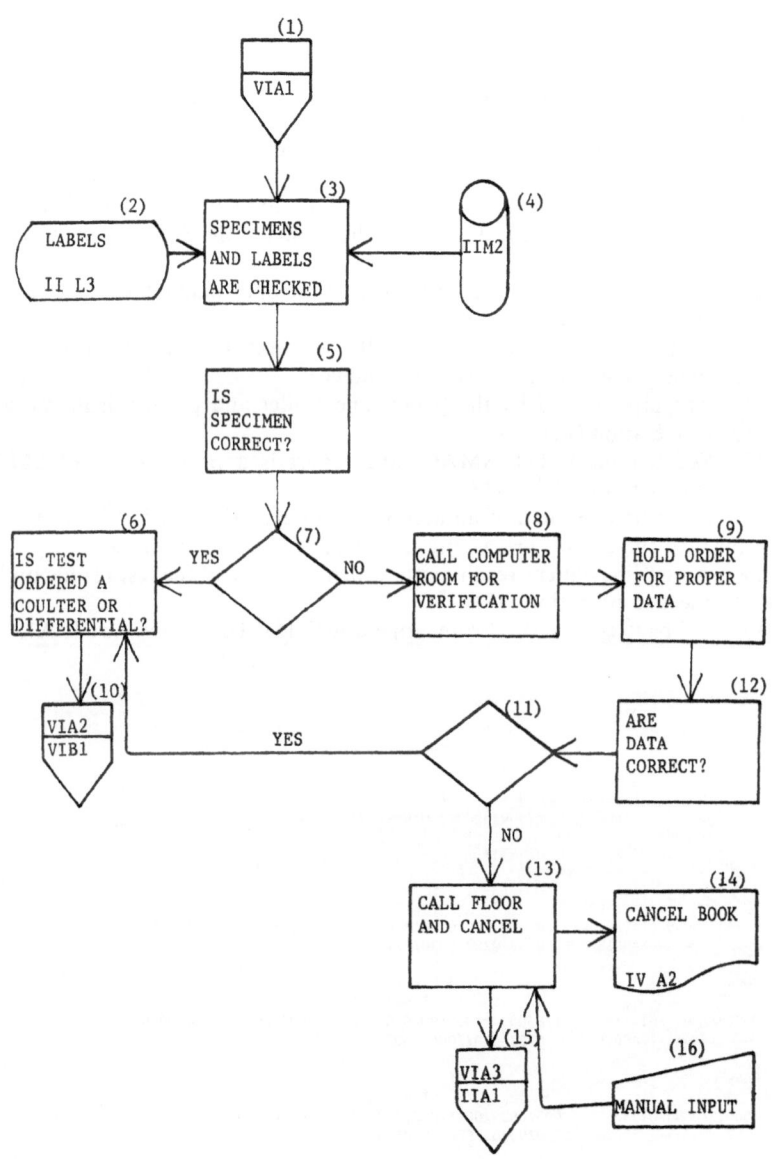

Flowchart VI A

Hematology

1. Off-page connector: From—location unspecified. To—operation (3).
2. Lab labels. See Exhibit II L3.
3. Specimens and labels are checked for accuracy. Connect to operation (5).
4. Specimen tube. Connect to operation (3).
5. Is specimen correct? Connect to operation (7).
6. Is test ordered a Coulter or differential? Connect to operation (10).
7. Decision: A—Yes, connect to operation (6). B—No connect to operation (8).
8. The computer room is called for verification of order. Connect to operation (9).
9. The order is held for proper data. Connect to operation (12).
10. Off-page connector: From—operation (10). To—Flowchart VI B1.
11. Decision: A—Yes, connect to operation (6). B—No, connect to operation (13).
12. Are data correct? Connect to operation (11).
13. The floor is called and the order canceled. Connect to operation (15).
14. Cancel book. See Exhibit IV A2.
15. Off-page connector: From—operation (15). To—Flowchart II A1.
16. The order is manually canceled on the system. Connect to operation (13).

FLOWCHART VIB

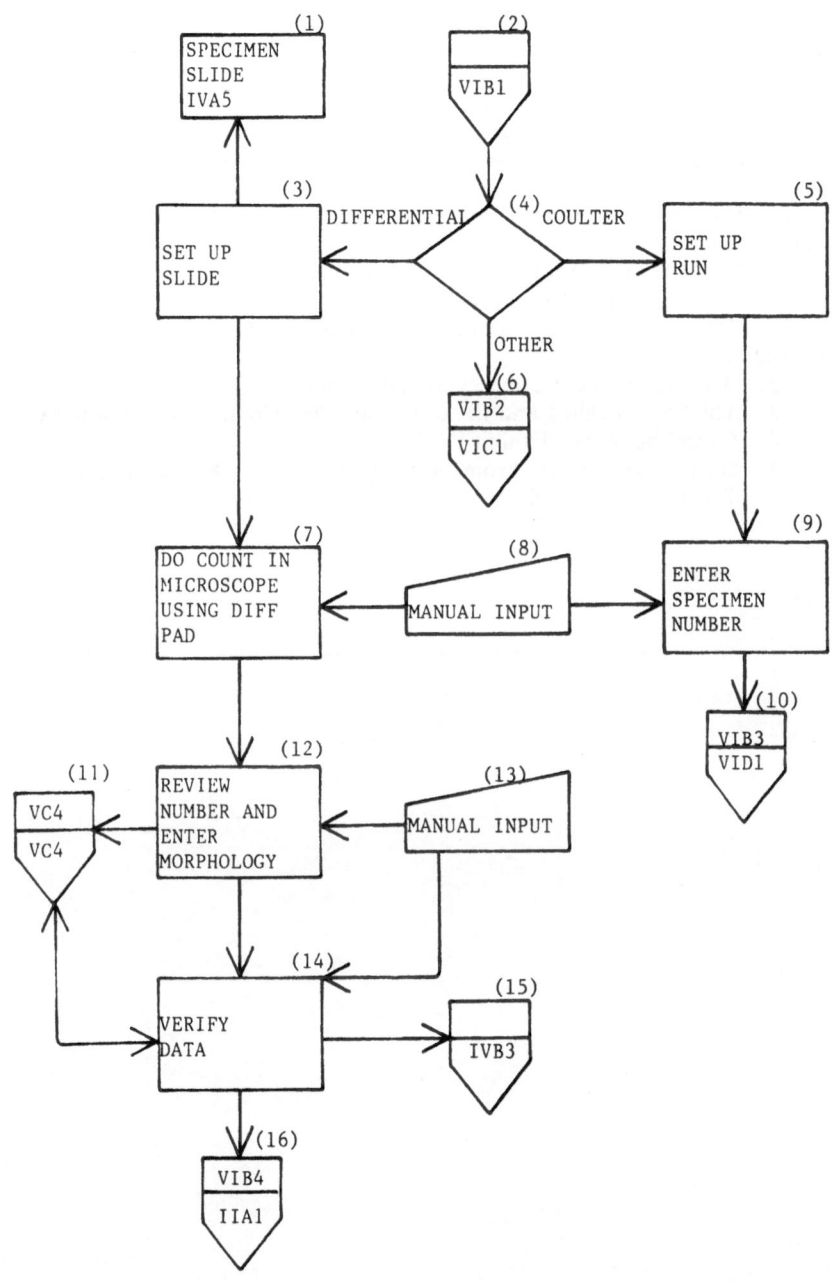

Flowchart VI B

1. Specimen slide. Connect to operation (3).
2. Off-page connector: From—location unspecified. To—operation (4).
3. The slide is set up for processing. Connect to operation (7).
4. Decision: A—Differential, connect to operation (3). B—Coulter, connect to operation (5). C—Other, connect to operation (6).
5. The run is set up on the Coulter. Connect to operation (9).
6. Off-page connector: From—operation (6). To—Flowchart VI C1.
7. A differential count is done on the microscope using the microprocessor diff pad. Connect to operation (11).
8. The specimen number and the count on the diff pad is manually entered. Connect to operations (7), (9).
9. The specimen number is entered on the terminal. Connect to operation (13).
10. Information may be entered into or called forth from the buffer. Connect to operation (14).
11. The technologist reviews the cell count and enters the morphology. Connect to operation (14).
12. The test results are manually entered into and verified on the system. Connect to operations (11), (14).
13. Off-page connector: From—operation (13). To—Flowchart VI D1.
14. The patient data is verified and the results become a part of the on-line patient result file. Connect to operation (16).
15. An on-line patient-result file contains all patient lab results. Connect to operation (14).
16. Off-page connector: From—operation (16). To—Flowchart II A1.

FLOWCHART VIC

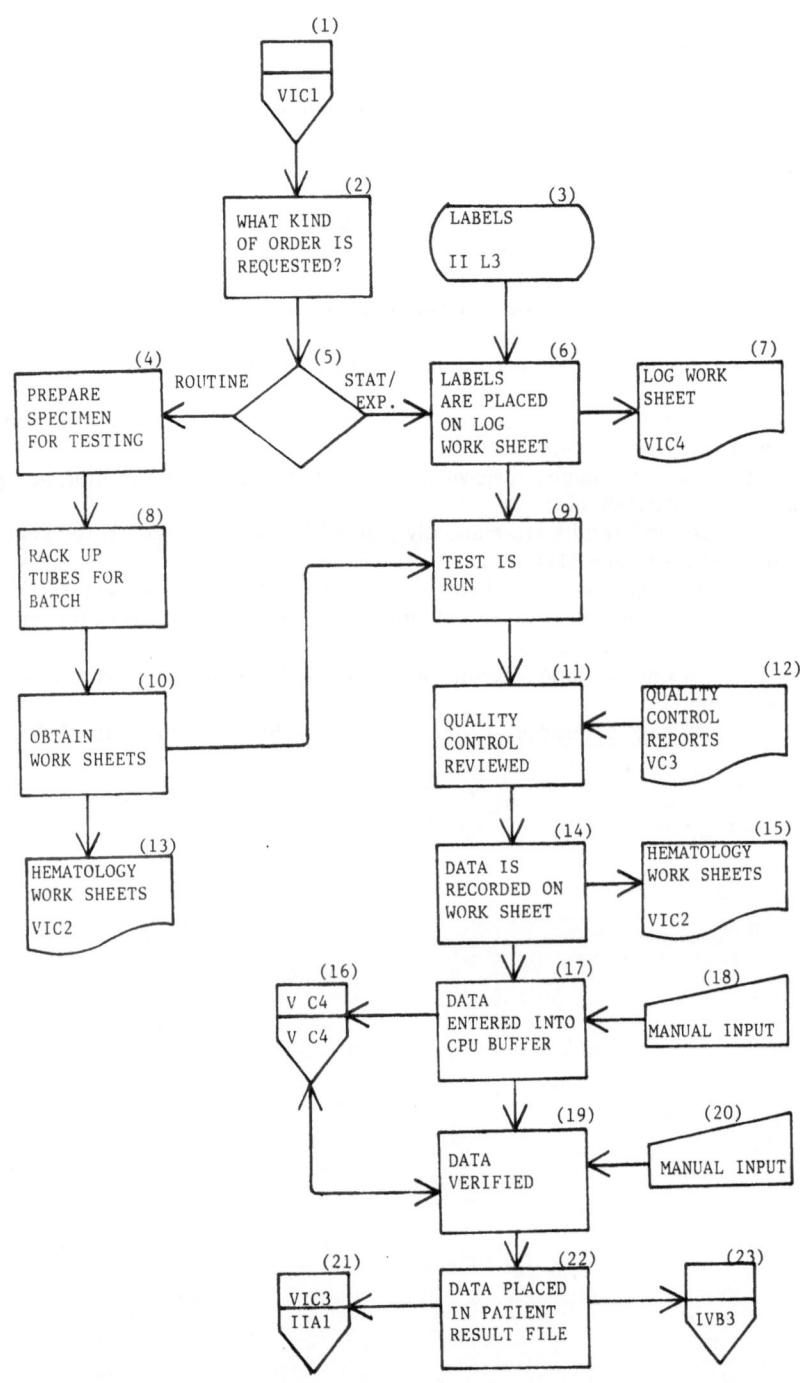

Flowchart VI C

1. Off-page connector: From—location unspecified. To—operation (2).
2. What kind of order is requested? Connect to operation (5).
3. Lab labels. See Exhibit II L3.
4. Prepare the specimen for testing. Connect to operation (8).
5. Decision: A—Routine, connect to operation (4). B—Stat or expedite, connect to operation (6).
6. Lab labels are placed on work sheets in Hematology log. Connect to operation (9).
7. See Exhibit VI C4. Hematology log sheet is a list of all patients for which lab work is done on a particular day. Connect to operation (6).
8. The tubes are racked up to be tested as a batch run. Connect to operation (10).
9. The test is run. Connect to operation (11).
10. The work sheets are obtained so test results may be recorded. Connect to operation (9).
11. The test results are reviewed against quality control normal values. Connect to operation (14).
12. Quality control reports. See Exhibit V C3.
13. See Exhibit VI C2. Hematology work sheets contain the patient name, specimen number, and a section to record test results. Connect to operation (10).
14. Test results are recorded on the Hematology work sheets. Connect to operation (17).
15. Hematology work sheets. See Exhibit VI C2.
16. Information may be entered into or called forth from the buffer. Connect to operation (19).
17. The date is entered into the test buffer. Connect to operation (16).
18. The test results are manually entered into the system. Connect to operation (17).
19. The test results are verified. Connect to operation (22).
20. The test results are manually verified on the system. Connect to operation (19).
21. Off-page connector: From—operation (22). To—Flowchart II A1.
22. Once verified, the data is placed in the patient result file. Connect to operation (21).
23. Results that have been run and verified are placed in a patient result file. Connect to operation (22).

Exhibit VI C2

PATIENT NAME	PATIENT NUM	SPEC.	TEST	IDENTIFICATION	REQ DATE
BXXX, MYRTIE L	H441B 280797	1077	998	INDICES CAL	07:45 07/12/76
		1077	002	HGB GM	07:45 07/12/76
		1077	003	HCT %	07:45 07/12/76
		1077	004	RBC 10X6/C	07:45 07/12/76
		1077	005	WBC 10X3/C	07:45 07/12/76
HXXXX, LESLIE S	H445B 308308	1080	006 DIFF		07:45 07/12/76
		1080	998	INDICES CAL	07:45 07/12/76
		1080	003	HCT %	07:45 07/12/76
		1080	004	RBC 10X6/C	07:45 07/12/76
		1080	005	WBC 10X3/C	07:45 07/12/76
RXXXXXXXX, BARBARA F	H451A 113682	1081	998	INDICES CAL	07:45 07/12/76
		1081	002	HGB GM	07:45 07/12/76
		1081	003	HCT %	07:45 07/12/76
		1081	004	RBC 10X6/C	07:45 07/12/76
		1081	005	WBC 10X3/C	07:45 07/12/76
GXXXXXX, LILLIE P	H453B 110702	1082	998	INDICES CAL	07:45 07/12/76
		1082	002	HGB GM	07:45 07/12/76
		1082	003	HCT %	07:45 07/12/76
		1082	004	RBC 10X6/C	07:45 07/12/76
		1082	005	WBC 10X3/C	07:45 07/12/76
		1082	998	INDICES CAL	07:45 07/12/76
		1082	002	HGB GM	07:45 07/12/76
		1082	003	HCT %	07:45 07/12/76
		1082	004	RBC 10X6/C	07:45 07/12/76
		1082	005	WBC 10X3/C	07:45 07/12/76
CXXXX, SHELLA M	H459C 305480	1084	006 DIFF		07:45 07/12/76
		1084	998	INDICES CAL	07:45 07/12/76
		1084	002	HGB GM	07:45 07/12/76
		1084	003	HCT %	07:45 07/12/76
		1084	004	RBC 10X6/C	07:45 07/12/76
		1084	005	WBC 10X3/C	07:45 07/12/76

Exhibit VI C2

HEMATOLOGY

7/14/76		RETIC CT		12	09:01

PATIENT NAME	SPEC	RESULT	TECH
RXXXXX, RICHARD	3068	------	----
CXXX, SHELLA M	3080	------	----
HXXXX, MAC S	3082	------	----
BXXXXXX, ANNIE	3087	------	----
BXXXX, VERA M.	3089	------	----

Exhibit VI C4

```
       0166
006 DIFF
KNIGHT, JOLEE E
A6168      1959683
19:00 10/12/76 309846

       0162
001 HEMOGRAM
EMELIO, MARY J.
H583A      1955152
18:30 10/12/76 306303

       0168
001 HEMOGRAM
SAMS, HENRY L.
EMRMX      00-0000
20:30 1/12/76 315143

       0158
001 HEMOGRAM
SZOKA, ENDRE JOSEPH
EMRMX      00-0000
22:00 10/12/76 315447
```

FLOWCHART VID

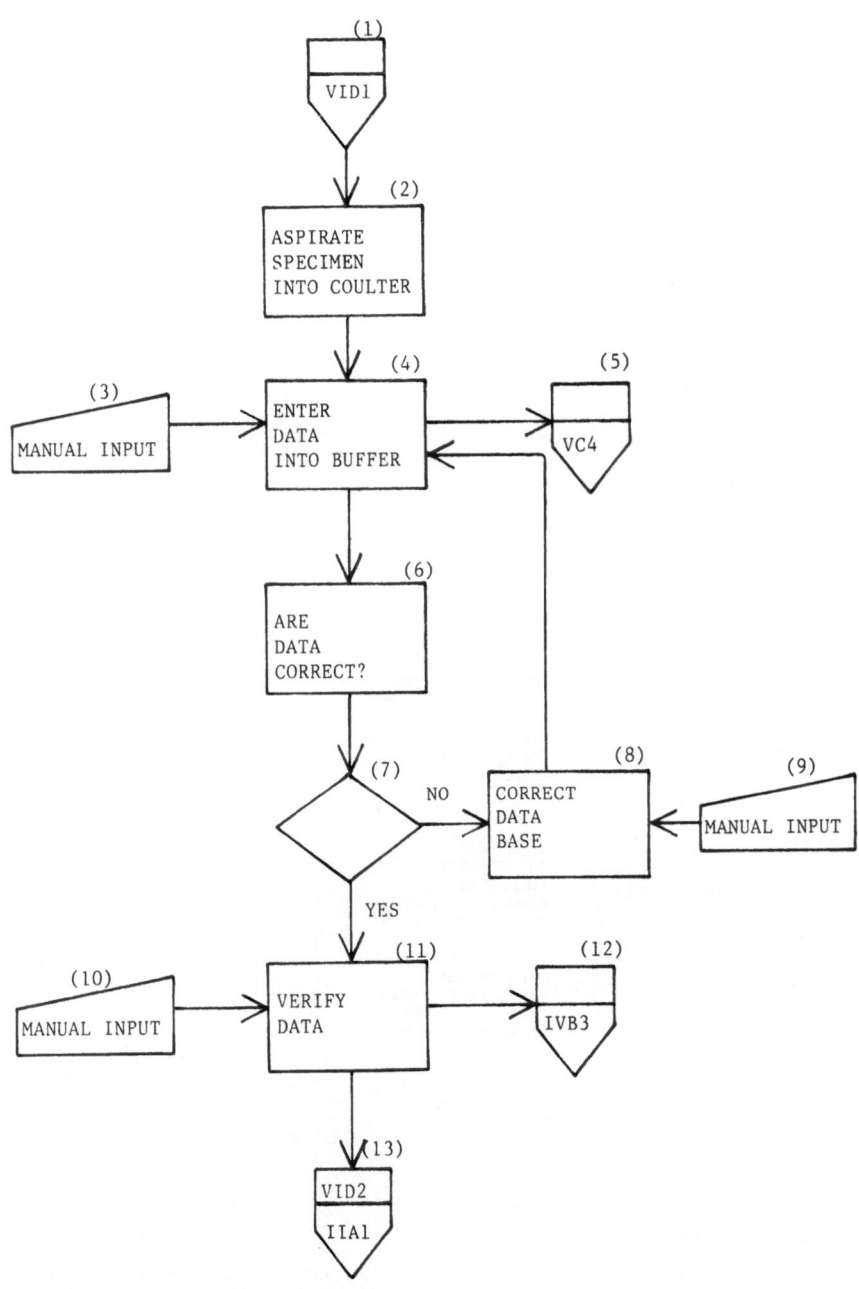

Flowchart VI D

1. Off-page connector: From—location unspecified. To—operation (2).
2. The specimen is aspirated into the Coulter. Connect to operation (4).
3. The test results are manually entered into the CPU buffer. Connect to operation (4).
4. The data is entered into the CPU buffer. Connect to operation (6).
5. The test results are stored in a CPU buffer until they are verified. Connect to operation (4).
6. Are data correct? Connect to operation (7).
7. Decision: A—Yes, connect to operation (11). B—No, connect to operation (8).
8. Correct the results previously entered into the buffer if necessary. Connect to operation (4).
9. The test results are manually corrected on the terminal. Connect to operation (8).
10. The results are verified manually on the system. Connect to operation (11).
11. The patient data is verified and the results become a part of the on-line patient-result file. Connect to operation (13).
12. On-line patient-result file. Connect to operation (11).
13. Off-page connector: From—operation (13). To—Flowchart II A1.

FLOWCHART VIIA   Level 2
MICROBIOLOGY

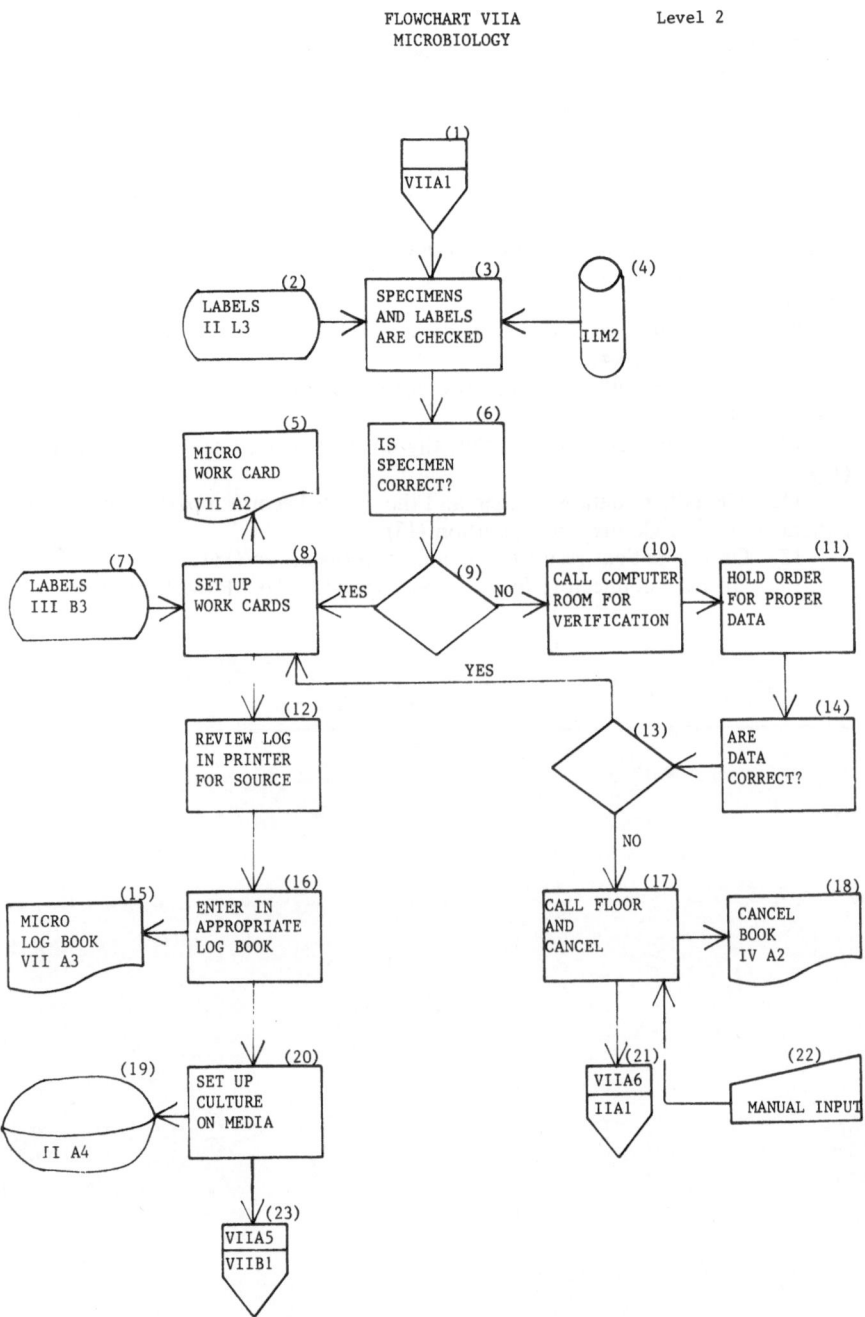

Flowchart VII A

Microbiology

1. Off-page connector: From—location unspecified. To—operation (3).
2. Lab labels. See Exhibit II L3.
3. Specimens and labels are checked for accuracy. Connect to operation (6).
4. Specimen tube. Connect to operation (3).
5. See Exhibit VII A2. The Microbiology work card is a handwritten record of patient test results. Connect to operation (8).
6. Is specimen correct? Connect to operation (9).
7. Lab labels. See Exhibit III B3.
8. Work cards are set up by attaching patient label, which contains patient name, medical record number, test, specimen number, location, and time. Work cards are filed until ready to post results. Connect to operation (12).
9. Decision: A—Yes, connect to operation (8). B—No, connect to operation (10).
10. The computer room is called for verification of lab work. Connect to operation (11).
11. The order is held for proper data. Connect to operation (14).
12. The log is reviewed in the printer to determine the source, or the body location of the specimen received. Connect to operation (16).
13. Decision: A—Yes, connect to operation (8). B—No, connect to operation (17).
14. Are data correct? Connect to operation (13).
15. See Exhibit VII A3. The patient name, medical record number, room number, specimen source, and specimen number are recorded in the Microbiology log book. Connect to operation (16).
16. Appropriate information is entered on patient in the log book. Connect to operation (20).
17. The floor is called and the lab work canceled. Connect to operation (21).
18. Cancel book. See Exhibit IV A2.
19. Microbiology media used for culture. Connect to operation (20).
20. A culture is set up on a medium to observe growth. Connect to operation (23).
21. Off-page connector. From—operation (21). To—Flowchart II A1.
22. The order is manually canceled on the system. Connect to operation (17).
23. Off-page connector: From—operation (23). To—Flowchart VII B1.

Exhibit VII A2

LAB NO.   DOB:

SPEC

TEST

COL CNT   PHYS. NOT:

MANN GAS INOS INDOL UREA MOT IL C IT H₂S GAS RHAM LYSIN

MORP MOTI OXID OF-G OF-M NITR CATA ARG 42°C SALT MR VP

TO C T P E SC AM CL K CD DX FD N TX FX GN CB B

LEWIS 70702

Exhibit VII A3
Specimen Log Book

6C179	Cox, Herbert	203090		—	2366
180	Kaufman, Mark	307436	7	—	2384
		Wed. June 30, 1976			
6C181	Agnett, Robert	306942			
6C182	Crook, JoAnne	301943	7		3215
6C183	Sizemore, Sandra	304739	4		3218
184	Richter, Karen	307260	4	—	3285
185	Cox, Herbert	203090	STCU		3340
186	Currier, Earl	261645	4	—	3345 0193at
		Thurs. July 1 1976			
7C1	Damon, Joshua	307545	737	CSF	4015
7C2	Kepler, Gregory	222857	5	CSF	4176
7C3	Huebo, Sarah	244660	3A		4242 4329
7C4	Blount, boy	303377	375	—	4328 0168at
7C5	Knight, P. June	307391	4	—	4344

FLOWCHART VIIB

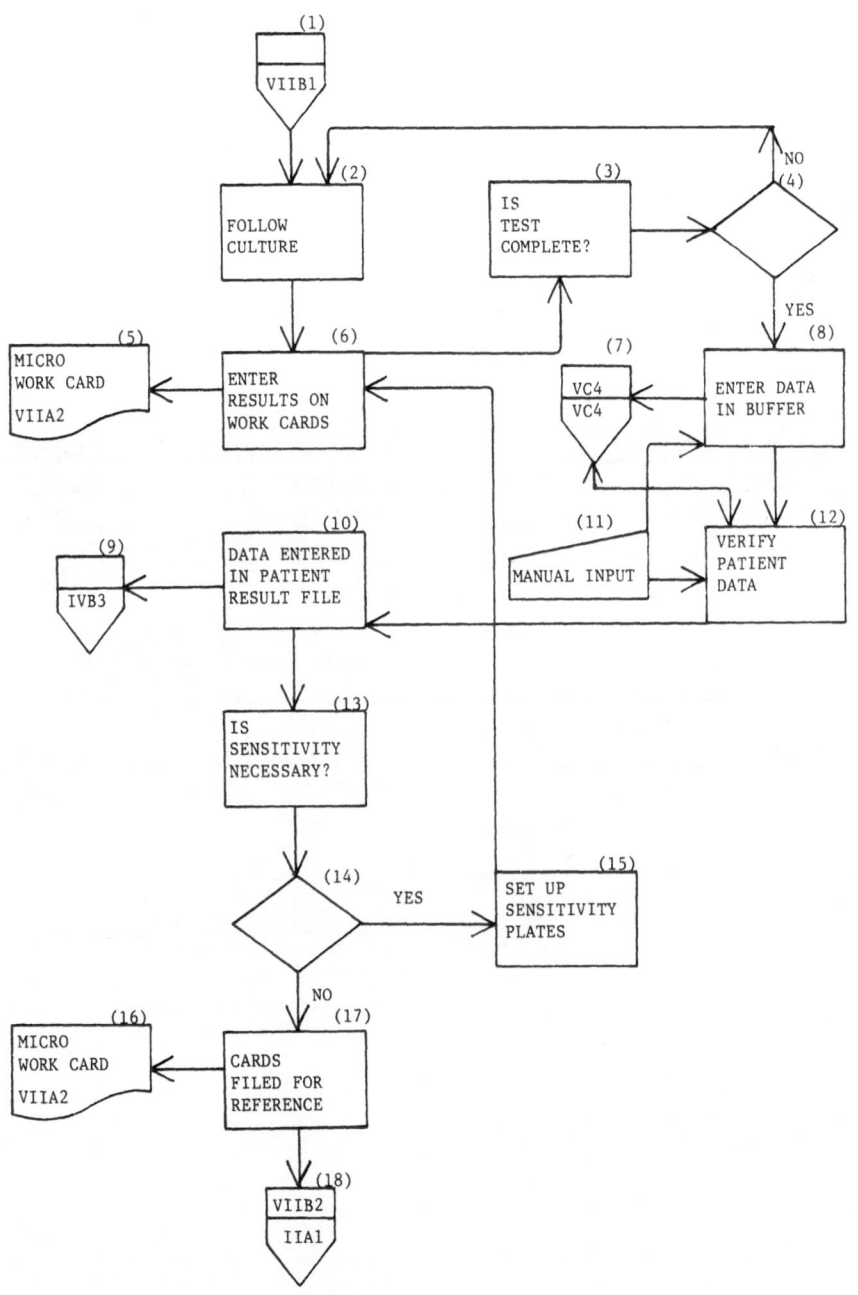

Flowchart VII B

1. Off-page connector: From—location unspecified. To—operation (2).
2. The culture is followed for one to four days for routine growth, four weeks for fungus, and six weeks for AFB. Connect to operation (6).
3. Is the test complete? Connect to operation (4).
4. Decision:—A Yes, connect to operation (8). B—No, connect to operation (2).
5. Microbiology work card. See Exhibit VII A2.
6. Test results are entered on work cards. Connect to operation (3).
7. Once the test results are entered into the CPU buffer, they are stored until verified. Connect to operations (8), (12).
8. The test results are entered into the CPU buffer. Connect to operation (12).
9. An on-line patient-result file contains all the verified test results. Connect to operation (10).
10. All verified test results are entered into a patient-result file. Connect to operation (13).
11. The test results are manually verified on the terminal. Connect to operations (8), (12).
12. The patient test results are verified. Connect to operation (10).
13. Is sensitivity necessary? Connect to operation (14).
14. Decision: A—Yes, connect to operation (15). B—No, connect to operation (17).
15. Certain organisms require sensitivity tests for antibiotics. The sensitivity plates are set up. Connect to operation (16).
16. Microbiology work card. See Exhibit VII A2.
17. Cards are filed for future reference. Connect to operation (18).
18. Off-page connector: From—operation (18). To—Flowchart II A1.

FLOWCHART VIIIA   Level 2
BLOOD BANK

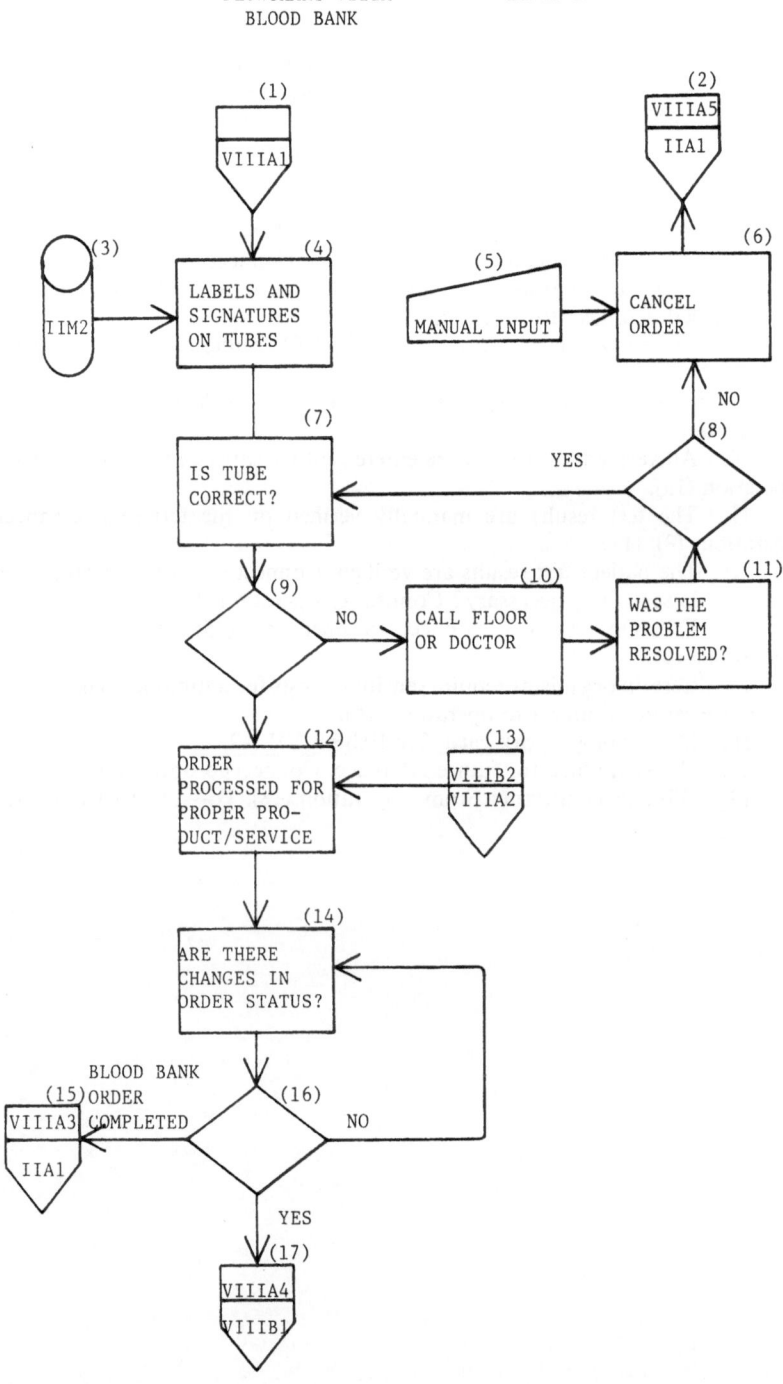

Flowchart VIII A

Blood Bank

1. Off-page connector: From—location unspecified. To—operation (4).
2. Off-page connector: From—operation (2). To—Flowchart II A1.
3. Specimen tube. Connect to operation (4)
4. The tubes must contain both a label and a signature. The signature is the person who drew the tube and must also contain the date drawn. Connect to operation (7).
5. The lab order is manually canceled on the system. Connect to operation (6).
6. Cancel the order. Connect to operation (2).
7. Is the tube correct? Connect to operation (9).
8. Decision: A—Yes, connect to operation (7). B—No, connect to operation (6).
9. Decision: A—Yes, connect to operation (12). B—No, connect to operation (10).
10. If there is any question about the tube, the floor or doctor is called. Connect to operation (11).
11. Was the problem resolved? Connect to operation (8).
12. The order is processed for proper product/service. Connect to operation (14).
13. Off-page connector: From—Flowchart VIII B1. To—operation (12).
14. Are there changes in order status? Connect to operation (16).
15. The Blood Bank order is complete, exit here. Connect to Flowchart II A1.
16. Decision: A—Yes, connect to operation (17). B—No, connect to operation (14). C—Blood Bank order complete, connect to operation (15).
17. Off-page connector: From—operation (17). To—Flowchart VIII B1.

FLOWCHART VIIIB   LEVEL 2
BLOOD BANK

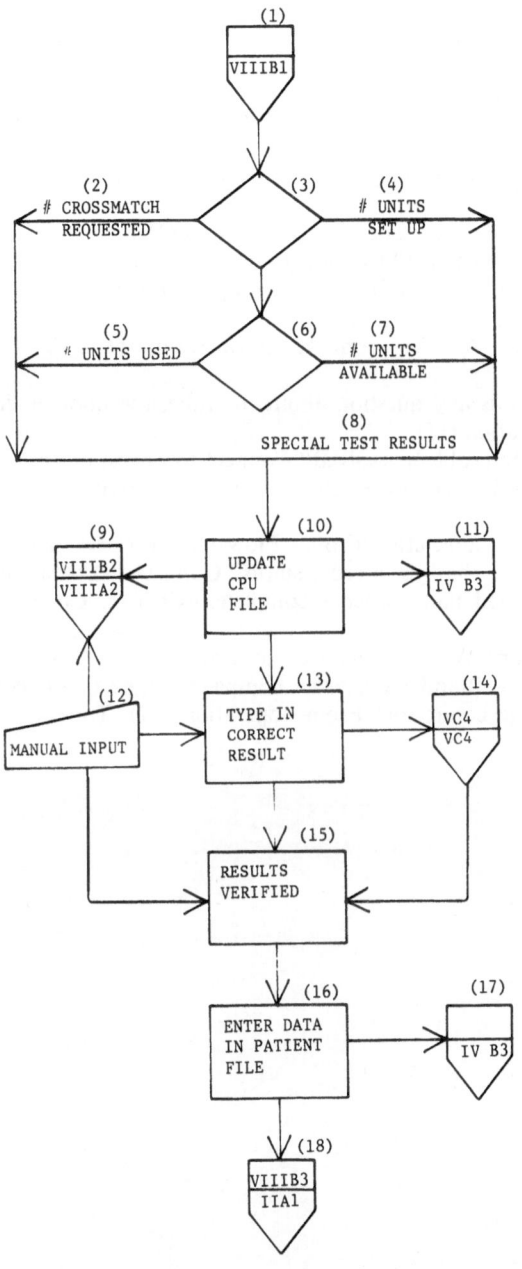

Flowchart VIII B

1. Off-page connector: From—location unspecified. To—operation (3).

2. The number of crossmatch requested are set up, usually crossmatch for each order. Connect to operation (10).

3. Decision: A—crossmatch request, connect to operation (2). B—number of units, connect to operation (4). C—proceed to next decision block.

4. Total number of units that are set up. Connect to operation (10).

5. Total number of units that are used. Connect to operation (10).

6. Decision: A—number of units used, connect to operation (5). B—number of units available, connect to operation (8). C—proceed to operation (7).

7. Total number of units that are available after order is processed. Connect to operation (10).

8. Special test results, such as direct Coombs, antibody identification, titres are entered. Connect to operation (10).

9. Off-page connector. From—operation (9). To—Flowchart VIII A2.

10. The CPU file is updated for number of units added or deleted. Connect to operations (9), (11), and (13).

11. An on-line patient-result file exists which contains all the test results on lab work. Connect to operation (10).

12. The total number of units of blood received and used are manually entered into the CPU file. Connect to operations (9), (13), and (15).

13. The correct test results are entered into the on-line patient-result file. Connect to operation (15).

14. The results, once entered, are stored in an on-line buffer until they are verified. Connect to operations (13), (15).

15. The tests results are verified. Connect to operation (16).

16. The data are entered into the on-line patient-result file. Connect to operation (18).

17. An on-line patient file exists which contains all the test results on lab work. Connect to operation (16).

18. Off-page connector: From—operation (18). To—Flowchart II A1.

FLOWCHART IXA   Level 2
IMMUNOLOGY

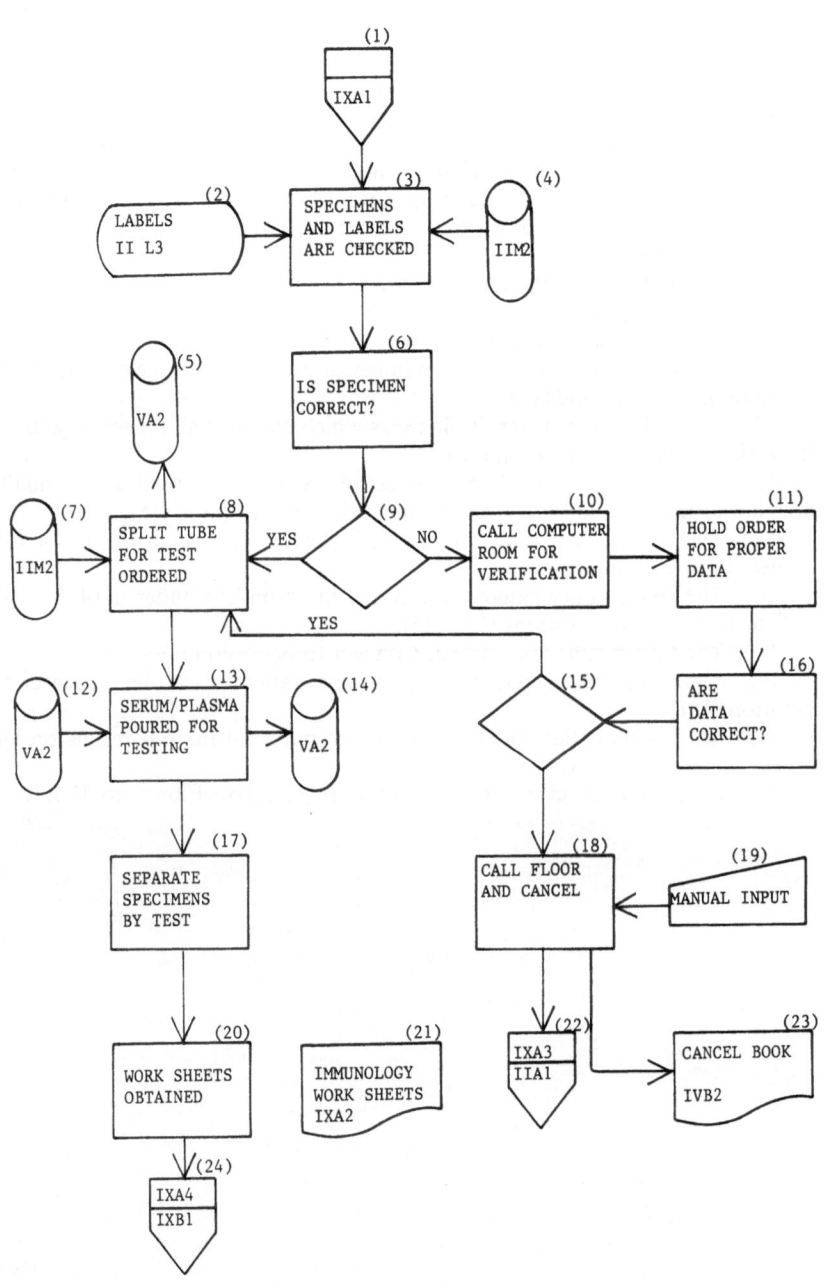

Flowchart IX A

Immunology

1. Off-page connector: From—location unspecified. To—operation (3).
2. Lab labels. See Exhibit II L3.
3. Specimens and labels are checked for accuracy. Connect to operation (6).
4. Specimen tube. Connect to operation (3).
5. Serum tube. Connect to operation (8).
6. Is specimen correct? Connect to operation (9).
7. Specimen tube. Connect to operation (8).
8. The tube is spun and the serum is placed in a new tube. Connect to operation (13).
9. Decision: A—Yes, connect to operation (8). B—No, connect to operation (10).
10. The computer room is called for verification. Connect to operation (11).
11. The order is held until the specimen is corrected. Connect to operation (16).
12. Serum tube. Connect to operation (13).
13. The serum/plasma is poured into separate tubes if more than one test is required. Connect to operation (17).
14. Serum tubes. Connect to operation (13).
15. Decision: A—Yes, connect to operation (8). B—No, connect to operation (18).
16. Are data correct? Connect to operation (15).
17. Specimen tubes are separated for processing by test. Connect to operation (20).
18. The floor is called and the tests canceled. Connect to operation (22).
19. The order is manually canceled on the system. Connect to operation (18).
20. Work sheets are obtained on each test. Connect to operation (24).
21. See Exhibit IX A2. Immunology work sheets contain patient name, medical record number, and a section to record test results. Connect to operation (20).
22. Off-page connector: From—operation (22). To—Flowchart II A1.
23. Cancel book. See Exhibit IV B2.
24. Off-page connector: From—operation (24). To—Flowchart IX B1.

Exhibit IX A2

06/27/76   INSULIN RIA   301   08:54

PATIENT NAME	SPEC NO.	FAST 120MN	10MIN 180NM	20MIN 240MN	30MIN 300MN	40MIN 360MN	50MIN	60MIN	TECH
KXXXXX, MICHAEL	2266	----- -----	----- -----	----- -----	----- -----	----- -----	-----	-----	-----
TXXXXXXXX, PATR	8371	----- -----	----- -----	----- -----	----- -----	----- -----	-----	-----	-----
SXXXX, JAMES	4413	----- -----	----- -----	----- -----	----- -----	----- -----	-----	-----	-----
GXXXXXXXXX, ROB	6239	----- -----	----- -----	----- -----	----- -----	----- -----	-----	-----	-----

Exhibit IX A2

9/13/76   HBS AG (AUST AG)   284   09:02

PATIENT NAME   SPEC   RESULT   TECH

FXXXXXX, FRAN   1045   ------   ----

AXXXX, ROBERT   1057   ------   ----

EXXXXXX, VERNO   1059   ------   ----

WXXXX, GRADY C   1069   ------   ----

BXXXXXX, BETTY   1111   ------   ----

WXXXXX, NANCY   1159   ------   ----

CXXXXXXX, LUCI   5237   ------   ----

AXXXX, LEWIS H   5284   ------   ----

RXXXX, FLORENC   5351   ------   ----

TXXXXXX, BARB   6148   ------   ----

WXXXXX, JANIS   7058   ------   ----

FLOWCHART IXB

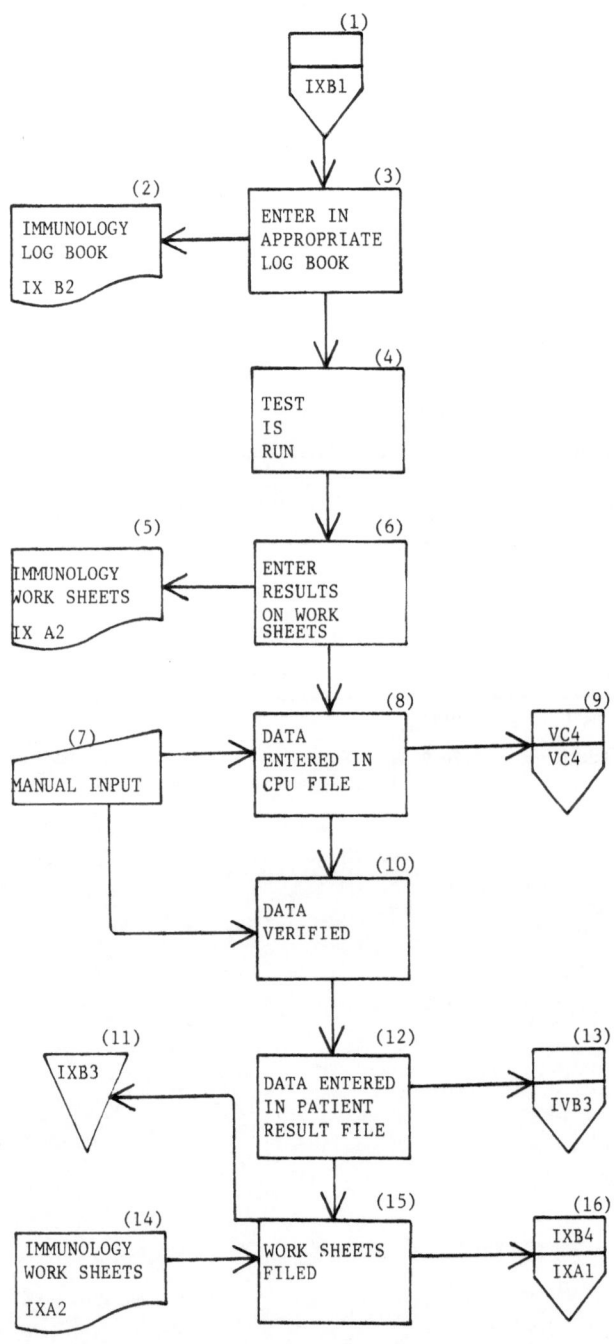

Flowchart IX B

1. Off-page connector: From—location unspecified. To—operation (3).
2. See Exhibit IX B2. Immunology log book contains such information as name, medical record number, and specimen number. Connect to operation (3).
3. There is a separate log book for each test run in Immunology. Connect to operation (4).
4. The test is run. Connect to operation (6).
5. Immunology work sheets. See Exhibit IX A2.
6. The test results are entered on the work sheets. Connect to operation (8).
7. The test results are manually entered into the CPU file. Connect to operation (8).
8. The data are entered into the CPU file. Connect to operation (10).
9. The results, once entered, are stored in an on-line buffer until they are verified. Connect to operation (8).
10. The data are verified on the Immunology terminal. Connect to operation (12).
11. The work sheets are filed in a file cabinet for future reference. Connect to operation (15).
12. The data are entered in the on-line patient result file. Connect to operation (15).
13. An on-line patient result file. Connect to operation (12).
14. Immunology work sheet. See Exhibit IX A2.
15. The work sheets are filed once all results are posted. Connect to operation (16).
16. Off-page connector: From—operation (16). To—Flowchart II A1.

Exhibit IX B2
HAA Log Book

Log#	Date	Patient	Hosp #	Spec #	Ward	Result	Notes
	1324	Alford, Robin	299089	1403	343	Neg ✓	
	1325	Spencer, Callie	152183	3157	OPCLC	Neg ✓	
	1326	O'Neal, Brantley	218786	2090	1039	(Neg) ✗	canceled per 3/69
	1327	Courson, Alex	700526	2174	462	Neg ✓	
	1328	Henderson, Dochia	260089	2288	H381	Neg ✓	
	1329	Trimble, Charles	290357	2290	H604	Neg ✓	
	1330	Hendershot, Fred	109529	2286	A321	Neg ✓	
	1331	Callaway, Augusta L.	292453	2260	H385	Neg ✓	
	1332	Vandervoorde, Babe	237912	2285	H535	Neg ✓	
	1333	English, Robert V.	300908	2258	H680	Neg ✓	
	1334	Perkins, Martha	264821	2196	OPC	Neg ✓	

FLOWCHART XA   Level 2
INFORMATION CONTROL AND PROCESSING

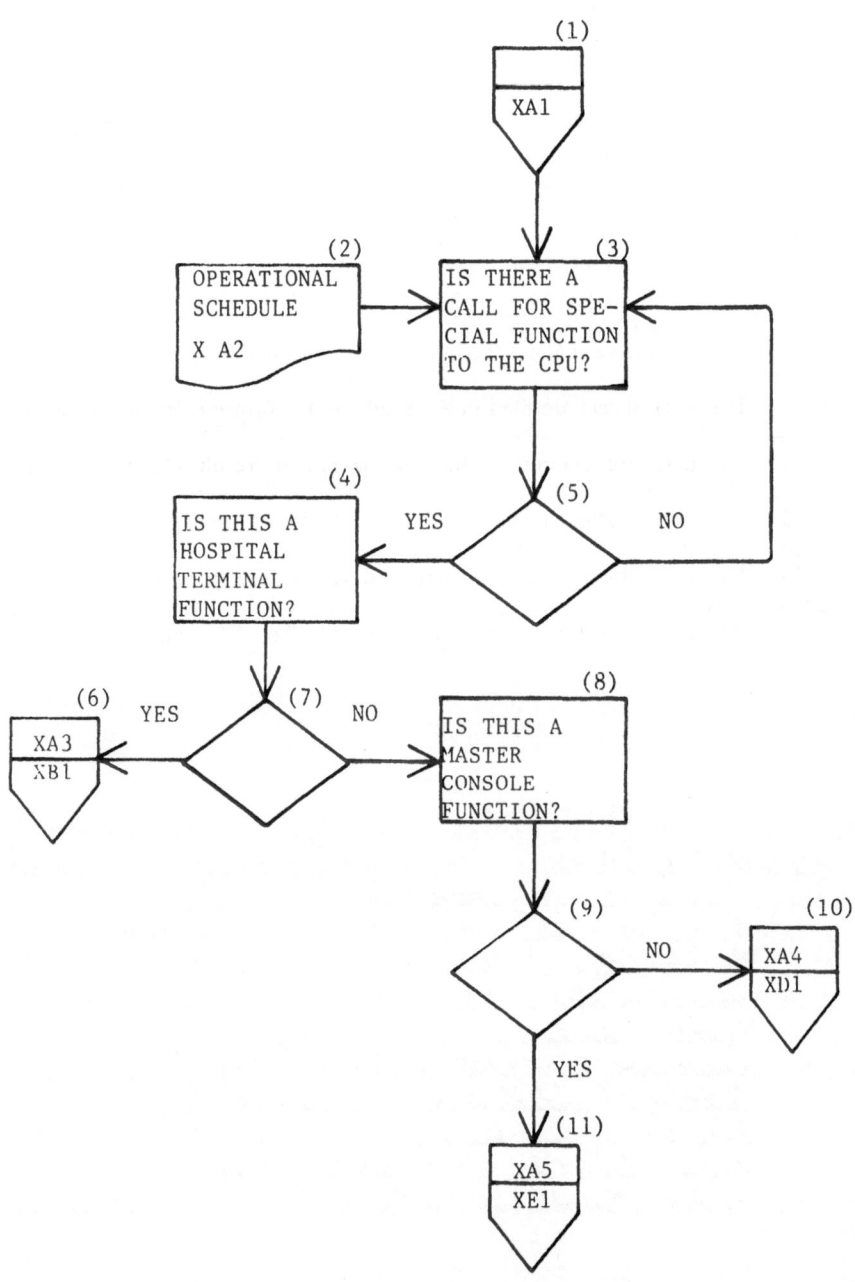

Flowchart X A

Information Control and Processing

1. Off-page connector: From—location unspecified. To—operation (3).
2. See Exhibit X A2. The operational schedule is a list of all computer activity, the time of day each task is run, and the operator who runs it. Connect to operation (3).
3. Is there a call for special function to the CPU? Connect to operation (5).
4. Is this a hospital terminal function? Connect to operation (7).
5. Decision: A—Yes, connect to operation (6). B—No, connect to operation (3).
6. Off-page connector: From—operation (6). To—Flowchart X B1.
7. Decision: A—Yes, connect to operation (11). B—No, connect to operation (8).
8. Is this a master console function? Connect to operation (9).
9. Decision: A—Yes, connect to operation (11). B—No, connect to operation (10).
10. Off-page connector: From—operation (10). To—Flowchart X D1.
11. Off-page connector: From—operation (11). To—Flowchart X E1.

Exhibit X A2   DATE _____

PROCEDURE SCHEDULE FOR COMPUTER OPERATIONS

TIME	PROCEDURE	TIME STARTED	TIME FINISHED	OPERATOR
7:30-8:30 A.M.	CONFIRM SPEC. (DRAW TEAM)			
8:30 A.M.	WORKSHEETS (NEW)			
	(1 part green, Chem., Hematology, Immunology, put in area baskets).			
8:45 A.M.	MASTER WORKSHEETS			
	(1 part green, Chem., Immun., B.B., put in area baskets).			
9:00 A.M.	UNFINISHED TEST REPT.			
	(1 part green, Chem., Immun., Microscopy, Anat. Path., B.B., Microbiology).			
9:20-9:30 A.M.	SMAC TAPES (STAT)			
	(place reports in SMAC room, notify tech. of report)			
10:20-10:30 A.M.	SMAC TAPES			
	(place reports in SMAC room, notify tech. of report)			
11.20-11:30 A.M.	SMAC TAPES			
	(place reports in SMAC room, notify tech. of report)			
12.00 P.M.	WARD REPORTS			
	(1 part green, deliver to floors)			
12:25 P.M.	COPY DRUM			
	(mag. tape, place in green cabinet on 2nd shelf, in upright position).			
12:35-12:45 P.M.	SMAC TAPES			
	(place reports in SMAC room, notify tech. of report)			
1:20-1:30 P.M.	SMAC TAPES			
	(place reports in SMAC room, notify tech. of report)			
2:20-2:30 P.M.	SMAC TAPES			
	(place reports in SMAC room, notify tech. of report)			
3:00 P.M.	WARD REPORT			
	(By DR# 083, 074, 069, 075, 110, 076, 080)			
3:20-3:30 P.M.	SMAC TAPES			
	(place reports in SMAC room, notify tech. of report)			
3:50 P.M.	UNFINISHED TEST REPT.			
	(Chemistry)			
4:00 P.M.	COPY DRUM			
	(Mag. tape, place in green cabinet on 2nd shelf on right on bottom of stack)			
4:10 P.M.	BILLING REPT. (Mon. only)			
	(Mag. tape, see instructions on next sheet, place in safe)			
4:20 P.M.	DAILY CHART REPORTS			
	(2 part green, deliver one to floors, others to "Dup. Daily Chart" basket)			
4:45-5:30 P.M.	SMAC TAPES			
	(place reports in SMAC room, notify tech. of report)			
7:00 P.M.	SMAC TAPES			
	(place reports in SMAC room, notify tech. of report)			
8:00 P.M.	SMAC TAPES			
	(place reports in SMAC room, notify tech. of report)			
9:45 P.M.	UNFINISHED TEST REPT.			
	(only by request)			
10:00 P.M.	COPY DRUM			
	(Run on mag. tape, place on 2nd shelf in green cabinet, in upright position)			
10:10 P.M.	BILLING REPORT			
	(See procedures below)			

Exhibit X A2   DATE _____

PROCEDURE SCHEDULE FOR COMPUTER OPERATIONS (CONT.)

TIME	PROCEDURE	TIME STARTED	TIME FINISHED	OPERATOR
10:15 P.M.	7-DAY CHARTS			

(Run on magnetic tape, printout on 2 part blue, deliver one to floors.
Put E.R., OPC and Discharge in Med. Records basket. Run one copy on
one part green, put in Gene's basket on area #49. Procedure for
diverting to tape drive is in the procedure manual).

11:55-12:05 A.M.   DO NOT DO ANYTHING BETWEEN THESE TIMES AS THE MACHINE IS PURGING.

12:05 A.M.   RESET SPECIMEN NO.
(Monday=1, Tuesday =2, Wednesday=3, Thursday=4, Friday=5, Saturday=6,
Sunday=7). Order a test to check for correct number for that day and
then order cancel the test.

12:30 A.M.   WARD REPORT
(Deliver 1 to floors, one part green).

3:00 A.M.   ARCHIVE ENTRY/MERGE
(Use 2707 for entries, use 1 part green, place print out in "Archive"
basket. Run an "Archive Print" every Sunday evening for Linda).

3:30 A.M.   COPY DRUM
(Run on mag. tape, place on 2nd shelf in green cabinet, upright to left).

4:00 A.M.   QUALITY CONTROL
(Cards are located in top basket behind CRT. In Computer Room. Run as
follows: Monday, Wednesday and Friday run Hyland I and II. On Tuesday
and Thursdays run Hyland I T/C, Hyland I, Hyland II. Run them in that order.
On Saturday run Hyland I, Hyland II. Do not run any Q.C. on Sunday).

4:45 A.M.   CENSUS REPORT
(2 part green, 1 to Admissions, 1 for Pharmacy).

5:50 A.M.   UNFINISHED TEST REPT.
(Hematology only, put in area basket).

6:15 A.M.   S.C.L. TUBES
(2 part green, x2)

6:25 A.M.   S.C.L. LABELS
(3-up labels, x2)

6:30 A.M.   COPY DRUM
(Mag. tape, put in green cabinet, 2nd shelf, in upright position).

BILLING PROCEDURE

1. Load tape to tape drive, make sure the ring is in. Check to make
   sure tape is loaded properly. Turn the power button on by depressing
   the power button. The light will come on. Depress the 'Load" button
   and "On-line" button before proceeding.
2. On 2707 depress "New" and Billing", check the display screen.
   Depress "New Line" and "Return".
3. If you have any problem with the first billing make sure you do a
   'Repeat". Never do two "News" in a row; if you do, you will wipe
   the billing. BE CAREFUL.
4. Place the tape in the safe for Don Guttinger.
5. On Mondays, billing will be done twice at 4:10 P.M. and 11:30 P.M.
   Tuesday-Sunday run at 11:30 P.M.

10/5/76

FLOWCHART XB

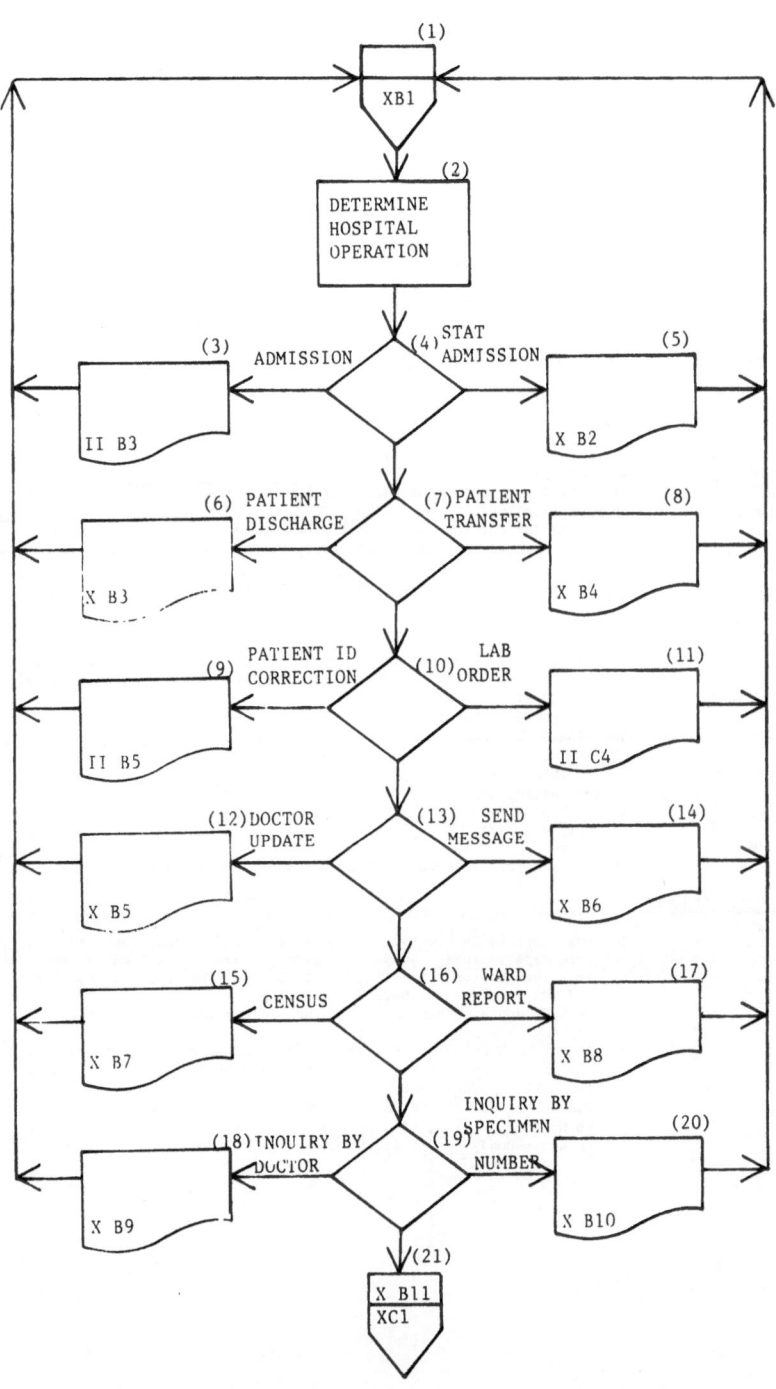

Flowchart X B

1. Off-page connector: From—location unspecified. To—operation (2).
2. The hospital terminal function is determined. Connect to operation (4).
3. Hardcopy of hospital admission. See Exhibit II B3. Connect to operation (1).
4. Decision: A—Admission, connect to operation (3). B—Stat admit, connect to operation (5). C—proceed to next decision block.
5. See Exhibit X B2. A stat admission is used to enter patients into the system before all admission information is available so lab work can be ordered. There is a hardcopy print-out of this procedure. Connect to operation (1).
6. See Exhibit X B3. A patient discharge is performed by the system. There is a hardcopy print-out of this procedure. Connect to operation (1).
7. Decision: A—patient discharge, connect to operation (6). B—patient transfer, connect to operation (8). C—proceed to next decision block.
8. See Exhibit X B4. A patient transfer is performed. There is a hardcopy print-out of this procedure. Connect to operation (1).
9. Hardcopy of patient ID correction. See Exhibit II B5. Connect to operation (1).
10. Decision: A—patient ID correction, connect to operation (9). B—lab order, connect to operation (11). C—proceed to next decision block.
11. Lab order. See Exhibit II C4. Connect to operation (1).
12. See Exhibit X B5. A doctor update is used to change doctors assigned to the patient. There is a hard copy print-out of this procedure. Connect to operation (1).
13. Decision: A—doctor update, connect to operation (12). B—send message, connect to operation (14). C—proceed to next decision block.
14. See Exhibit X B6. One terminal can contact another by special number to transmit free text messages. Connect to operation (1).
15. See Exhibit X B7. A census is a listing of patients by floor and room number. There is a hardcopy print-out of this procedure. Connect to operation (1).
16. Decision: A—census, connect to operation (15). B—ward report, connect to operation (17). C—proceed to next decision block.
17. See Exhibit X B8. A ward report is a listing of patient tests ordered and the results since the last daily chart report. This can be done by doctor number or ward. There is a hardcopy print-out of this procedure. Connect to operation (1).
18. See Exhibit X B9. An inquiry by doctor is a hardcopy print-out of all the patient assigned to a particular doctor. Connect to operation (1).
19. Decision: A—inquiry by doctor, connect to operation (18). B—inquiry by specimen number, connect to operation (20). C—proceed to operation (21).
20. See Exhibit X B10. An inquiry by specimen number shows all unfinished results for a patient. Connect to operation (1).
21. Off-page connector: From—operation (21). To—Flowchart X C1.

Exhibit X B2

```
** READY
STAT ADMIT, USER ID:  00,  08:39  10/12/75,  STATION 12


MR#:  665544
NAME:  SXXXXXXX, JXXXXXXXXX  OK?  Y
SEX·    M   OK?  Y
AGE·    23Y   OK?  Y
ROOM:  EMRMX      OK?  Y
ENTRY OK?   Y

          ---------- 08:40   ENTRY ACCEPTED
```

Exhibit X B3

```
**READY


DISCHARGE,  USER ID 00,  14:17   10/13/75,  STATION  12

MR#:  123456    OK?  Y   BXXXXXX, JXXXXX G.  32Y  M  H541D  OK?  Y
ADMIS#:  1234567   10/13/75
ENTRY OK?   Y


          --------------14:17  ENTRY ACCEPTED.
```

Exhibit X B4

```
** READY

TRANSFER,  USER ID. 00, 14:14   10/13/75,  STATION 12


MR#.  123455    OK?  Y  BXXXX, JXXXXX  G.  32Y  M  H541C  OK?   N
ROOM:  H541D    OK?  Y
ENTRY OK?   Y
          ------------ 14:15  ENTRY ACCEPTED
```

Exhibit X B5

```
**READY
DR. UPDATE  , USER ID:  22,  14:11  09/12/76 , STATION 12


MR#  948014    OK? Y  GXXXXXX, JANICE  25Y  F WF02 OK? Y
 DR#:  250 260 231 241
ZXXXXXXX, J W SXXXXXXXXX, R  SXXXXXXX, W RXXXXXX, WILL  OK? Y
 DR#:  250.253.
ZXXXXXXX, J W KXXXXXXXXXX, T  OK? Y
 ENTRY OK? Y
```

Exhibit X B6

```
LAB ORDER  , USER ID:  22,  13:45    09/11/76    ,     STATION 12

MR#  345610   OK?  Y
NAME:  MXXXXXXXX, PAULA     WF02    22    ,  13:45    09/11/76  OK?  Y
DR#:   250 260 231 241
PROBLEM:  LOW FEVER  OK?  Y
T#   649  MISC ROUTINE CUL   OK?  Y  STAT:  N  EXP#  Y
    EXPEDITE TRANSPORT--ONLY FOR UNLISTED SOURCE-LABEL SOURCE + TYPE MSG
MSG:  LEFT EAR
ENTRY OK?  Y                            2250      DONE
 T#
**READY
```

Exhibit X B7

```
ROOM:  WF07?  OK?  Y


MEDICAL        LIST CENSUS         07/02/76      10:51

WF07

A406
299384   HXXX, RAYMOND S      32Y M REJECT-TR-KIDNEY    A406A

A409
309584   SXXXXXX, GERTRUDE C   54Y F NONE GIVEN         A409A

A415
106843   SXXXX, SOPHIE I       63Y F 284               A415B
103847   CXXXX, GENE M         49Y F NEUROMEYPATHY      A415A

A417
013847   SXXXX, ROOSEVELT *    62Y M CHEST PAIN         A417B

ZZZZZ

A418
302937   BXXXXX, FRANCES E     54Y F HORNES SYNDROME    A418B
307284   SXXXX, VELMA M        40Y F NOT GIVEN          A418A

MEDICAL        LIST CENSUS         07/02/76      10·51

A419
004837   GXXXX, DORIS L        48Y F HYPERPARATHY       A419A

A421
302947   RXXXXXXX, KAREN M     32Y F SUBARO HEMMORAGE   A421B
304837   MXXXXX, ELNORA U      39Y F CHF                A421A

H435
306281   SXXXX, PATRICIA A     29Y F RETINAL EMBOLUS    H435B
306154   WXXXXXX, HELEN J      53Y F REFLUX EXOPH       H435A

H439
305483   MXXXX, WILLIE *       69Y M PLEURAL EFFUSION   H439D
304958   MXXXXXX, LEROY R      69Y M MALABSO            H439C
307903   HXXXX, VINCENT E      70Y M S.O.E.             H439B

ZZZZZ

H441
304851   NXXX, JOHNNIE MAE     59Y F OBS JDCE           H441A
091393   WXXXXXXX, ESTEL, M    76Y F DEHYDRATION        H441B

H445
303958   GXXXXX, LOU L         69Y M WT LOSS-MALAB      H445B

MEDICAL        LIST CENSUS         07/02/76      10:51
```

Exhibit X B8

WARD REPORT , USER ID: 22, 14:31   09/03/76 , STATION 12

TYPE: 001
AXXXXXX, S C OK? Y

MEDICAL   WARD REPORT   09/03/76   14:32   PAGE 1

H441B   GXXXXXXXX, LOU *   MEDICAL RECORD # 312515

```
HEMOGRAM                    09/03/76    00:00
  HGB  GM            10.8* GM            09/03/76    00:00
  HCT  %             34.1* PERCENT       09/03/76    00:00
  RBC  10X6/CMM      3.68* 10X6/CMM       09/03/76    00·00
  WBC  10X3/CMM      12.4* 10X3/CMM       09/03/76    00:00
  MCV  CUB MIC         93  CUB MIC        09/03/76    00:00
  MCH MC MC GM       29.3  MC MC GM       09/03/76    00:00
  MCHC %             31.7* PERCENT       09/03/76    00:00
PT CONTROL SEC       10.8  SEC            09/03/76    13·00
PT SEC               13.8  SEC            09/03/76    13:00
PTT CONTRL SEC         30  SEC            09/03/76    13:00
PTT SEC                32  SEC            09/03/76    13:00
SGPT     IU/L    REQUEST RECEIVED         09/03/76    00:00
VDRL             REQUEST RECEIVED         09/03/76    00:00
HBS AG (AUST AG)  REQUEST RECEIVED        09/03/76    00:00
RETIC CT         REQUEST RECEIVED         09/03/76    00:00
ESR              REQUEST RECEIVED         09/03/76    00:00
PLAT CT 10X3 CUM REQUEST RECEIVED         09/03/76    00:00
DIFF             REQUEST RECEIVED         09/03/76    00·00
MG     MG/DL     REQUEST RECEIVED         09/03/76    00:00
CPK   MIU/ML     REQUEST RECEIVED         09/03/76    00·00
AMYLASE   IU/L    REQUEST RECEIVED        09/03/76    00:00
SGOT     IU/L    REQUEST RECEIVED         09/03/76    00:00
ALK PHOS    IU/L REQUEST RECEIVED         09/03/76    00:00
D BIL   MG/DL    REQUEST RECEIVED         09/03/76    00:00
T BIL   MG/DL    REQUEST RECEIVED         09/03/76    00:00
ALBUMIN GM/DL    REQUEST RECEIVED         09/03/76    00:00
T PROT  GM/DL    REQUEST RECEIVED         09/03/76    00:00
CALCIUM MG/DL    REQUEST RECEIVED         09/03/76    00:00
GLUCOSE MG/DL    REQUEST RECEIVED         09/03/76    00:00
ADLT TYPTS BUN CR REQUEST RECEIVED        09/03/76    13:00
HEMOGRAM         REQUEST RECEIVED         09/03/76    13:00
REPORT COMPLETE
```

Exhibit X B9

```
**READY
INQUIRY-DOCTOR    , USER ID:  22, 14:15  09/11/76 , STATION  12


DR#:   250.
ZXXXXXXX, J W  OK? Y

        049613   SXXXXX, HARRIET     LOW FEVER          WF02

      --------
DR#:
      REPORT COMPLETE
```

Exhibit X B10

```
**READY
INQUIRY-SPECIMEN, USER ID:  22,   13:41    09/02/76 , STATION  12



ACQ#:  2166     MXXXX, ARTHUR J  OK?  Y  BURN  H541B  951
BXXXXXXX, H G

  4320  603  URINE CULTURE            09/02  00:00
  4289  625  BURN WOULD CULT          09/02  12:45
  4283  625  BURN WOULD CULT          09/02  12:45
  3396  619  CATH TIP CULTURE         09/01  21:00
  3141  426  17-KETOSTERO-24U         09/01  10:30
  3141  425  17-OH 24U                09/01  10:30
  2166  427  CATECHOL-24U             08/31  09:45


REPORT COMPLETE


      ------------
ACQ#:
```

FLOWCHART XC

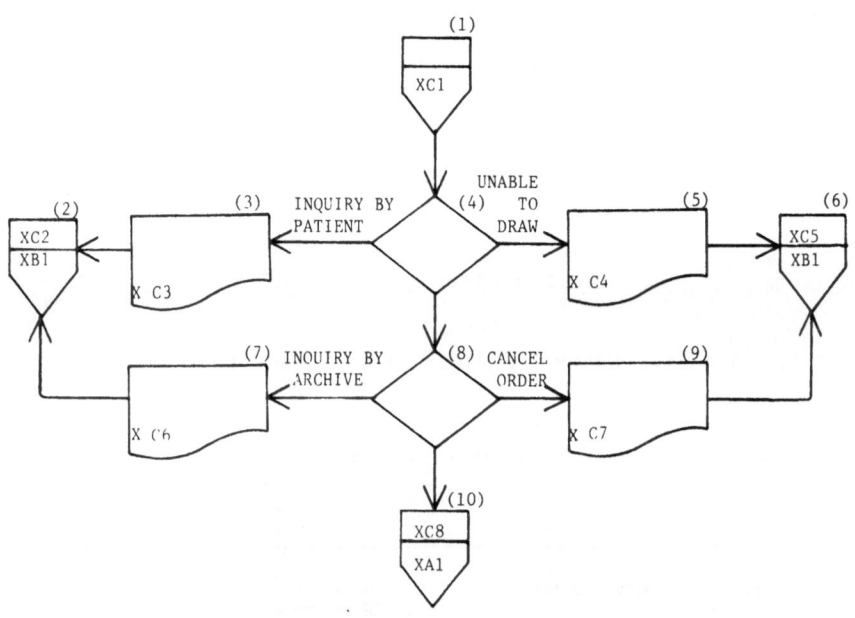

Flowchart X C

1. Off-page connector: From—location unspecified. To—operation (4).
2. Off-page connector: From—operation (2). To—Flowchart X B1.
3. See Exhibit X C3. An inquiry by patient is a hardcopy print-out, of all finished and unfinished test results. These can be called LIFO or FIFO, and the number required can be specified. Connect to operation (2).
4. Decision: A—inquiry by patient, connect to operation (3). B—unable to draw, connect to operation (5). C—proceed to next decision block.
5. See Exhibit X C4. Unable to draw is a postponement of blood drawing until the next blood collection. Connect to operation (6).
6. Off-page connector: From—operation (6). To—Flowchart X B1.
7. See Exhibit X C6. An inquiry by archive is a listing of a particular patient's hospital visits and the microfilm location (by cartridge and page number) where all laboratory work may be found. Connect to operation (2).
8. Decision: A—inquiry by archive, connect to operation (7). B—cancel order, connect to operation (9). C—proceed to operation (10).
9. See Exhibit X C7. Cancel order is the means by which an order may be taken out of the system and credited to the patient's account. Connect to operation (6).
10. Off-page connector: From—operation (10). To—Flowchart X A1.

Exhibit X C3

```
**READY
INQUIRY-PATIENT , USER ID:  03 , 14:33  07/07/77 , STATION 12


MR#  138365  OK?  Y  AXXXXX, HARVEY   H466A  OK?  Y
 TYPE:  095  ADLT LYTS BUN CR  OK?  Y
LIF/FIF?  L 02  OK?  Y

            NA   MEQ/L        138  MEQ/L              07/07  07:45
            NA   MEQ/L        138  MEQ/L              07/06  21:45
            K MEQ/L           4.3  MEQ/L              07/07  07:45
            K MEQ/L           4.4  MEQ/L              07/06  21:45
            CL MEQ/L         109*  MEQ/L              07/07  07:45
            CL MEQ/L         108*  MEQ/L              07/06  21:45
            CO2  MEQ/L         20*  MEQ/L             07/07  07:45
            CO2  MEQ/L         20*  MEQ/L             07/06  21:45
            BUN  MG/DL         75*  MG/DL             07/07  07:45
            BUN  MG/DL         73*  MG/DL             07/06  21:45
            CREATININE MG/DL  2.6*  MG/DL             07/07  07:45
            CREATININE MG/DL  2.6*  MG/DL             07/06  21:45

REPORT COMPLETE
TYPE:  080  CREATININE MG/DL  OK?  Y
LIF/FIF?  F 03  UK?  Y

            CREATININE MG/DL  2.7*  MG/DL             07/06  09:00
            CREATININE MG/DL  2.6*  MG/DL             07/06  21:45
            CREATININE MG/DL  2.6*  MG/DL             07/07  07:45

REPORT COMPLETE
TYPE:    ALL  OK?  Y
LIF/FIF?      OK?  Y

    1116  631  PLEURAL CAV ASP          07/04  14:45
    4247  598  BLOOD CULTURE            07/07  12:15

REPORT COMPLETE
TYPE:  000  OK?  Y
LIF/FIF?  L 99  OK?  Y

            K MEQ/L           4.3  MEQ/L              07/07  07:45
            CREATININE MG/DL  2.6*  MG/DL             07/07  07:45
            BUN MG/DL          75*  MG/DL             07/07  07:45
            CO2  MEQ/L         20*  MEQ/L             07/07  07:45
            CL MEQ/L         109*  MEQ/L              07/07  07:45
            NA   MEQ/L        138  MEQ/L              07/07  07:45
```

Exhibit X C4

UNABLE TO DRAW , USER ID: 33, 15:08   10/19/76 , STATION 12

ACQ#: 2080 SXXXXX, DOLLIE MA OK? Y

        2080   010 PLAT CT 10X3 CUM   10/19 07:15

REPORT COMPLETE
HOLD T# 010 PLAT CT 10X3 CUM OK? Y
REASON: PATIENT GONE

HOLD T#

Exhibit X C6

MR#:   121212

SXXXXXX, AL A   MALE

DATE	AGE	PROBLEM	CART	PAGE	I/O
10/23/74	23	CHEST PAIN	0002	0001	O
12/23/74	23	MYOCARDIAL INFAR	0001	0001	I

REPORT COMPLETE

Exhibit X C7

MR#   121212   OK? Y   GXXXX, RALPH R   ERMA OK? Y

          0000 002   HGB   02/03 00:00
          0011 018   G6PD U/GHB/MIN   02/03 12:30
          2011 598   BLOOD CULTURE   02/03 12:15
          0008 298   DIGOXIN RIA   02/03 12:15
          0007 002   HGB   02/03 12:15
          0006 001   HEMOGRAM   02/03 12:15

REPORT COMPUTER
CANC T#: 002 HGM   OK? Y

CANC T#: 018 G6PD SCREEN   OK? Y

CANC T#: 001 HEMOGRAM OK? Y

FLOWCHART XD

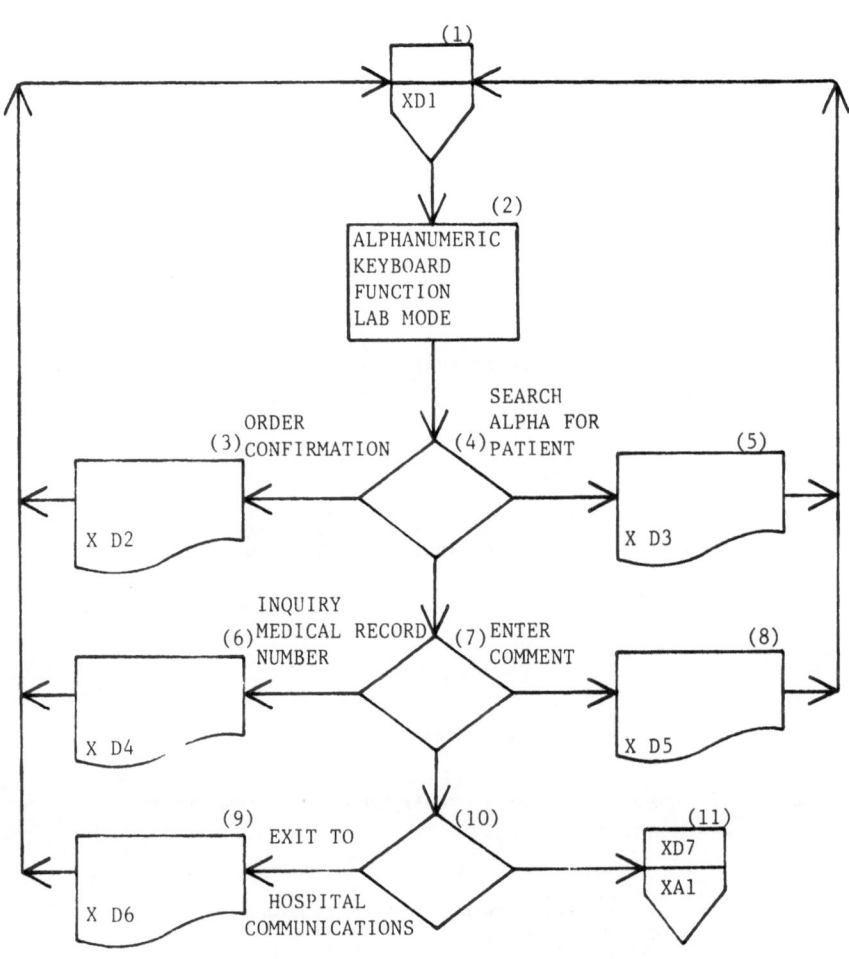

Flowchart X D

1. Off-page connector: From—location unspecified. To—operation (2).
2. The alphanumeric keyboard functions are performed in the computer room by typing in a code command for each position. Connect to operation (4).
3. See Exhibit X D2. An order confirmation gives the specimen check-in time and initiates the ordering of lab labels. Connect to operation (1).
4. Decision: A—order confirmation, connect to operation (3). B—alpha search for patient, connect to operation (5). C—proceed to next decision block.
5. See Exhibit X D3. Alpha search for a patient gives one an access to the patient's records when a medical record number is not known or is incorrect. It provides the full name, medical record number, and room number. Connect to operation (1).
6. See Exhibit X D4. An inquiry on the medical record number provides lists of all results for a specific test, all results since the last chart report plus all unfinished reports, and all unfinished tests. Connect to operation (1).
7. Decision: A—inquiry by medical record number, connect to operation (6). B—enter comment, connect to operation (8). C—proceed to next decision block.
8. See Exhibit X D5. The comment function is the mechanism for entering results for a test which is not numeric; for example, Anatomic Pathology, electrophoresis, Microbiology. Connect to operation (1).
9. An exit to hospital communications is the software access to nursing terminal operations. Connect to operation (1).
10. Decision: A—exit to hospital communications, connect to operation (9). B—proceed to operation (11).
11. Off-page connector: From—operation (11). To—Flowchart X A1.

Exhibit X D2

```
**READY
**READY
OFF-LINE
U 3238 2
ENTRY ACCEPTED
U 3240 2 11 30
ENTRY ACCEPTED
U 3247 2 11 30 07 06 77
ENTRY ACCEPTED
```

Exhibit X D3

```
MSG:
**READY
**READY
OFF-LINE
          S WXXXXXXX
WXXXXXXX, BILLY M              316111      EMRMM
WXXXXXXX, HATTIE               201095      OPCLO
WXXXXXXX, MICHAEL              201677      OPCLK
WXXXXXXX, CWAYNE A             162223      A606B
WXXXXXXX, ALFREDA              003112      OPCLO
WXXXXXXX, BURDETTE             297207      DISCH
WXXXXXXX, RALPH *              314826      H562D
WXXXXXXX, CAROLYN              204850      OPCLO
WXXXXXXX, KATHY                000000      DISCH
WXXXXXXX, MICHAEL L.           000000      DISCH
WXXXXXXX, ROULNEY D            000000      DISCH
WXXXXXXX, BOY *                000000      DISCH
```

Exhibit X   D4

```
I  31559 000
INQUIRY              315995   SXXXX, MARIE B        H461B   10/20/76
     3386  582 INDIA INK                          10/20  22:15
     3368  575 FUNGUS CULTURE                     10/20  21:00
     3367  649 MISC ROUTINE CUL                   10/20  20:45
     3366  583 AFB STAIN                          10/20  20:45
     3365  584 DIR GRAM STAIN                     10/20  20:45
     3364  598 BLOOD CULTURE                      10/20  20:45
     3347  157 IRON PROFILE                       10/20  17:30
     3347  140 PROTEIN-ELECTRO                    10/20  17:30
     3385  576 AFB CULTURE                        10/20  22:15
     3383  601 CSF CULTURE                        10/20  22:15
     3384  583 AFB STAIN                          10/20  22:15
     0179  010 PLAT CT 10X3 CUM                   10/20  00:00
     3343  603 URINE CULTURE                      10/20  00:00
     3390  598 BLOOD CULTURE                      10/20  22:45
```

Exhibit X   D5

```
C 0170 827 NO SERUM VALUE FOR CLEARANCE
ENTRY ACCEPTED
C 0170 827 !
ENTRY ACCEPTED
```

FLOWCHART XE

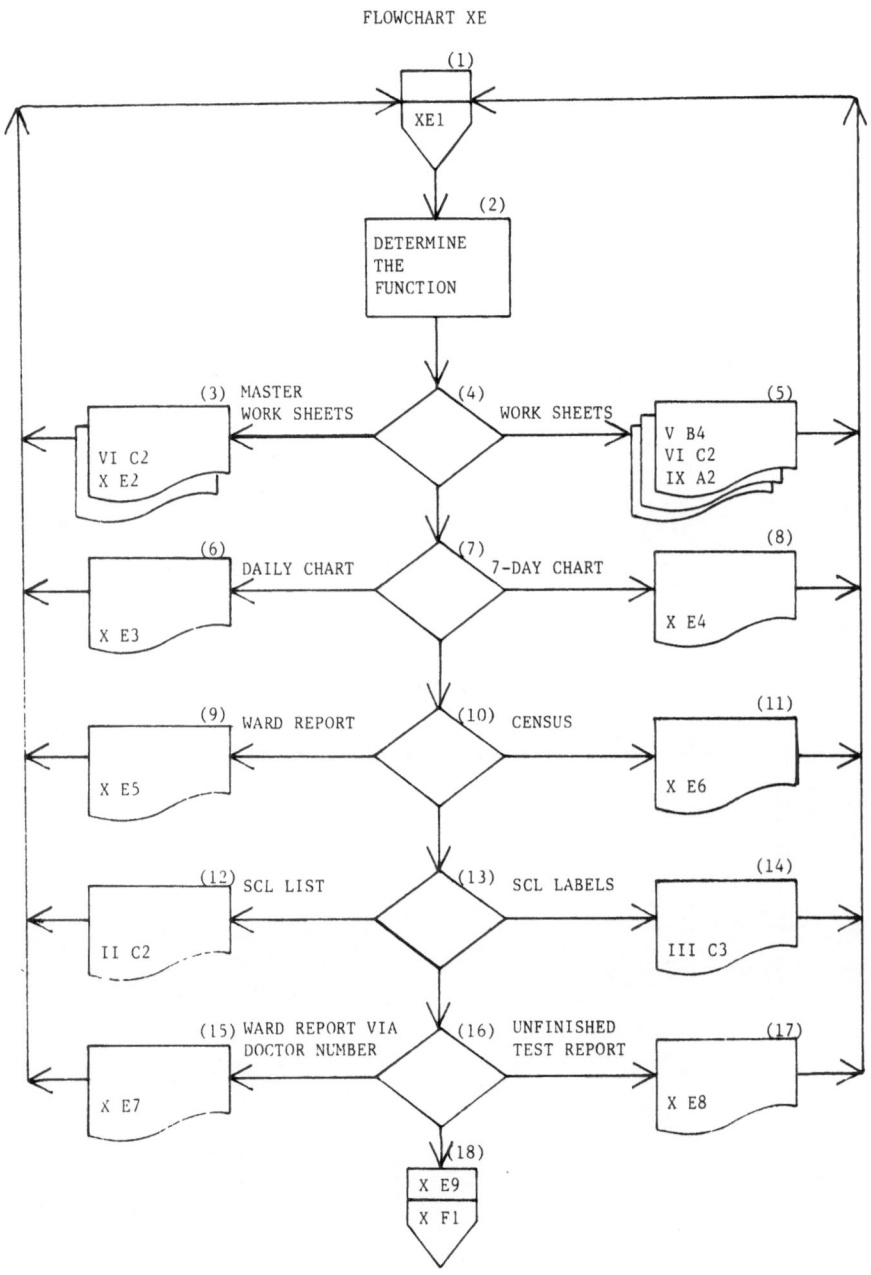

Flowchart X E

1. Off-page connector: From—location unspecified. To—operation (2).
2. The function is selected. Connect to operation (4).
3. Master work sheets. See Exhibit V1 C2 and X E2. Connect to operation (1).
4. Decision: A—master work sheets, connect to operation (3). B—work sheets, connect to operation (5). C—proceed to next decision block.
5. Work sheets. See Exhibit V B4, VI C2, and IX A2. Connect to operation (1).
6. See Exhibit X E3. A daily chart is a print-out of all the tests completed since the last seven-day chart. It contains all pertinent information on the patient and is distributed to the individual floors daily. Connect to operation (1).
7. Decision: A—daily chart, connect to operation (6). B—seven-day/final chart, connect to operation (8). C—proceed to next decision. block.
8. See Exhibit X E4. A seven-day contains all tests and results on a particular patient since the last seven-day chart. The last seven-day chart is called a final chart if the patient has been discharged from the hospital. Connect to operation (1).
9. See Exhibit X E5. The ward report shows all patients who have lab work since the last daily chart and contains room number, lab order, time of order, and all test results. Connect to operation (1).
10. Decision: A—ward report, connect to operation (9). B—census, report, connect to operation (11). C—proceed to next decision bloc.
11. See Exhibit X E6. A census report shows all patients presently in the hospital, clinics, or emergency room. A copy is sent to admissions and pharmacy. Connect to operation (1).
12. SCL list. See Exhibit III C2. Connect to operation (1).
13. Decision: SCL list, connect to operation (12). B—SCL labels, connect to operation (14). C—proceed to next decision block.
14. SCL labels. See Exhibit III C3. Connect to operation (1).
15. See Exhibit X E7. A ward report via doctor number is a listing of all patient results by doctor. Connect to operation (1).
16. Decision: A—ward report via doctor number, connect to operation (15). B—unfinished test report, connect to operation (17). C—proceed to operation (18).
17. See Exhibit X E8. An unfinished test report is a listing of all tests ordered for which results have not been entered. This is run once a day and given to the chief technologist for departmental audit. Connect to operation (1).
18. Off-page connector: From—operation (18). To—Flowchart X F1.

Exhibit X E2

```
MASTER              WORKSHEET    BLOOD BANK      06/23/76    09:32    PAGE 1

PATIENT NAME        PATIENT NUM      SPEC  TEST  IDENTIFICATION   REQ DATE


AXXXXXX, CHARLES W   A394B  294756   4021  859   065 ORDERED/AVA   07:45  06/23/76
                                     4021  858       USED/Q.AD.U.  07:45  06/23/76

HXXXXX, KATHERINE E  A345B  302948   4023  859   365 ORDERED/AVA   07:45  06/23/76
                                     4023  858       USED/Q.AD.U.  07:45  06/23/76

PXXXXX, HILDA F      A365C  495837   4024  859   365 ORDERED/AVA   07:45  06/22/76
                                     4024  858       USED/Q.AD.U.  07:54  06/22/76

JXXXX, MABEL         H455A  416911   5096  354   ANTIBODY SC       08:15  06/17/76
```

Exhibit X E3

```
SHANDS TEACHING*HOSPITAL/CLINICS              LABORATORY CHART REPORT

WARD:  3-WING              DAILY          CHART REPORT          PAGE 1

NAME:  MXXXXXX, JEANNE E                  MEDICAL RECORD #283948

ROOM:  A375A    35Y  F  00  DR:  WXXXX, E R

PROBLEM:  MORBID OBESITY


TEST            LIMITS        05/18    05/19
                             17:15    08:00
HEMATOLOGY
HEMOGRAM
    HGB   GM      12-16       16.3*
    HCT   %       34-47       49.6*
    RBC 10X6/CMM  4.20-5.20   5.74*
    WBC 10X3/CMM  4-11        9.6
    MCV   CUB MIC 79-99       86
    MCH MC MC GM  27-31       28.4
    MCHC  %       32-36       32.9
PT CONTROL SEC                         10.8
PT SEC            0-14                  10.1
PTT CONTROL SEC                         29
PTT SEC           20-40                 26
```

Exhibit X E4

SHANDS TEACHING*HOSPITAL/CLINICS   LABORATORY CHART REPORT

WARD: 7th PEDS   FINAL -- CHART REPORT   PAGE 1

NAME: JXXXXXX, MELISSA   MEDICAL RECORD   395837

ROOM: H394B 05Y   F   00   DR: FXXXX, R   07:54   17/26/76

PROBLEM: ILL

TEST		LIMITS	07/23 14:15	07/24 16:24	07/25 14:22
CHEMISTRY					
CL	MEQ/L	95-105	107*	105	106*
C02	MEQ/L	24-32	32	30	28
BUN	MG/DL	10-20	21*	30*	41*
CREA	MG/DL	0.7-1.4	1.4	1.6*	1.8*
URIC AC	MG/DL	2.5-8	6.8	8.9	7.0

Exhibit X E5

5-A WING   WARD REPORT   09/25/76   12:26   PAGE 1

A507B EXXXXX, DELORES *   MEDICAL RECORD # 485736

    URINE CULTURE   REQUEST RECEIVED   09/25/76 09:00
    URINE CULTURE   REQUEST RECEIVED   09/23/76 00:00
    URINALYSIS   REQUEST RECEIVED   09/23/76 00:00

A507A AXXXXXX, MARSHA A   MEDICAL RECORD # 847365

    DIFF   REQUEST RECEIVED   09/25/76 00:00
    HEMOGRAM   REQUEST RECEIVED   09/25/76 00:00
    MISC ROUTINE CUL   REQUEST RECEIVED   09/21/76 20:45
    MISC ROUTINE CUL   REQUEST RECEIVED   09/21/76 20:45

A514B GXXXX, JEFF E   MEDICAL RECORD # 495836

    HBS AG (AUST. AG NEG   09/23/76 17:15

A515B SXXXXXX, RICKY E   MEDICAL RECORD # 4837560

    URINE CULTURE   URINE-CLEAN CAT NO GROWTH   09/24/76 09:15
    URINE CULTURE   TEST COMPLETE   09/24/76 09:15

A516A CXXXX, JOHN   MEDICAL RECORD # 573655

    URINE CULTURE   REQUEST RECEIVED   08/28/76 16:30
    CAT TIP CULTURE   REQUEST RECEIVED   09/24/76 11:00
    BLOOD CULTURE   REQUEST RECEIVED   09/20/76 07:45

A517B TXXXXX, MARK A   MEDICAL RECORD # 583758

    MISC ROUTINE CUL   REQUEST RECEIVED   09/23/76 14:15

A518B NXXX, PAMELA C   MEDICAL RECORD # 843791

    CATH TIP CULTURE   FOLEY CATH TIP   IN SUBCULTURE   ECOL 1
    CATH TIP CULTURE   FOLEY CATH TIP   ECOL1 S   TETRACYCLINE   09/22/76
    CATH TIP CULTURE   FOLEY CATH TIP   ECOL1 S   AMPICILLIN   09/22/76
    CATH TIP CULTURE   FOLEY CATH TIP   ECOL1 S   KANAMYCIN   09/22/76
    CATH TIP CULTURE   FOLEY CATH TIP   ECOL1 S   CARBENICILLIN   09/22/76

Exhibit X E6

3-AWING	LIST CENSES	06/29/76	08:43

```
A312
306039    GXXXX, FRANK              54Y M REFLUX ESOPH      A312B
307037    BXXXXXXX, DELL L          63Y M CA RECTUM         A312A


A314
307201    MXXXX, GEORGE H           BOY M TIC               A314A
305955    AXXXX, BENNIE L           26Y M BAL HYPERTEN      A314B


ZZZZZ

A316


A320
213375    TXXXXX, BEVERLY A         18Y F NONE GIVEN        A320B


A321
271635    CXXXXXX, GEORGIA          60Y F CARC BREAST       A321A


A322
300965    TXXXXX, MAURICE           36Y M SARC-L AXILLA     A322B


A323
244660    GXXXX, SARAH A            43Y F LBP               A323A


ZZZZZ
```

Exhibit X E7

```
MEDICAL        WARD REPORT                    09/14/76        14:16      PAGE 1
DOCTOR:  SXXXXXX, CHARLES


H439D     CXXXXXXX, LUCILLE C                 MEDICAL RECORD # 263543

   CHOL    MG/DL          227  MG/DL          09/10/76  13:15
   TRIG    MG/DL           56  MG/DL          09/10/76  13:15
   CATH URINE CULT    REQUEST RECEIVED        09/14/76  12:00


H439C     EXXXXX, RUBY L                      MEDICAL RECORD # 311879

HEMOGRAM                          09/17/76  08:00
   HGB  GM          9.3*  GM                  09/14/76  08:00
   HCT  %          29.2*  PERCENT             09/14/76  08:00
   RBC  10X6/CMM   3.37*  10X6/CMM            09/14/76  08:00
   WBC  10X3/CMM    7.3   10X3/CMM            09/14/76  08:00
   MCV  CUB MIC      87   CUB MIC             09/14/76  08:00
   MCH MC MC GM    27.6   MC MC GM            09/14/76  08:00
   MCHC %          31.8*  PERCENT             09/14/76  08:00
NA MEG/L           137    MEQ/L               09/14/76  08:00
K MEG/L            5.5*   MEQ/L               09/14/76  08:00
CL MEQ/L           107*   MEQ/L               09/14/76  08:00
CO2  MEQ/L          15*   MEQ/L               09/14/76  08:00
BUN  MG/EL          53*   MG/DL               09/14/76  08:00
CREATININE MG/DL   7.4*   MG/DL               09/14/76  08:00
URIC AC  MG/DL     5.5    MG/DL               09/14/76  08:00
CALCIUM  MG/DL     8.5    MG/DL               09/14/76  08:00
PO4  MG/DL         3.5    MG/DL               09/14/76  08:00
GLUCOSE  MG/DL      92    MG/DL               09/14/76  08:00
T BIL    MG/DL     0.2    MG/DL               09/14/76  08:00
D BIL    MG/DL     0.1    MG/DL               09/14/76  08:00
TOT  LDH  IU/L     173    MIU/ML              09/14/76  08:00
SGOT     IU/L       19    IU/L                09/14/76  08:00
SGPT     IU/L        7    IU/L                09/14/76  08:00
AMYLASE  IU/L      246*   IU/L                09/14/76  08:00
   E1 ALB GM/DL    3.0*   GM/DL               09/01/76  08:15
   ALPHA-1 GM/DL   0.2    GM/DL               09/01/76  08:15
   ALPHA-2 GM/DL   0.6    GM/DL               09/01/76  08:15
   BETA    GM/DL   0.7    GM/DL               09/01/76  08:15
   GAMMA   GM/DL   1.9*   GM/DL               09/01/76  08:15
URINALYSIS BILI    NEG                        09/13/76  18:45
   SP/GR-U        1.013                       09/13/76  18:45
   PH-U           6                           09/13/76  18:45
   PROT-U QUAL    3+                          09/13/76  18:45
   GLUC-U QUAL    TRACE                       09/13/76  18:45
   KETONES-U      NEG                         09/13/76  18:45
   HGB-U          NEG                         09/13/76  18:45
   WBC-U          2-5                         09/13/76  18:45
   OTHER-U        OCC EPITH CELL              09/13/76  18:45
```

Exhibit X E8

```
UNFINISHED TEST REPORT   MICROSCOPY       10/28/76      12:58      PAGE 1

PATIENT NAME             PATIENT NUM      SPEC. TEST   IDENTIFICATION  REQ DATE

BXXXXXXX, HELEN J        H356A 138573     3252   400 URINALYSIS   14:00  10/26/76

BXXXXXXX, REBEC          H356B 947515     3262   400 URINALYSIS   14:15  10/26/76

DXXXX, IRIS M            H368A 428178     3018   400 URINALYSIS   13:00  10/25/76

LXXXXX  BOY              H342C 682965     3110   400 URINALYSIS   14:30  10/26/76

HXXXXXX, STEPH           H892B 395867     3263   400 URINALYSIS   13:00  10/26/76

MXXX, CORA M             H886C 396830     3029   400 URINALYSIS   00:00  10/25/76
```

FLOWCHART XF

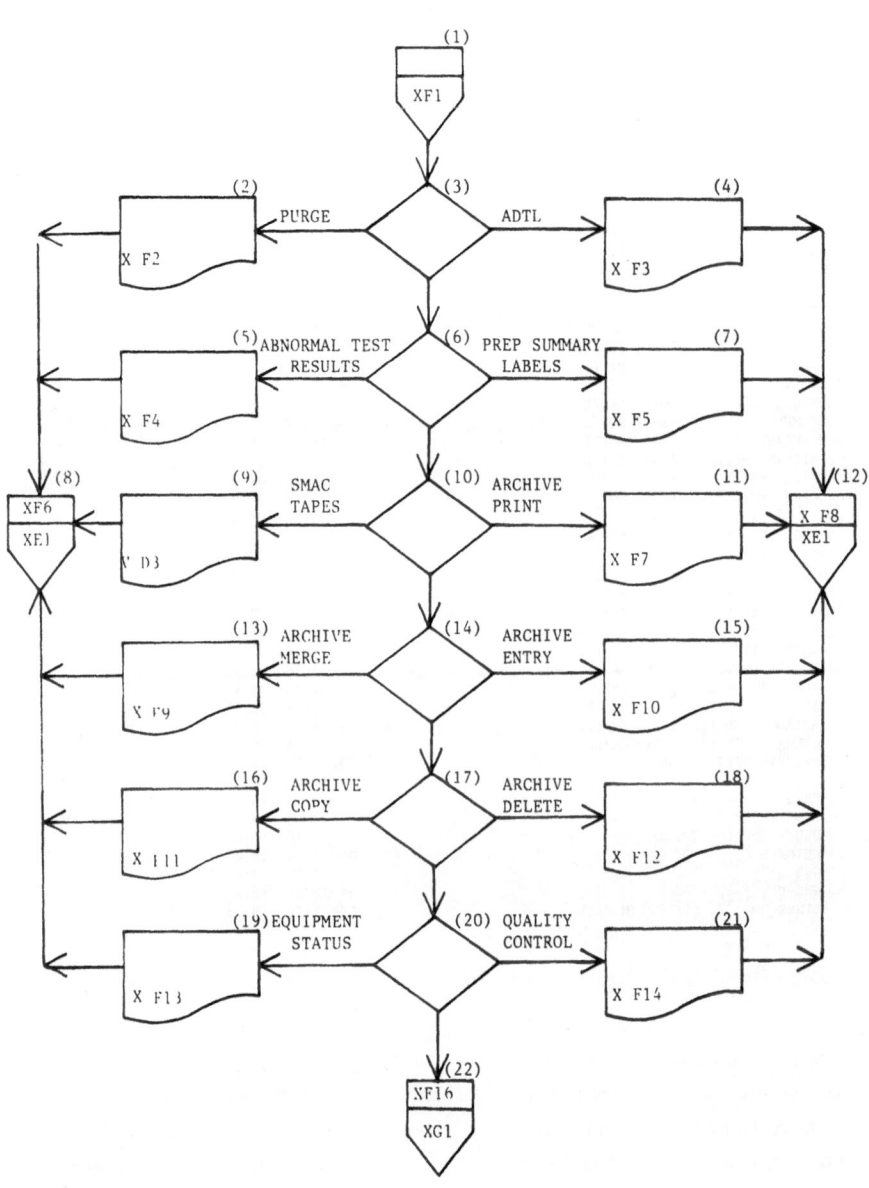

Flowchart X F

1. Off-page connector: From—location unspecified. To—operation (3).
2. See Exhibit X F2. A purge is a report of all results printed on the seven-day charts and removed from the patient's file. Results are purged if: 1. a patient has more than 126 results, 2. a patient has been inhouse for 28 days or multiples thereof, and 3. a patient has been discharged. This report is printed upon request. Connect to operation (8).
3. Decision: A—purge, connect to operation (2). B—ADTL, connect to operation (4). C—proceed to next decision block.
4. See Exhibit X F3. The ADTL is a daily report which contains all patient admissions, discharges, and transfers. This report is printed upon request. Connect to operation (12).
5. See Exhibit X F4. An abnormal test result shows data outside normal limits. Connect to operation (8).
6. Decision: A—abnormal test result, connect to operation (5). B—prep summary labels, connect to operation (7). C—proceed to next decision block.
7. See Exhibit X F5. A prep summary label tells one how much sample, in milliliters, is required to run a test. These labels are printed upon request. Connect to operation (12).
8. Off-page connector: From—operation (8). To—Flowchart X E1.
9. SMAC tapes. See Exhibit V D3. Connect to operation (8).
10. Decision: A—SMAC tape, connect to operation (9). B—archive print, connect to operation (11). C—proceed to next decision block.
11. See Exhibit X F7. Archive entries are in the permanent file. It contains such information as name, medical record number, sex, age, problem, date of admission, inpatient or outpatient status, and the cartridge and page number where the patient's charts are located. Connect to operation (12).
12. Off-page connector: From—operation (12). To—Flowchart X E1.
13. An archive merge is the mechanism for taking the temporary archive file and merging it with the permanent archive and printing an update to the permanent file on the line printer. Connect to operation (8).
14. Decision: A—archive merge, connect to operation (13). B—archive entry, connect to operation (15). C—proceed to next decision block.
15. An archive entry is a two-part procedure for entering pertinent information on a patient into the archive package. Connect to operation (12).
16. An archive copy is the new archive copy minus the last merge. It takes the backup permanent archive file and copies it to the archive permanent file. Connect to operation (8).
17. Decision: A—archive copy, connect to operation (16). B—archive delete, connect to operation (18). C—proceed to next decision block.
18. An archive delete allows a patient to be deleted from the file. Connect to operation (12).
19. Equipment status is the process whereby the line printer can be diverted to the alternate printer and the alternate printer can be diverted to the magnetic tape. Connect to operation (8).
20. Decision: A—equipment status, connect to operation (19). B—quality control, connect to operation (21). C—proceed to operation (22).
21. Quality control reports can be printed upon request. Connect to operation (12).
22. Off-page connector: From—operation (22). To—Flowchart X G1.

Exhibit X F2

PURGE RESULTS

306038   CXXXXXXX, SOPHIEA   1958720   19Y F   DISCHARG   10/10/76

```
          1   HEMOGRAM                         10/11/76  08:45
          5     WBC   10X3/CMM       18.3  10X3/CMM          10/11/76  08:45
          4     RBC   10X6/CMM       2.61  10X6/CMM          10/11/76  08:45
          2     HGB   GM              8.3  GM                10/11/76  08:45
          3     HCT   %              25.2  PERCENT           10/11/76  08:45
        997     MCV   CUB  MIC         90  CUB MIC           10/11/76  08:45
        996     MCH   MC  MC  GM     29.5  MC  MC  GM         10/11/76  08:45
        995     MCHC  %              32.9  PERCENT           10/11/76  08:45
          3     HCT   %              26.6  PERCENT           10/12/76  09:15
        642   ENDOMETRIAL CUL     ENDOMETRIUM IN SURCULTURE   HAEMOPHILUS VAGI
        642   ENDOMETRIAL CUL     TEST COMPLETE              10/10/76  16:30
        604   CATH URINE CULT     URINE-CATH  NO GROWTH                10/11/76
        604   CATH URINE CULT     TEST COMPLETE              10/11/76  12:15
```

234556   WXXXXXXXX, PAT A   00-0000   17Y F   EMERG   10/16/76

```
          1   HEMOGRAM                         10/16/76  02:45
          5     WBC   10X3/CMM        7.9  10X3/CMM          10/16/76  02:45
          4     RBC   10X6/CMM       4.18  10X6/CMM          10/16/76  02:45
          2     HGB   GM             11.7  GM                10/16/76  02:45
          3     HCT   %              35.5  PERCENT           10/16/76  02:45
        997     MCV   CUB  MIC         85  CUB MIC           10/16/76  02:45
        996     MCH   MC  MC  GM     28.0  MC  MC  GM         10/16/76  02:45
        995     MCHC  %              33.0  PERCENT           10/16/76  02:45
        444   QUAL HCG                         10/16/76  02:45
        753     SP/GR-U             1.026                    10/16/76  02:45
        754     HCG-QUAL            NEG                       10/16/76  02:45
         78     CO2  MEQ/L            26  MEQ/L              10/16/76  02:45
         77     CL  MEQ/L           105  MEQ/L              10/16/76  02:45
         76     K MEQ/L             3.8  MEQ/L              10/16/76  02:45
         75     NA  MEQ/L           143  MEQ/L              10/16/76  02:45
         79     BUN  MG/DL            9  MG/DL              10/16/76  02:45
         80     CREATININE  MG/DL  0.7  MG/DL              10/16/76  02:45
         84     GLUCOSE MG/DL       201  MG/DL              10/16/76  02:45
        130     AMYLASE    IU/L     132  IU/L               10/16/76  02:45
        591   GC CULTURE          ENDOCERVIX  CULTURE NEG    NEISSERIA GONORR
        591   GC CULTURE          TEST COMPLETE              10/16/76  03:00
```

315721   EXXXXX, SHERRY L   1960555   19Y F   DISCHARG   10/17/76

```
          3   HCT %                39.4  PERCENT            10/18/76  07:45
```

315721   SWTLLEY, MILDRED   1960830   61Y F   SURG INT   10/13/76

```
          0                        138                       10/13/76  18:15
          0                         38                       10/13/76  18:15
          0                        100                       10/13/76  18:15
          0                         29                       10/13/76  18:15
          0                         12                       10/13/76  18:15
          0                          8                       10/13/76  18:15
          0                        188                       10/13/76  18:15
```

Exhibit X F3

```
                  ADTL   REPORT        ADMIT                        07/21/76

307010   AXXXXX, SIDNEY E             1908505 H561C   00 M 19Y  SYBAVITIS L-KN
510                                   07/19/76  10:40

249962   SXXX, DWIGHT L               1908588 H561B   00 M 26Y  INFECTER OSTEO
510                                   07/19/76  10:41

268179   KXXX, LEWIS                  SS-0000 OPCLU   00 M 75Y  NOT GIVEN
794                                   07/19/76  10:43

106354   HXXXXXX, DEBBIE R            1908561 A634A   00 F 12Y  NONE GIVEN
999                                   07/19/76  10:45

308855   KXXXXXXXX, JOAN              00-0000 OPCLO   00 F 23Y  DIABETES
223                                   07/19/76  10:53

308858   KXXXXXXX, MARGUERITE         MM-0000 EMRMX   00 F 64Y  LUMPIN THROAT
657                                   07/19/76  10:54

308803   WXXXXX, RICHARD N.           00-0000 EMRMX   00 M 43Y  KIDNEY
514                                   07/19/76  10:55

308848   BXXXXXX, KATHY J             1908898 A312B   00 F 05Y  W/BT-CLS HUMERUS
510                                   07/19/76  10:56
```

Exhibit X F4

```
6-A WING              ABNORMAL RESULTS        09/04/76              PAGE 1

H360A  35Y  F  OODXXXXXX, JUDY M.          ILL          MEDICAL RECOR 451783

        ALBUMIN GM/DL       3.5  GM/DL
        ALBUMIN GM/DL       3.5  GM/DL
        ALK PHOS  IU/L       40  IU/L
        TOT LDH  IU/L        85  MIU/ML
        SGOT IU/L            51  IU/L


A618A  15Y  M  OOBXXXXXX, BARNEY JR.       ORT          MEDICAL RECOR 476931

        BUN   MG/DL          36 MG/DL
        SGPT  IU/L          140 IU/L
        CPK   MIU/ML         86 MIU/ML


H359C  03D  M  OO   BOY                    NEWBORN      MEDICAL RECOR 621893

        BUN MG/DL            92  MG/DL
        CREA MG/DL          9.3  MG/DL


H655A  69Y  F  OOFXXXXXX, JULIA, M.        ORT          MEDICAL RECOR 402861

        BUN    MG/DL          8  MG/DL
        URIC AD MG/DL       1.6  MG/DL


H658B  52Y  M  OOBXXXXXX, HOWARD C.        ILL          MEDICAL RECOR 692714

        NA    MEQ/L         128  MEQ/L
```

Exhibit X F5

			H271A	FXXXXXXXX, DAVID	395714	
3168	3168	3168	GREEN	152 FIBRINO MG/DL	1.OCC PLASMA	3168
3168	3168	3168	GRAY	84 GLUCOSE MG/DL	0.6CC BLOOD	3168
			OB/GYN	PREPARATION SUMMARY	08/26/75	
			H321B	MXXXXX, BONNIE	391137	
3241	3241	3241	RED-7	77 CL MEQ/L	0.6CC BLOOD	3241
3241	3241	3241	RED-7	78 CO2 MEQ/L	0.6CC BLOOD	3241
3241	3241	3241	RED-7	79 BUN MG/DL	0.6CC BLOOD	3241

Exhibit X F7

015284 WXXXXXXXX, BERTHA M   F   55   0001   0039   12/05/75   I
MALIG. DEGURERAT

016395 MXXXXXXX, LUELLA *   F   32   0001   0024   11/27/75   I
FX HYGOID BONE

016395 MXXXXXXX, LUELLA *   F   32   0001   0022   11/26/75   I
FX HYBOID/BONE

016395 MXXXXXXX, LUELLA *   F   32   0001   0020   11/25/75   I
FX HYGOID/BONE

016739 WXXXXXXXX, CINDY *   F   15   0002   1995   12/21/75   I
IUP

018611 KXXXXX, BILLYRAY *   M   15   0001   0026   12/02/75   I
SHUNT MALFORMATI

021498 CXXXXX, CORA *   F   30   0001   0051   12/09/75   I
MIGRANES

023885 CXXXXXXX, DAVID W   M   14   0002   2036   12/22/75   I
GAP OBSTRUCTION

024668 TXXXX, CAROLYN *   F   34   0003   0248   12/04/75   I
PEL/MAS POSS/AB

024391 MXXXXX, DILLON *   M   44   0001   0047   12/05/75   I
CH SINUSITIS

028534 FXXXX, MARY N   F   50   0001   2071   12/06/75   I
S/P OBS BYPASS

028585 FXXXXXX, DOROTHY F   F   63   0002   2039   12/21/75   I
NOT KNOWN

028764 WXXX, LAWRENCE WALDO   M   45   0001   0045   12/03/75   I
BASTRITIS

029084 FXXXXXX, CLANZEL V   F   39   0002   2002   12/21/75   I
SEVERE DYSPLASIA

029749 TXXXXX, DOSHIE B   F   58   0002   1781   12/20/75   I
CELLULITUS

032827 JXXXX, MARTHA N   F   21   0001   0062   11/22/75   I
IUP

033747 AXXXXXX, WOODROW W   M   63   0002   2049   12/21/75   I
CORNEAL ULCER

035676 HXXXXX, JOHN B   M   51   0001   2078   12/03/75   I
ILL

FLOWCHART XG

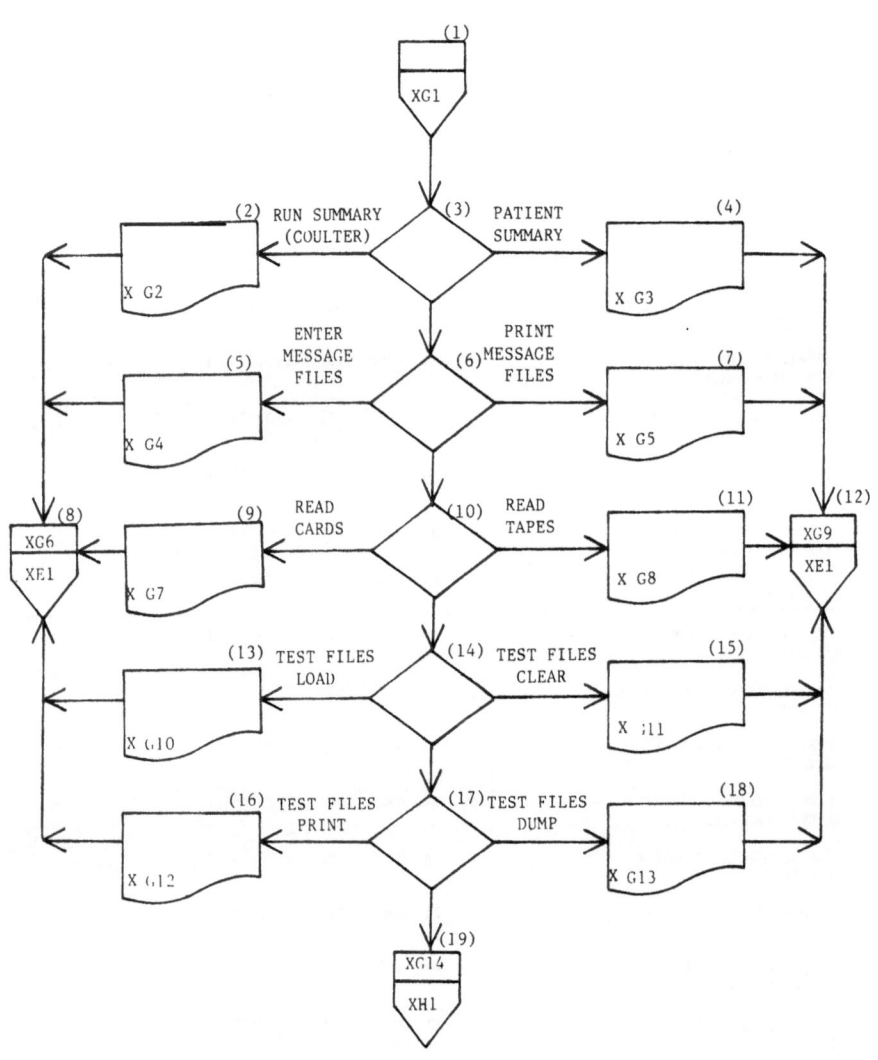

Flowchart X G

1. Off-page connector: From—location unspecified. To—operation (3).
2. See Exhibit X G2. A run summary is a report which gives a listing of all tests with results, by specimen number, which were run on the Coulter. This is printed upon request. Connect to operation (8).
3. Decision: A—run summary, connect to operation (2). B—patient summary, connect to operation (4). C—proceed to next decision block.
4. See Exhibit X G3. A patient summary is a complete patient laboratory chart. This report is printed upon request. Connect to operation (12).
5. Enter message files enables one to change a message within the file. Connect to operation (8).
6. Decision: A—enter message file, connect to operation (5). B—print message file, connect to operation (7). C—procees to next decision block.
7. The message file is a list of standard messages the machine uses for output. This is printed upon request. Connect to operation (12).
8. Off-page connector: From—operation (8). To—Flowchart X E1.
9. Read cards enables one to read cards through the mark sense reader. Connect to operation (8).
10. Decision: A—read cards, connect to operation (9). B—read tapes, connect to operation (11). C—proceed to next decision block.
11. Read tapes enables one to read magnetic tapes. Connect to operation (12).
12. Off-page connector: From—operation (12). To—Flowchart X E1.
13. Load test files from cards or magnetic tape. Connect to operation (8).
14. Decision: A—load test file, connect to operation (13). B—clear test files, connect to operation (15). C—proceed to next decision block.
15. Clear test files function. Connect to operation (12).
16. Test files may be printed out in a special format—used mainly for reference. Connect to operation (8).
17. Decision: A—test files print, connect to operation (16). B—test file dump, connect to operation (18). C—proceed to operation (19).
18. Dump test files prints the file in numeric code the way the machine uses the cards—coded values are used instead of messages. Connect to operation (12).
19. Off-page connector: From—operation (19). To—Flowchart X H1.

Exhibit X G2

RUN SUMMARY   MG

RUN: 1   08:47   11/04/76   TECH

CUP	SPEC.	TP	ALB	CA	CHOL	GLU	BUN	URIC	CRT	BILI	ALK-P	LDH	SGOT
1	EMPT	0.0	0.0		0	0	0	0	0.0	0	0.0	0	0.0
2	EMPT	0.0	0.0		0	0	0	0	0.0	0	0.0	0	0.0
3	EMPT	0.0	0.0		0	0	0	0	0.0	0	0.0	0	0.0
4	EMPT	0.0	0.0		0	0	0	0	0.0	0	0.0	0	0.0
5	EMPT	2.4	3.6		93	10	22	16	4.5	0	3.5	88	5.0
6	0004	6.6	21.2		48	42	0	0	0.0	0	0.0	0	0.0
7	EMPT	5.1	6.4		111	0	45	53	0.1	0	8.3	86	6.3
8	0004	0.5	0.0		100	193	0	0	0.0	0	0.0	0	0.0
9	0168	4.6	3.8		101	33	7	9	6.8	0	2.7	30	6.9
10	0002	9.9	33.0		93	135	0	0	0.0	0	0.0	0	0.0
11	0172	4.0	4.0		104	20	7	4	3.2	0	4.9	61	6.9
12	0003	5.1	46.9		42	18	0	0	0.0	0	0.0	0	0.0
13	0169	2.9	7.2		85	9	51	66	0.0	0	8.2	41	6.7
14	EMPT	0.0	0.0		0	74	0	0	0.0	0	0.0	0	0.0
15	0171	2.9	7.2		85	9	51	66	0.0	0	8.2	41	6.7
16	EMPT	0.0	0.0		0	74	0	0	0.0	0	0.0	0	0.0
17	0170	4.2	3.7		106	24	11	8	5.1	0	2.7	64	6.7
18	0003	3.0	41.4		62	86	0	0	0.0	0	0.0	0	0.0
19	0177	4.0	3.6		103	26	13	6	2.9	0	4.1	36	5.8
20	0003	8.3	16.4		24	19	0	0	0.0	0	0.0	0	0.0
21	0179	3.9	4.0		103	20	11	6	6.1	0	4.9	10	7.4
22	0002	6.5	35.0		38	7	0	0	0.0	0	0.0	0	0.0
23	0166	4.5	5.2		86	30	145	0	3.5	0	5.1	74	7.0
24	0036	4.8	0.0		93	69	0	0	0.0	0	0.0	0	0.0
25	0187	3.9	4.0		96	30	6	3	4.1	0	4.2	27	6.3
26	0003	9.9	0.0		34	12	0	0	0.0	0	0.0	0	0.0
27	0190	3.4	3.3		95	30	14	6	6.5	0	1.6	90	5.6
28	0019	7.6	29.8		61	20	0	0	0.0	0	0.0	0	0.0
29	0192	5.5	7.5		110	20	24	17	9.0	0	3.4	97	7.9
30	0004	0.6	27.6		35	9	0	0	0.0	0	0.0	0	0.0
31	3246	4.2	4.0		96	30	14	7	6.2	0	4.2	08	7.8
32	0002	7.4	25.9		110	115	0	0	0.0	0	0.0	0	0.0
33	3054	4.2	3.9		100	29	25	9	3.8	0	3.6	90	7.1
34	0002	4.4	13.2		29	24	0	0	0.0	0	0.0	0	0.0
35	EMPT	2.6	3.7		94	11	22	16	4.6	0	3.5	99	5.1
36	0004	6.8	21.3		50	45	0	0	0.0	0	0.0	0	0.0
37	EMPT	5.2	6.6		111	0	45	53	0.2	0	8.2	95	6.3
38	0004	0.8	49.3		100	195	0	0	0.0	0	0.0	0	0.0
39	EMPT	0.0	0.0		0	0	0	0	0.0	0	0.0	0	0.0
40	EMPT	0.0	0.0		0	0	0	0	0.0	0	0.0	0	0.0
AV		5.1	16.8		78	46	29	17	6.1	0	4.4	20	6.8

Exhibit X G3

Patient Summary

SHANDS TEACHING*HOSPITAL/CLINICS   LABORATORY CHART REPORT

WARD: MEDICAL   7 DAY   CHART REPORT   PAGE 1

NAME: WALDON, ROSE L   MEDICAL RECORD #187434

ROOM: H480A   66Y F 00   DR: KHAKOO, RASHIDA   08:50   11/04/76

PROBLEM: UGI BLEEDER

TEST		LIMITS	11/01 17:45	11/01 19:00	11/01 22:30	11/02 07:45	11/03 07:30
HEMATOLOGY							
HEMOGRAM							
HGB	GM	12-16	5.1*	4.3*	10.3*	11.0*	11.5*
HCT	%	37-47	17.6*	15.2*	29.7*	33.3*	34.9*
RBC	10X6/CMM	4.20-5.20	2.18*	1.88*	3.57*	3.97*	4.15*
WBC	10X3/CMM	4-11	19.2*	16.9*	23.4*	18.8*	15.1*
MCV	CUB MIC	79-99	81	81	83	84	84
MCH	MC MC GM	27-31	23.4*	22.9*	28.9	27.7	27.7
MCHC	%	32-36	29.0	28.3	34.7	33.0	33.0
DIFF-POLY		50-75	67				67
BANDS	%	0-7	7				3
LYMPHS	%	25-45	23				25
MONDS	%	0-10	3				5
NRBC	%		5				

MORPHOLOGY			
	11/01	17:45	OVALOCYTES
	11/01	17:45	MOD MICRO
	11/01	17:45	MOD HYPO
	11/01	17:45	MKD ANISO
	11/01	17:45	PLAT NORM
	11/03	07:30	MOD ANISO
	11/03	07:30	MOD POIK
	11/03	07:30	PLAT NORM
	11/03	07:30	MOD POLY
	11/03	07:30	MOD MACRO
	11/03	07:30	OVALOCYTES
	11/03	07:30	TEAR DROP CELLS
	11/03	07:30	TARGET CELLS

TEST	LIMITS			
PT CONTROL SEC		10.7		
PT SEC	0-14	11/01 17:45		SCLOTTED FLOOR CALLED
		12.4		
PTT CONTRL SEC		32		
PTT SEC	20-40	11/01 17:45		SCLOTTED FLOOR CALLED
		28		
TT CONTROL SEC		15.8		
TT SEC	10-25	10.8		
PLAT CT 10X3 CUM	140-440		495.0	

FLOWCHART XH

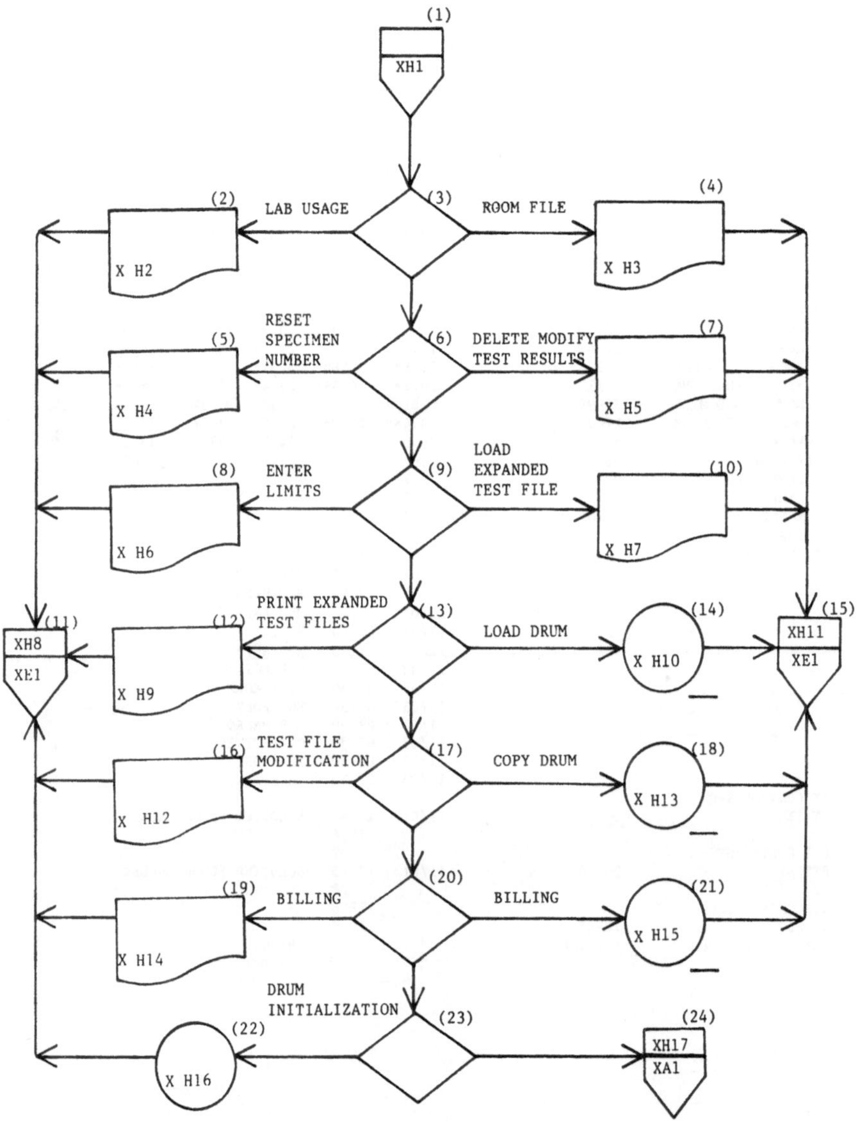

(1)
XH1

(2) LAB USAGE (3) ROOM FILE (4)
X H2   X H3

(5) RESET (6) DELETE MODIFY (7)
SPECIMEN   TEST RESULTS
NUMBER
X H4   X H5

(8) ENTER (9) LOAD (10)
LIMITS   EXPANDED
TEST FILE
X H6   X H7

(11) PRINT EXPANDED (13) LOAD DRUM (14) (15)
XH8   (12) TEST FILES   XH11
XE1   X H10   XE1
X H9

(16) TEST FILE (17) COPY DRUM (18)
MODIFICATION
X H12   X H13

(19) BILLING (20) BILLING (21)
X H14   X H15

DRUM
INITIALIZATION (23) (24)
(22)   XH17
X H16   XA1

Flowchart X H

1.   Off-page connector: From—location unspecified. To—operation (3).

2.   See Exhibit X H2. The lab usage report gives all tests requested grouped by eight different cost centers by lab. This report is printed upon request. Connect to operation (11).

3.   Decision: A—lab usage, connect to operation (2). B—room file, connect to operation (4). C—proceed to next decision block.

4.   See Exhibit X H3. The room file report gives a listing of all the wards in the hospital with rooms for the appropriate ward. This report is printed upon request. Connect to operation (15).

5.   The specimen number is reset every day. Connect to operation (11).

6.   Decision: A—reset specimen number, connect to operation (5). B—delete, modify test results, connect to operation (7). C—proceed to next decision block.

7.   Delete, modify test results is the mechanism for deleting or modifying test results via medical record number once results have been entered and verified. Connect to operation (15).

8.   Enter limits allows the limits for a test to be changed; for example, normal/upper/lower limits, normal age/sex limits. Connect to operation (11).

9.   Decision: A—enter limits, connect to operation (8). B—load expanded test file, connect to operation (10). C—proceed to next decision block.

10.   Load expanded test file reads the Hollerith cards into the proper location in the file structure. Connect to operation (15).

11.   Off-page connector: From—operation (11). To—Flowchart X E1.

12.   Print expanded test file shows the English translations. Connect to operation (11).

13.   Decision: A—print expanded test file, connect to operation (12). B—load drum, connect to operation (14). C—proceed to next decision block.

14.   Load drum takes the previous copy of magnetic tape and puts the information in the drum. Connect to operation (15).

15.   Off-page connector: From—operation (15). To—Flowchart X E1.

16.   Test file modification allows one to change the ten parameters of a test (although they are not changeable in the master and subtests). Connect to operation (11).

17.   Decision: A—test file modification, connect to operation (16). B—copy drum, connect to operation (18). C—proceed to next decision block.

18.   Copy drum puts the system copy to magnetic tape. Connect to operation (15).

19.   Billing is printed of all patient billing information since the last billing report. Connect to operation (11).

20.   Decision: A—billing, connect to operation (19). B—billing tape, connect to operation (21). C—proceed to next decision block.

21.   A billing tape is made which contains all the patient billing information since the last billing tape (usually one per day). Connect to operation (15).

22.   Drum initialization is the process which zeros out all patient files not affecting the programs and reference file. Connect to operation (11).

23.   Decision: A—drum initialization, connect to operation (22). B—proceed to operation (24).

24.   Off-page connector: From—operation (24). To—Flowchart X A1.

Exhibit X H2

LAB USAGE REPORT   CHEMISTRY   11/04/76

TEST NAME	OUT/P	PEDS	SURGE	ICU/R	MEDIC	OB/GY	NURSE	PSYCH	CA	TOTAL
ADLT LYTS BU	145	213	906	105	494	121	20	83	6.0	12522
NA MEQ/L	9	3	60	31	12	8	10	6	1.0	139
K MEQ/L	31	4	82	37	15	9	9	6	1.0	193
CL MEQ/L	7	2	52	13	11	8	10	6	1.0	109
CO2 MEQ/L	9	0	46	14	10	8	9	6	1.0	102
BUN MG/DL	94	8	74	23	14	26	7	15	1.0	261
CREATININE M	90	5	32	23	13	8	7	6	1.0	184
URIC AC MG/D	67	16	30	60	55	7	3	30	1.0	268
CALCIUM MG/D	102	56	98	200	267	6	4	23	1.0	756
PO4 MG/DL	63	14	30	118	83	4	2	14	1.0	328
GLUCOSE MG/L	145	94	332	78	243	264	9	54	1.0	1219
T PROT GM/D	43	7	88	149	60	53	0	14	1.0	414
ALBUMIN GM/D	58	10	82	143	63	49	1	16	1.0	422
CHOL MG/DL	30	3	7	68	39	1	1	3	1.0	152
TRIG MG/DL	24	3	7	66	33	1	1	3	1.0	138
T BIL MG/D	85	11	87	286	67	13	7	24	1.0	580
D BIL MG/D	44	4	81	211	56	11	3	21	1.0	431
ALK PHOS	129	12	97	109	90	23	7	29	1.0	496
TOT LDH IU/L	53	6	113	92	83	13	6	16	1.0	382
SGOT IU/L	159	23	124	143	125	27	16	45	1.0	662
SGPT IU/L	141	7	79	126	77	22	8	25	1.0	485
PED LYTE,BUN	0	19	15	479	3	0	0	6	6.0	3132
NA MEQ/	0	0	0	17	0	0	0	0	3.0	51
K MEQ/	0	0	2	21	0	0	0	0	3.0	69
CL MEQ/	0	0	0	8	0	0	0	0	4.0	32
CO2 MEQ/	0	0	0	7	0	0	0	0	4.0	28
BUN MG/D	0	0	0	11	0	0	0	0	4.0	44
PEDS CREATIN	0	0	0	10	0	0	0	0	4.0	40
OSMOLALITY	0	1	44	7	16	2	0	0	10.0	700
MG MG/D	24	5	27	31	63	7	0	9	13.0	2158
CALCITONIN	1	0	0	0	0	0	0	0	6.0	6
PEDGLUC MG/D	0	10	0	66	3	0	0	0	4.0	316
2HR-PC MG/DL	50	2	5	1	5	34	0	0	4.0	388
3-HOUR-GTT	17	0	0	2	3	0	0	2	20.0	480
5-HOUR-GTT	1	0	0	0	1	0	1	5	28.0	224
RAPID IV GTT	0	0	0	0	0	0	0	5	28.0	140
ACETONE MG/D	2	8	8	1	7	1	0	2	10.0	290
ACID PHOS IU	13	1	12	0	11	1	1	6	4.0	180
AMYLASE IU	40	93	57	21	130	1	1	10	22.0	7766
CEPULO MG/D	2	0	0	1	3	0	0	0	19.0	114
COPPER MCG/D	2	0	0	1	1	0	0	0	6.0	24
R-G6PD U/GHB	1	0	0	1	0	0	0	0	10.0	20
L AMIN PEP I	6	0	0	5	19	0	0	2	22.0	704
LIPO-ELECTRO	2	0	0	1	7	0	0	6	26.0	416
PROTEIN-ELEC	26	1	4	3	48	4	0	7	15.0	1395
ALCOHOL MG/D	1	24	0	0	0	1	0	0	49.0	1274
BARB MG/D	0	7	0	0	0	0	0	0	44.0	308
LEAD MCG/DL	2	0	2	1	2	0	0	0	6.0	42
SALICY MG/D	15	8	0	0	1	0	2	2	12.0	336
AMMONIA MCG/	0	0	1	12	1	1	0	0	39.0	585
BROMIDE MG	0	0	0	0	2	0	1	0	15.0	45
BSP % RE	1	0	2	0	6	0	0	7	11.0	176
CAROT MCG/D	7	0	0	7	23	0	0	0	8.0	296
LACTIC AC M	0	0	1	1	0	0	0	0	27.0	54
FIBRINO MG/D	1	0	3	1	0	6	0	0	28.0	308
PL HGB MG/D	0	0	1	0	5	0	0	0	15.0	90

Exhibit X H3

Room File

```
01 OR/REC R 2 051
   H225
02 3-AWING  7  005
   WF03     A300    A301    A302    A303
   ZZZZ     A309    A310    A311    A312
   A314     ZZZZ    A316    A320    A321
   A322     A323    ZZZZ    A324    A325
   A326     A327    A328    ZZZZ    A329
   A330     A331    A332
03 LABOR RM 5  025
   WF02     3-LR    3PAS    ZZZZ
04 OB/GYN   5  007
   WF04     H339    H341    H343    H345
   ZZZZ     H347    H349    H360    H362
   H363     ZZZZ    H365    H366    H367
   H378     H380    ZZZZ    H381    H382
   H383     H384    H385    ZZZZ    H387
   ZZZZ     ZZZZ    ZZZZ    ZZZZ    ZZZZ
   H374
05 NURSERY  3  063
   H359
06 PRETMIE  3  039
   H375
07 MEDICAL  4  007
   WF07     A406    A409    A415    A417
   ZZZZ     A418    A419    A421    H435
   H439     ZZZZ    H441    H445    H449
   H451     H453    ZZZZ    H459    H460
   H462     H464    H470    ZZZZ    H473
   H477     H478    H479    H480    ZZZZ
   H481     H482    H483    H484    H485
   ZZZZ     H487    APAS
08 ICU/CCU  4  011
   WF08     H461    H465    ZZZZ    ZZZZ

09 CRC/RENL 4  015
   WF09     A414    A416    A423    A424
   ZZZZ     A426    A429    A431    A433
   A434     ZZZZ    APAS
10 OPTHAMOL 2  005
   WF10     A517    A519    A521    A522
   ZZZZ     A524    A526    A527    A528
   A529     ZZZZ    A530    A531    A532
   A533     A534    ZZZZ    A535
11 SURG/SPL 2  008
   WF11     H535    H539    H541    H545
   ZZZZ     H549    H551    H553    H559
   H560     ZZZZ    H561    H562    H563
   H564     H565    ZZZZ    H573    H577
   H578     H579    H580    ZZZZ    H581
   H582     H583    H584    H585    ZZZZ
   H587     5PAS    ZZZZ    ZZZZ    ZZZZ
   H574
12 SURG INT 2  013
   H660     H661    H665    ZZZZ
13 SURGICAL 2  009
   WF13     H635    H639    H641    H645
   ZZZZ     H649    H651    H653    H673
   H677     ZZZZ    H678    H679    H680
```

APPENDIX *IV*

The Shands System Files

INTRODUCTION

The construction of a laboratory communication system requires an extensive series of files. These data repositories are used by a host of programs which perform the services required. Because of the extensive nature of these files, only representative samples can be shown.

MASTER TEST FILES

The master laboratory test file is the core reference area and lists all tests the laboratory performs. In this file are included: subtests (if any), normal limits (age and sex if applicable), reject limits, sample types needed for patient service, type of blood, and the number of tubes required.

Master test file description (reading from right to left) for coding
1.   Internal test number or physical position of test within test file
HEMOGRAM   Test name
001   External test number—test number for request and result entry

NLLM:0000	Normal lower limit
NULM:0000	Normal upper limit
	4 digit decimal place predefined
1 PURPLE	1: number of specimen tubes required (1/4 tube can be drawn; system will calculate and print to the nearest whole tube); PURPLE: blood-tube type
000	CAP workload factor
RLLM:0000	Reject lower limit
RULM:0000	Reject upper limit
	Age/sex limits take priority; if not coded, then the program goes to the singular normal range. If the result is outside normal limits, it will be starred (*). If there is a reject limit revealed, the machine will not accept the result, but will print "result reject." Other: if the sample is not blood, then it is listed as other.
998	External test numbers for subtest of a master test
INDICES	
CALCS	Name for the subtest of a master test
Internal Test 3.	
	Age/sex pointers for age/sex limits are correlated to establish the table for hospital laboratory work. The age and sex of the patient is determined from the patient file, the program inspects Table 3 for pointers to the limit pointer file. The limit-pointer file references the corresponding actual limit file for an internal test number.
	The limit pointer file reads from left to right, starting with age category 00 (limit, 48) and incrementing by one for the next column.
GM	Reporting units

TEST FILES

06/30/78		HEMATOLOGY		Page: 01
1. Hemogram	001 NLLM:0000	NULM:0000		1 PURPLE
	RLLM:0000	RULM:0000		000
998	INDICES CALC			
002	HGB GM			
003	HCT %			
004	RBC 10X6/CMM			
005	WBC 10X3/CMM			
2. Coulter-S	707 NLLM:0000	NULM:0000		000
	RLLM:0000	RULM:0000		
005	WBC 10X3/CMM			
004	RBC 10X6/CMM			
002	HGB GM			
003	HCT %			
998	INDICES CALC			

3. HGB GM   002 NLLM:000.0   NULM:000.0 GM   1 PURPLE
                        RLLM:000.0   RULM:000.0   000

    LIMIT PNTS: LIMITS

00:	48	48	48	50		48	020.0	016.0
04:	50	50	50	50		50	016.0	012.0
08:	52	52	52	52		52	018.0	014.0
12:	52	52	50	50		54	000.0	000.0
16:	48	48	48	50		56	000.0	000.0
20:	50	50	50	50		58	000.0	000.0
24:	50	50	50	50		60	000.0	000.0
28:	50	50	50	50		62	000.0	000.0

4. HCT %   003 NLLM:000.0   NULM:000.0 Percent 1 PURPLE
                        RLLM:000.0   RULM:000.0   000

    LIMITS PNTS: LIMITS

00:	48	48	48	50		48	062.0	052.0
04:	50	50	50	50		50	047.0	037.0
08:	52	52	52	52		52	052.0	042.0
12:	52	52	50	50		54	000.0	000.0
16:	48	48	48	50		56	000.0	000.0
20:	50	50	50	50		58	000.0	000.0
24:	50	50	50	50		60	000.0	000.0
28:	50	50	50	50		62	000.0	000.0

5. RBC 10X6/CMM 004 NLLM:00.00   NULM:00.00 10X6/ 1 PURPLE
                        RLLM:00.00   RULM:00.00 CMM   000

    LIMIT PNTS: LIMITS

00:	48	48	48	50		48	06.50	05.20
04:	50	50	50	50		50	05.20	04.20
08:	52	52	52	52		52	06.20	04.50
12:	52	52	50	50		54	00.00	00.00

EXPANDED TEST FILES

The expanding test files provide additional information for specimen processing and floor communication. Each is an exact match, test for test, with the master test files.

Provided expanded test file description (reading from right to left)

HEMOGRAM	Test name
001	Master test file number
TERMINAL 00	Designated lab terminal that will receive the request and the message from the floors
CAP:	College of American Pathology work load units (four digit number with one decimal point)
VERIFY:	A means by which a specimen number is assigned; if YES, the system will always assign a specimen number at the time of order; everything other than a blood bank order will have a YES if NO, a specimen number is only assigned if the test is ordered expedite or stat

ØLL—Not operational
ØUL—Not operational

VOL: The amount of sample required to perform the test, represented in milliliters

TYPE: Type of sample needed for test; the system will accept 10 different sample types, which are listed in the message file, e.g., BLOOD

LABELS: Number of prep summary labels required for lab work, set up in multiples of three minilabels

ROUTN: The user receives a message when ordering a routine or expedite procedure. This is restricted to a 72 character message or nine eight-character segments

STAT: The user receives a message when ordering a stat test. This is restricted to a 72 character message or nine eight-character specimens,
               e.g., *U DO COLLECTION: 5ML VER TUBE RQ: DELSTAT LAB H400*
               131 132   133 134   135 136 0 0 0

EXPANDED TEST FILES

08/30/76   HEMATOLOGY   Page: 1
1. Hemogram   001   Terminal 00   CAP: 5.0   Verify: NO
    QQL:00   QUL:00   VOL:1.0   Type: Blood   Labels: 0
ROUTN:
    0   0   0   0   0   0   0   0   0   0
STAT:
U do collection: 5ml Ver tube RQ/Delstat LAB H400
    131   132   133   134   135   136   0   0   0   0
2. Coulter-S   707   Terminal 00   CAP: 0.0   Verify: NO
    QQL:00   QUL:00   VOL:1.0   Type: Plasma Labels: 0
ROUTN:
Invalid order#: Press*No*Recheck order form
    112   113   114   161   162   163   0   0   0   0
STAT:
Invalid order#: Press*No*Recheck order form
    112   113   114   161   162   163   0   0   0   0
3. HGB GM   002   Terminal 00   CAP: 5.0   Verify: NO
    QLL:00   QUL:00   VOL:1.0   Type: Blood   Labels: 0
    0   0   0   0   0   0   0   0   0   0
STAT:
U do collection: 5ml Ver tube RQ:Delstat LAB H400
    131   132   133   134   135   136   0   0   0   0
4. HCT %   003   Terminal 00   CAP: 3.0   Verify: NO
    QQL:00   QUL:00   Vol:1.0   Type: Blood   Labels: 0
ROUTN:
    0   0   0   0   0   0   0   0   0   0

STAT:
U do collection: 5ml Ver tube RQ: Delstat LAB H400
  131   132   133   134   135   136   0   0   0   0
5. RBC 10X5/CMM 004 Terminal 00   CAP: 15.0   Verify: NO
    QQL:00   QUL:00   VOL:1.0   Type: Blood   Labels: 0
ROUTN:
   0   0   0   0   0   0   0   0   0   0
STAT:
U do collection: 5ml Ver tube RQ: Delstat LAB H400
  131   132   133   134   135   136   0   0   0   0

MESSAGE FILE

The message file contains standard words the machine uses to output information. Without listing all data, the following areas are covered:

1. Doctor number and names'
2. Interactive messages
3. Messages which correspond to particular numbers in the expanded test file
4. Predetermined messages for standard program use
5. Terminal messages
6. Test names
7. Standard message for each lab
8. Test units
9. Ward names
10. Hospital service names
11. Report messages

ROOM FILE

The room file is a list of all rooms and expansion space by ward.

The following is an explanation of the characters and numbers used in the file—reading from left to right by major header.

Room file description:
01	Designates ward number
OR/REC R	Denotes ward name that will be printed on reports
2	Service code—there are a total of eight cost centers within the hospital
051	Maximum number of patients per room

H225	Specific room number(s) allowed
WF03	Ward file coding for calling a census report for the entire ward
ZZZ	Spare room numbers inserted for expansion

ROOM FILE

01 OR/REC R 2 051
    H225

02 3-AWing 7 005

WF03	A300	A301	A302	A303
ZZZZ	A309	A310	A311	A312
A314	ZZZZ	A316	A320	A321
A322	A323	ZZZZ	A324	A325
A326	A327	A328	ZZZZ	A329
A330	A331	A332		

03 Labor RM 5 025

WF02	3–LR	3PAS	ZZZZ

04 Ob/Gyn 5 007

WF04	H339	H341	H343	H345
ZZZZ	H347	H349	H360	H362
H363	ZZZZ	H365	H366	H367
H378	H380	ZZZZ	H381	H382
H383	H384	H385	ZZZZ	H387
ZZZZ	ZZZZ	ZZZZ	ZZZZ	ZZZZ
H374				

05 Nursery 3 063
    H359

06 Preemie 3 039
    H375

07 Medical 4 007

WF07	A406	A409	A415	A417
ZZZZ	A418	A419	A421	H435
H439	ZZZZ	H441	H445	H449
H451	H453	ZZZZ	H459	H460
H462	H464	H470	ZZZZ	H473
H477	H478	H479	H480	ZZZZ
H481	H482	H483	H484	H485
ZZZZ	H487	APAS		

08 ICU/CCU 4 011

WF08	H461	H465	ZZZZ	ZZZZ

09 CRC/Renl 4 015

WF09	A414	A416	A423	A424
ZZZZ	A426	A429	A431	A433
A434	ZZZZ	APAS		

10 Opthamol 2 005

WF10	A517	A519	A521	A522
ZZZZ	A524	A526	A527	A528
A529	ZZZZ	A530	A531	A532
A533	A534	ZZZZ	A535	

11 Surg/SPL 2 008

WF11	H535	H539	H541	H545
ZZZZ	H549	H551	H553	H559
H560	ZZZZ	H561	H562	H563
H564	H565	ZZZZ	H573	H577
H578	H579	H580	ZZZZ	H581
H582	H583	H584	H585	ZZZZ
H587	5PAS	ZZZZ	ZZZZ	ZZZZ
H574				

12 Surg INT 2 013

H660	H661	H665	ZZZZ

13 Surgical 2 009

WF13	H635	H639	H641	H645
ZZZZ	H649	H651	H653	H673
H677	ZZZZ	H678	H679	H680

The Emergency System

INTRODUCTION

The Emergency Manual is located on all floors proximal to the communication system terminals. In case of system failure, three plans are referenced and can be activated. Selection of plan A, B, or C is dependent on the type of system failure, the potential repair time, and the time of day. The selection of plan A, B, or C is made by the operating staff of the hospital at the time of system interruption.

Plan A is used from 7 AM to 12 PM and allows the laboratory to correct all system problems. Plan B extends from 12 PM to 4 AM and requires nursing service to assist in the blood drawing by providing orders that have been lost in the computer. Plan C is the worst case and is operated between 4 AM and 7 AM. This requires massive laboratory and nursing backup to quickly construct the morning draw list and provide the specimens.

MANUAL LABORATORY SYSTEM
PLAN A

The main laboratory-computer system is totally disconnected from floor operation for an unknown reason. During this period of time we will

419

use our manual backup system, and the service and retrieval of information will be greatly slowed. Virtually every area of the hospital will be affected in some way, and we are attaching a specific description sheet to describe how each one of the areas in the hospital will function in manual mode.

We would like to encourage all physicians to minimize their orders and calls for stat information during this period. This will facilitate our laboratory operations and minimize delays for critical data. Our staff will be on hand around-the-clock to try to handle the problems that will develop, and to make sure that no patient is inconvenienced during this time. We thank you in advance for your cooperation and consideration, and hope to work closely with you during this unfortunate period.

A. Outpatient Clinic

The outpatient clinic will use its standard order forms and transmit these to the clinic area, making sure to enter the clinic designator along with all appropriate age and sex parameters for each patient. The reports returning to the outpatient clinic will be provided on an order sheet on which the laboratory data will be reported. This will be stamped with a special notification saying: "FINAL REPORT, DO NOT DESTROY."

B. Inpatient Blood Drawing

Our computer system will be unable to provide blood-drawing lists, and we therefore request that all orders for AM pick-up be kept in one location on the floor or ward area so that the blood-drawing team can draw directly from the laboratory order sheets in the morning. Each order sheet should show the proper, legibly-written, floor location along with the appropriate patient identification. If more than one area of the laboratory is to be used for a single patient, such as hematology and chemistry, a separate order sheet should be made out for each area. This will make it easier to report the results and process the specimens. The order sheets for each patient should be stapled together and kept in a central basket until the blood drawing team arrives to procure the specimen. Along with the order sheet should be several addressographed labels stapled to the sheets so that these can be transferred directly to the tubes for subsequent handling. Reports from the laboratory on a stat basis will be called to you and those that are routine will be

delivered in the evening. They will all be stamped with a special code saying, "FINAL REPORT, DO NOT DESTROY."

For specimens drawn by physicians on an inpatient basis, these should be transported directly to the lab area with an order sheet, making sure that the floor and patient identification is visible. These reports will be processed in identical fashion to that described in the previous paragraph.

C. Emergency Room

Specimens coming from the emergency room will use the standard order form along with the appropriate identification of the patient and a stamp marked ER. Stat and emergency results will be called to the area and routine reports can be expected in the evening of that same day.

D. Medical Records

Medical records will receive cumulatives and handwritten reports stamped with "FINAL REPORT, DO NOT DESTROY," which should be kept as part of the patients' permanent records. This data *will not* be repeated by the computer system at a later time.

MANUAL LABORATORY SYSTEM
PLAN B

A. Outpatient Clinic

(See Plan A)

B. Inpatient Blood Drawing

The system has lost the blood drawing list. All blood drawing orders for AM pickup must be collected from the holding basket on the floor, and labels must be made before 06:30. Nurses, aides, and students will need to assist in this emergency. Each order sheet should show the proper legibly-written floor location along with the appropriate patient identification. If more than one area of the laboratory is to be used for a single patient, such as hematology and chemistry, a separate order sheet should be made our for each area. This will make it easier to report the

results and process the specimens. The order sheets for each patient should be stapled together and kept in a central basket until the blood drawing team arrives to procure the specimen. Along with the order sheet should be several addressographed labels stapled to the sheets so that these can be transferred directly to the tubes for subsequent handling. Reports from the laboratory on a stat basis will be called to you, and those that are routine will be delivered in the evening. They will all be stamped with a special code saying, "FINAL REPORT, DO NOT DESTROY."

For specimens drawn by physicians on an inpatient basis, these should be transported directly to the lab area with an order sheet, making sure that the floor and patient identification is visible. These reports will be processed in identical fashion to that described in the previous paragraph.

C. Emergency Room

(See Plan A)

D. Medical Records

(See Plan A)

MANUAL LABORATORY SYSTEM
PLAN C

A. Outpatient Clinic

(See Plan A)

B. Inpatient Blood Drawing

The computer has failed before a blood drawing list was printed. Laboratory techs are assigned to come to the floor and help collect the order sheets and labels necessary to acquire all required specimens. All nursing personnel should assure their prompt access to this information. All additional blood drawing orders should be kept in one location on the floor or in the ward area so that the blood drawing team can draw

directly from the laboratory order sheets the following morning. Each order sheet should show the proper floor location, legibly written, along with the appropriate patient identification. If more than one area of the laboratory is to be used for a single patient, such as hematology and chemistry, a separate order sheet should be made out for each area. This allows easier reporting of the results and processing of the specimens. The order sheets for each patient should be stapled together and kept in a central basket until the blood drawing team arrives to procure the specimen. Several addressographed labels should be stapled to the order sheets for transfer directly to the tubes before handling. Reports from the laboratory on a stat basis will be called directly to the originator, and those that are routine will be delivered in the morning. All will be stamped with a special code saying: "FINAL REPORT, DO NOT DESTROY."

Specimens drawn by physicians on an inpatient basis should be transported directly to the lab area with an order sheet that has visible floor and patient identification. These reports will be processed in identical fashion to that described in the previous paragraph.

C. Emergency Room

(See Plan A)

D. Medical Records

(See Plan A)

Subject Index

A

Admission, 23, 63–74
  audit trail, 71
  critique, 73, 74
  discharge, 67, 72
  flowcharts, 270–274
  format, general admission data,
    64, 65
  processing patients needing lab
    work, 70
  space, 70, 71
  stat, 65
  terminal, 65, 66
  transfer, 68, 71
  types of patients, 63, 64
Age–sex table, 56
Anatomic, 180–183
  chart report, 183
  flowcharts, 326–334
  mark sense card (cytology), 181,
    182
  order form, 181
  routine order, 86
  terminal, 181
  unfinished test report, 181

Archive system, 106, 107, 213,
    217–223
  microfilm, 217–219
  microfilm computer interface,
    219–223
Assembler language, 9

B

Backup system, 203–207
  down time greater 24 hours, 206
  down time less 24 hours, 205,
    206
  hardware, 203, 204
  manual system, 205
  spare parts, 204
Bed control files, 53, 69
Billing, 214–216
  tape, 214–215
  interface to hospital system, 216
Blood bank, 172–179
  chart reports, 174, 175
  mark sense card, 175–178
  order form, 83, 173
  personnel, 175

Blood bank—*continued*
  specimen handling, 173, 366–367
  terminal, 173, 174
  unfinished test report, 174
Blood drawing, routine morning,
    87, 124, 128

C

Cabling, 41, 42
Census, hospital, 67, 68, 101, 102,
    212
Chemistry, 131–143
  chart report, 138, 139
  equipment, 125, 131
  flowcharts, 334–348
  mark sense, 141, 142
  order form, 83, 132
  personnel, 140
  quality control, 141
  referral labs, 141
  routine order, 86
  SMAC interface, 135
  specimen preparation, 132
  terminal, 134, 135
  worksheets, 133, 134
Communication lines, 41, 42
Comparative systems, 244–246
Computer center, 184–196
  down time, 201
  future design, 193
  new programs, 196
  noise, 196
  operational schedule, 187–190
  personnel, 184, 186
  physician problems, 192
  schedules, 186
  service, 195, 196, 199–202
  software maintenance, 201, 202
  specimen handling, 192–194
  system halt, 191
  system loop, 191, 192
  system reports, 187, 191, 194, 195
  training, 186, 187
Computer, laboratory, 38–42
  cabling, 41, 42
  power supply, 38–41
Computer output microfilm,
    219–223

Contracts, 31–33, 229–231, 250–258
  lease agreements, 250–258
Coulter S, 146–148
Cytology (see anatomic)

D

Departmental requirements, 224–229
  control, 225
  orientation to house staff, 226
  start up and training, 225–226
  vendors, 226–229
Differential cell counter, 147, 148
Discharge, patient, 67
Distributed processing network, 3–21
  hardware requirements, 5–8
  software requirements, 9–11
Doctor draws, 128, 129
Doctor, reports, 60, 210
Documentation, 51
  overview, 5

E

Emergency order, 87, 92, 292–295,
    302, 303
Emergency room, 23, 43, 75–79
  daily reports, 78
  files, 53
  forms, 76
  specimen reporting system, 77
  terminal, 77, 78
Epidemiology, 164
Expedite order, 86–88
  specimen number, 93, 120

F

File housekeeping, 9, 99–102, 192
File structure, 35, 51–60
Files, 53–62, 90, 192, 259–261,
    412–418
  doctors, 60
  documentation of laboratory
    procedures, 259–261
  expanded test, 56–59, 414–416
  general files, 53, 54
    room numbers, 53
    terminal matrix files, 54

instruments, 59
lab areas, 60
maintenance, 61, 62, 192
master, 55, 56, 412–414
  age–sex, 56
  subtest, 55
  test files, 55, 413–414
message, 90
room, 416–418
special, 59–61
worksheets, 60
Flowcharts, 51, 262–411
  admission, 270–274, 302–303
  doctors orders, 268, 274–285
  information control and
      processing, 374–411
  introduction, 262–264
  order process, 286
    dialysis, 296–299
    emergency, 292–295, 303–303
    floors, 286–291
    OB, 300–301
    outpatient laboratory, 304–307
  overview flowchart, 266–267
  problem statement, 265
  specimen processing, 308
    anatomic, 326–334
    blood bank, 366–367
    chemistry, 334–347
    hematology, 348–357
    immunology, 368–373
    outpatient clinic, 320–322
Forms, 34, 43, 44, 81–90
  blood bank order form, 83
  chemistry order form, 82
  emergency room, 76
  hematology order form, 83, 144
  immunology order form, 83
  information contained on order
      form, 81
  microbiology order form, 84
  microscopy order form, 83
  outpatient order form, 85
Functions outline, 245–246
Future plans, 240–244
  accomplishments to date, 243
  library, 241–242
  "normal value" statistics, 242
  on-line versus off-line, 241
  terminals, 242–243

H
Hardware, 5–9, 31, 203, 204
  configuration, 197–199
  requirements, 5–8
Hematology, 144–153
  abnormal test report, 148
  chart report, 148–150
  equipment online, 144
  flowcharts, 348–357
  mark-sense card, 152
  order form, 83, 144
  personnel, 150
  routine order, 86
  terminal, 146
  unfinished test report, 148
  worksheets, 145, 146
Hospital data processing
    requirements, 20, 21
Hospital patient number, 69, 70

I
Immunology, 165–171
  abnormal test report, 168
  chart report, 168, 169
  flowcharts, 368–373
  mark-sense cards, 169, 170
  order form, 84
  personnel, 169
  quality control, 169
  routine order, 86
  specimen handling, 166, 368–373
  terminals, 166
  unfinished test report, 168
  worksheets, 166, 167
Implementation of lab systems,
    230–239
  case history, 231–237
  education, 238–239
  physician, problems with, 237–239
  staff, 230
Information control and processing,
    374–411
  lab mode functions, 388–398
  operation schedule, 376–377
  types of reports, 378–387
Installation, 38
  cable, 41, 42
  evaluation, 42–45

Installation—*continued*
  power, 38–41
  staff, 45, 47
Insurance verification, 97, 98

L

Labels, mini, 58
Laboratory, 29, 60–62, 95–115,
  184–187
  computer room personnel, 184–187
  nursing station interface, 95–115
  problems, 29
  worksheets, 60–62
Laboratory/nursing station interface,
  95–115
Laboratory order, 57–59, 81–90
  cancel order, 129
  emergency order, 87
  expedite order, 86, 87, 120
  microbiology, 155
  morning blood drawing, 87, 124,
    128
  nursing station, 97
  routine order, 86, 120
  stat order, 87–119

M

Maintenance, 61, 62, 199–205
  file, 61, 62
  hardware records, 200
  service contract, 204, 205
  system, 199–202
Mark sense cards
  blood bank, 175–178
  chemistry, 141
  cytology, 182, 183
  hematology, 152
  immunology, 169, 170
  manual systems, 205
  microbiology, 162–164
Medical records, 69–99, 217
Microbiology, 154–164
  flowcharts, 358–365
  message function, 155
    chart report, 159–161
    epidemiology, 164
    mark sense cards, 162–164
    personnel, 161

reporting card, 156
  specimen preparation, 155–157
  terminals, 157–159
  unfinished test report, 159
  order, 155
  order forms, 84
  routine order, 86
Microscopy, 334–348
  order form, 83
Morning blood-drawing, 87
Multiplexer/concentrator, 6, 8
Multiprocessor, 4

N

Network, distributed, 3–21
Noise, 110, 196
  computer center, 196
  noise specifications for hospitals,
    110
  terminal, 152
Nursing station, 23, 43, 91, 92
  interface with lab, 95–115
  new prototype smart terminal,
    110–115
  personnel, 92, 95–97, 107, 108
  reports, 98–107
  space, 109
  specimen handling, 107
  terminal, 96, 97, 109
  terminal noise, 110

O

Operational schedule, 187–190
Order form, 81
  anatomic, 181
  blood bank, 173
  chemistry, 83, 132
  general short form, 44
  hematology, 144, 145
  immunology, 165
  microbiology, 155
  outpatient, 117
Order, laboratory, 57–59, 97
Ordering cycle, 87, 88, 91, 92
  physician critique, 92
  physician interface, 91
Outpatient clinic, 53, 116–118
  files, 53

Outpatient, clinical laboratory, 23
  order form, 85
  specimens, 130

P

Patient laboratory history, 106, 107
Patient number, 69, 70
Personnel, 45–47, 80
  computer room, 184–187
  emergency room, 79
  laboratory, 125, 127, 140, 161,
    169, 175
  nursing station, 92, 95–97, 107, 108
  schedules, 186
  training, 186, 187
Physician, 91
  laboratory/computer room, 185,
    192
Power supply (UPS), 38–41
Printer (see terminal)
Printer noise, 152
Processor, central, 4
PSRO audit, 120, 121

Q

Quality control, 99–101, 109, 123,
    141, 151, 169
  audit trails, 90, 91, 109, 123
  chemistry, 141
  hematology, 151
  immunology, 169

R

Reliability, system, 197–199
Reporting system, 25
  emergency, 76–78
  manual, 25–27
Reports, 98–107, 194, 195, 208–213
  ADTL, 209–210
  archive, 213
  census, 101, 102, 187, 212
  correct patient data files, 211
  daily chart, 98, 100, 117, 121, 138,
    139, 148, 159, 168, 169,
    187–191, 208
  disc copy, 210
  doctor, 60, 98–107

doctor reports, 210–211
  inquiry, 102–106
    abnormal test reports, 137,
      148, 168, 209
    by patient, 103, 104
    by physician, 102
    by specimen number, 105, 106
    unfinished test reports, 136,
      148, 159, 168, 181
    seven day/final charts, 99, 100,
      187–191, 209
    SMAC paper tape, 209
    ward, 98, 99, 105, 208
    worksheets, 211
Response time, 5, 20, 30, 42, 43
  high speed CRT, 70, 97
Routine order, 86–88
  specimen handling, 93, 120

S

Security, system, 108
Service, 199–201
SMAC, 135
SNOMED, 183
Software, 9–11, 31, 155
  halts, 191
  loops, 191, 192
  maintenance, 201, 202
  new programs, 196
Specimen handling, 119–130,
    308–321
  audit trail, 123, 124
  blood draw, 128, 310–311,
    314–315
  check-in-timing, 121, 123
  chemistry, 132
  computer room, 192–194
  doctor draw, 128
  hematology, 145
  immunology, 166
  labels, 124
  outpatient clinic, 320–322
  problems, 126
Specimen numbers, 93, 119, 120,
    123, 124
Staff (see personnel)
STAT, 65, 87–93, 119, 120, 129
  stat admission, 65
  stat order, 87, 88, 92, 129

STAT—*continued*
  stat specimen numbers, 93, 119,
    120
Surgical pathology (see anatomic)
System, backup (see backup system)
System, equipment list, 198, 199
System failure, 191–206, 419–422
  downtime, 201
  emergency manual, 419–422
  greater than 24 hours, 206
  halts, 191
  hardware record, 100
  less than 24 hours, 205, 206
  loops, 191, 192
  service, 199–202
System objectives, 30
System planning, 34–37
  files, 35
  forms, 34
  inspection, 37
  supplies, 34
System reliability, 197–199
System reports (see reports)
System study, 28–31, 37
  laboratory problems, 29, 126
  pert chart, 35, 36

T

Terminals, 5–7, 242–243
  admission area, 65, 66
  chemistry, 134, 135
  CRT (cathode ray tube), 70, 71,
    76, 77
  evaluation, 42, 43
  failure, 109
  fixed format, 158, 166, 167, 173,
    174
  fixed remote (see also nursing
    station or laboratory), 9

function matrix, 54
  immunology, 166
  laboratory, 9
  location of terminals in the
    hospital (matrix), 54, 71
  noise, 96, 110, 152
  nursing station, 9, 96, 97
  portable, 6–8
  reliability, 110–115
  smart (ideal), 5, 8, 110–115
  speed, 97
Test files, 55, 56, 61, 62
  expanded, coding, 56
  maintenance, 61, 62
  master, coding, 55
Tests, cancellation, 129
Training, 47, 125, 127, 186, 187
  manuals, 47
  personnel, 125, 127, 186, 187
  tapes, 47
Transfer patients, 68, 71

U

UPS (uninterruptable power supply),
  38–41

V

Vendors, 32, 226–229

W

Worksheets, 60–62, 133, 134, 145,
  146, 166, 167, 211
  chemistry, 133, 134
  hematology, 145, 146
  immunology, 166, 167
  laboratory, 60–62